Barbara Cous

Easy.
Tasty.
Healthy.

Delicious everyday recipes
all free from gluten, dairy,
sugar, soya, eggs & yeast

Thorsons

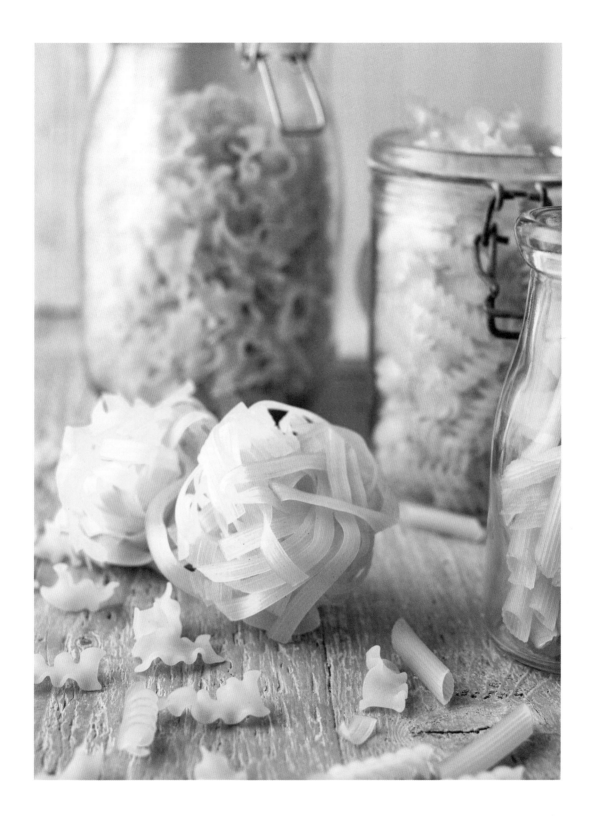

Contents

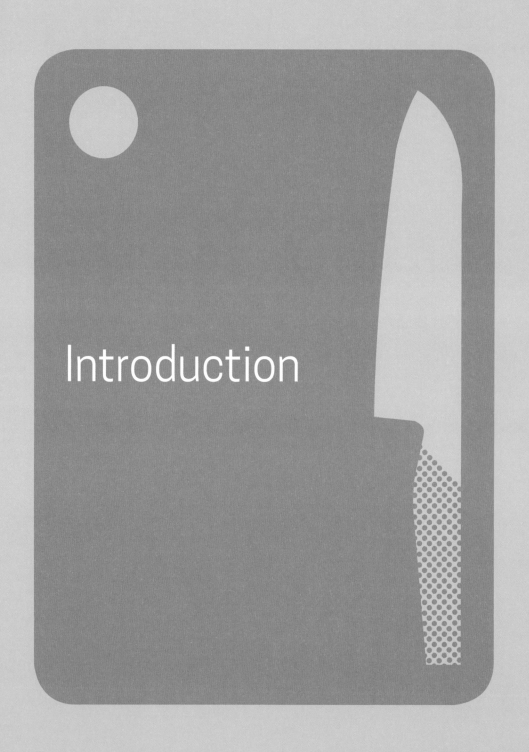

Introduction

Easy, Tasty, Healthy is all about eating for good health – how to achieve this and make it part of your life. It isn't a 'diet', as such, more a way of living that will help keep you slim, fit and full of vitality.

This book is not an extreme approach to 'free from' eating using specialist health foods, but a practical guide full of easy, delicious recipes and advice on how to make healthy choices for day-to-day cooking and meal planning.

Over the years, many diet books have hit the headlines only to disappear soon afterwards because they are difficult to adhere to and don't fit in with everyday life. We're told about the benefits of a low-fat or low-carbohydrate diet, but cutting out sustaining foods will just leave you with cravings and can lead to deficiencies in the long run. We need a balance of protein, fats and carbohydrates in order to obtain all the essential nutrients to keep us healthy. Diets are fine in the short term, but most people put weight back on once they return to their normal regime. The approach in this book enables you to eat heartily, to snack if you are hungry and to have treats when you need them. It's a way of eating that you can follow for the rest of your life and never feel deprived.

Wholefoods form the basis of the recipes in this book – 'real' foods with nothing added to them, such as vegetables, fruit, nuts, seeds, beans, pulses, fish and meat. By eating foods in their natural state, we automatically cut out processed foods and any chemical additives such as flavourings and preservatives. This is the key to a healthy diet, one shared by the world's longest-living people.

Although wholefoods are the way to go, there are some that our bodies have more difficulty dealing with, often leaving us feeling under par. Of the wholefoods that impinge most on our health, gluten- and dairy-based items come top of the list, with soya, eggs and yeast close behind. In this book I have created recipes that draw upon a wide range of delicious wholefoods while avoiding these common triggers.

FAST FOOD CAN BE GOOD FOR YOU

Feeding ourselves and our families isn't easy. We all juggle with a lack of time, temptation from processed food that is readily available (but not always healthy) and sometimes the sheer boredom of having to think up yet another meal. How to produce healthy, tasty food quickly is the aim of this book.

On page 19 is a table of ingredients that you'll find useful for making the recipes in these pages. The list isn't extensive, nor are the ingredients difficult to find – they're mostly just basics, many of which you probably already have.

It's also a good idea to try to be organised with your cooking, whether this means planning your menus for the week or just having an idea for what to cook the next day. When my children were young and I was working full time, I used to assemble ingredients for cooking the following evening to ensure I was always a day ahead of myself. I might prepare a casserole and some potatoes for baking one night, ready to pop into the oven when I got back from work the following evening. This was in the days before I had an oven timer or slow cooker. All I needed to do then was prepare a salad or some fresh vegetables to go with the casserole and potatoes and while they were cooking I could think about what to make for supper the next day. It meant that I could quickly pop the meal on to cook when I returned home, then see to the boys without feeling pressured. It still gives me a lovely relaxed feeling knowing that food is cooking while I get on with other things.

The recipes in this book have been designed to be time and labour saving. They include lots of 'pop it in a pan' recipes as well as whole meals you can cook in the oven. The soups involve a quick bubble and a blitz and can be made in minutes. There are pastas and pâtés made from store cupboard ingredients. In other words, you can eat well without spending forever in the kitchen or at the supermarket.

Double Up and Save Time

If I'm making a casserole, I find it just as easy to make enough for six or eight rather than just for the two of us. This means that I can freeze the extra for those nights when I know I won't have time or I just don't feel like cooking. There are lots of recipes that can be doubled and the extra portions popped in the freezer, so try to get into the habit of cooking in bulk.

Aim to Have Leftovers

I always like to cook with the aim of having leftovers whenever possible. I know that in an ideal world we would eat freshly prepared food at every meal, but time is short and it's far better to eat homemade leftovers, in my view, than resort to ready-made meals or takeaways.

If I cook potatoes, for instance, I like to have some left over for the following day. There are so many wonderful ways to use them, as you will see in the 'Love your Leftovers' chapter (pages 190–205). If I cook a joint of meat, I prefer to cook more than enough so that we can have a second-day roast or incorporate it in another meal.

Save Time, Don't Sweat

My favourite time-saving suggestion is to miss out the frying/sweating stage from recipes. I don't brown meat for casseroles, sweat vegetables for soup or sear joints before cooking in the oven. This is not only a healthier way of cooking (it stops free radicals from being produced), but it saves time and washing up. It means that generally you just throw everything into the pot and cook. I promise you won't notice the difference, as there are enough tasty ingredients in these recipes.

More Flavour, Fewer Steps

A friend of mine who hates cooking said that she always looks for recipes with the fewest ingredients. As far as I'm concerned, fewer ingredients mean less flavour. What I look for are enough ingredients to add depth and intensity of flavour, but using the shortest method possible; it's the making that takes the time. If you have all the ingredients to hand, it doesn't take very long to throw a selection of them into a pot. If all you have to do is let it bubble away for a few minutes on the hob or leave it in the oven for a few hours, then you have great-tasting food with very little effort – my sort of cooking.

EAT YOUR WAY TO GOOD HEALTH

Most people, when asked, know the principles of healthy eating – consume more fruit and vegetables, less saturated fat, sugar and salt, etc. What they find difficult is putting this into practice, especially when no help is at hand. Occasionally I buy a 'healthy eating' magazine and look hopefully at the recipes included. But the cakes are still sugar laden and meals still lacking in vegetables. They send out very mixed messages – just like processed foods labelled 'healthy' or 'low fat' that are actually filled with hidden sugar.

In order to eat more healthily, we need to concentrate on good food. We can't get away with filling up on poor-quality ingredients.

Manufacturers tend to be less interested in consumer health than in making money – the cheaper the ingredients they use, the more profit they make. Cheap ingredients, however, mean less healthy ingredients, such as fat and sugar, with lots of chemical additives to manipulate the way the food tastes. The best way to eat healthily is to avoid processed foods and buy ingredients in their raw state to make your own meals. You then know exactly what goes into them.

Of course, there are some healthy ready-prepared foods out there. Use them by all means, but don't be conned – read the labels on the packaging. When sugar-free, supposedly healthy snack bars first came on to the scene, I was impressed – but when my blood sugar started to dip after eating them, I suddenly figured out what was going on. The manufacturers were simply using sugar made from other ingredients such as rice or vegetables, rather than sugar cane, and so their bars were just as sweet and over-processed as many others; they just sounded healthier.

Let Food Be Your Medicine

Our bodies need good nutrition in order to work properly. Vitamins, minerals, fats, carbohydrates and protein are nutrients that we need in sufficient amounts to function optimally. Unfortunately, much of what we eat today is devoid of nutrients. What's more, we are ingesting toxic substances from the additives in food as well as from the air we breathe, the alcohol we drink and the drugs we take – including over-the-counter remedies. Because of the lack of nutrients, our bodies are becoming less able to rid themselves of these harmful substances and so are unable to work as efficiently as they should. Ill-health becomes the norm.

Every cell in your body is like a miniature factory with a particular job to do. This may be to pass on a message or produce a substance needed for a certain reaction to take place. But if the factory is full of waste products (toxicity) and lacking in the raw materials it needs (nutrients), each cell is unable to function properly. This paves the way for health problems and often a vicious circle where more drugs are taken to help treat the symptoms.

The aim of good nutrition is to build a better cell or factory and hence body. Body cells are continually being replaced. A blood cell lasts for 60–120 days, so in 3–4 months your whole bloodstream is completely renewed. In a year, all your bones are replaced, constructed entirely from the nutrients that you eat. This means that although improved nutrition will have some immediate benefits, you will have to wait for months, or even years, for your body to reach its full potential for optimum health.

It's not unlike a neglected house plant: if you start feeding and watering it, the leaves will perk up a bit from the improved nutrition, but you have to wait for the old leaves to die off and new ones to grow before you get a really healthy plant. In the same way, you can't do a three-day detox and expect miracles to happen. Building good health is about changing the way you eat long term.

My first book, *Cooking Without*, goes into detoxification in greater depth and talks about the reasons for avoiding wheat, dairy, yeast and so on. This book moves on from there to concentrate on some of the latest information about diet and health.

SUGAR – PURE, WHITE AND DEADLY

We need sugar to give us energy, to fuel our cells and to feed our brains so that we can think, but sugar in the concentrated form found in biscuits and cakes, or in other over-processed foods, is not the right kind. Any carbohydrate-based foods such as grains, beans and pulses or vegetables are broken down into simple sugars by the digestive process, but it takes much longer to break down sugar from, say, chickpeas or porridge than from a biscuit.

White sugar was originally part of a piece of sugar cane or sugar beet and in that form we would have to chew our way through a lot of fibre to release a small amount of sugar. However, once the sugar cane or beet is processed and the sugar used in various foods, we can eat large amounts very easily. Anyone who has ever made treacle toffee or jam will know that you start with a big pan of sugar that soon boils down to a much smaller amount, so that by the time you eat your sweet or spoonful of jam, you are probably consuming the equivalent of a 3-metre piece of sugar cane. Hard to imagine, but it's true.

In other words, nature doesn't package foods in a way that we can overdose on sugar. Even if you are really hungry and you are offered apples to eat, you may munch your way through a couple – but after that you would be fed up of munching. The sugar in the apples would then have to be broken down from the fibre before being released into your bloodstream. Not an instant process.

Balancing Your Blood Sugar

If you look at the diagram opposite, you will see that there is an optimum range that our blood sugar should stay within. If we eat sugar in the form of complex carbohydrates (vegetables, beans and pulses or wholegrains), then sugar will be released from these gradually and the level in the bloodstream will stay within the green zone. It will rise and fall a little as we eat and become hungry again, but provided we eat sufficient of the right kind of food at regular intervals, it will stay within an acceptable range.

But what happens if we eat sugary and over-processed foods? These include not just sugar but also white bread, cakes, biscuits, alcohol (fermented sugar), soft drinks, sweets and many breakfast cereals, as well as seemingly good foods containing hidden sugars. In fact

BALANCING YOUR BLOOD SUGUR

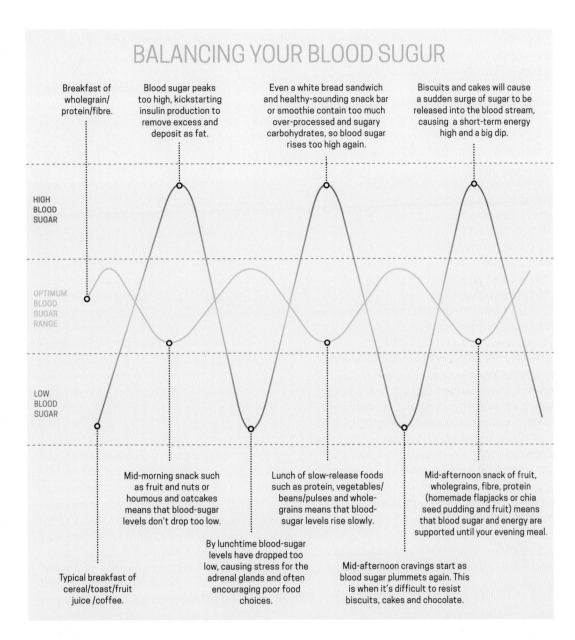

Breakfast of wholegrain/protein/fibre.

Blood sugar peaks too high, kickstarting insulin production to remove excess and deposit as fat.

Even a white bread sandwich and healthy-sounding snack bar or smoothie contain too much over-processed and sugary carbohydrates, so blood sugar rises too high again.

Biscuits and cakes will cause a sudden surge of sugar to be released into the blood stream, causing a short-term energy high and a big dip.

HIGH BLOOD SUGAR

OPTIMUM BLOOD SUGAR RANGE

LOW BLOOD SUGAR

Mid-morning snack such as fruit and nuts or houmous and oatcakes means that blood-sugar levels don't drop too low.

Lunch of slow-release foods such as protein, vegetables/beans/pulses and whole-grains means that blood-sugar levels rise slowly.

Mid-afternoon snack of fruit, wholegrains, fibre, protein (homemade flapjacks or chia seed pudding and fruit) means that blood sugar and energy are supported until your evening meal.

By lunchtime blood-sugar levels have dropped too low, causing stress for the adrenal glands and often encouraging poor food choices.

Mid-afternoon cravings start as blood sugar plummets again. This is when it's difficult to resist biscuits, cakes and chocolate.

Typical breakfast of cereal/toast/fruit juice /coffee.

the supermarket shelves are filled with these kind of products, food in a manufactured state that our grandparents wouldn't recognise. Highly processed and sugary foods cause our blood sugar to rise quickly; it's why we get a sudden lift or boost of energy from eating them. But this sudden rise is dangerous for the body, so it produces insulin to remove some of the sugar and store it as fat. Our blood-sugar levels then drop below normal (see diagram) and we are left feeling hungry, lethargic or craving sugar and stimulants such as coffee or cigarettes. Stimulants work by kicking our adrenal glands to release an emergency supply of energy, a bit like whipping a flagging horse and just as counterproductive. Eating over-processed and sugary foods means that we are on a roller-coaster ride of highs and lows, which as well as affecting our physical health can also impinge on our mood and behaviour, leading to great swings from euphoria to depression, hyperactivity to exhaustion, clear thinking to mental fog.

Forget Fat – Sugar is the New Enemy

At last, the problems caused by sugar are starting to be recognised. For many years fat has been blamed for the rise in obesity and other health problems, but little attention has been paid to sugar. Unfortunately, when John Yudkin warned of the dangers of sugar in his book *Pure, White and Deadly* back in 1972, he was largely ignored. If you ask most people if they eat a lot of sugar they will say they don't, as they tend to think of grains in a bowl. But while sales of loose sugar have declined, our consumption has in fact trebled over the past 50 years. We are eating sugar but don't realise it, because it is hidden in prepared products, from soups and sauces to pizza, crisps, ready meals, bacon and bread. Each week the average Briton consumes well over 100 teaspoons of added sugar, often without knowing it. Sometimes we are misled because the word 'sugar' does not appear on the label. Instead, manufacturers are cleverly using other names for what is basically sugar and often making it from healthy-sounding food such as fruit, vegetables and milk. One of the worst offenders is corn. This seemingly innocent ingredient is transformed into high-fructose corn syrup (HFCS) by the food industry and because it is cheap to make it is frequently used in ready-prepared food.

Many of the low-fat foods on the market have been adding to the problem, as they are often manufactured with extra sugar to make them palatable. It's the same with commercially produced 'free from' foods: remove gluten and you need something to bind ingredients in bread and cakes, so extra sugar is used. Other forms of sugar, some of which are used as supposedly healthy alternatives to sugar, such as agave syrup, maple syrup and honey, are still made up of glucose and fructose. A simple sugar is a simple sugar and its consumption needs to be limited on a daily basis for our health's sake.

Excess Sugar a Slow Killer

In its many forms, sugar is broken down mainly into fructose or glucose or a combination of these (depending on the food) as it passes through the body. If sugar is naturally present in foods this is generally less of a problem, as the sugar needs to be released from the food before it enters the body and this takes time. It becomes more of an issue when food is over-processed or high in added sugar, as there is nothing to prevent it from entering the body in a rush.

When too much glucose enters the body, it quickly raises the sugar levels in the bloodstream, which prompts the pancreas to start pumping out insulin in response. Over time, excess sugar consumption exhausts the pancreas so that eventually it is no longer able to produce sufficient insulin. This is the beginning of type 2 diabetes, but it is also the forerunner of other major health problems, from high blood pressure and cholesterol to heart attacks, strokes and Alzheimer's disease.

When fructose enters the body, it does not cause a sudden rise of sugar in the bloodstream like glucose because it is first processed by the liver. This may sound like a good thing – but when too much fructose is consumed, the liver can't convert it fast enough for the body to use as energy, so instead it is transformed into fat that is then released into the bloodstream as triglycerides or stored in the liver. Non-alcoholic fatty liver disease from eating too much fructose is now superseding fatty liver disease (cirrhosis) caused by excess alcohol consumption. Excess fat in the bloodstream leads to health problems such as heart attacks and strokes and, of course, obesity when deposited in the body.

Don't Go Overboard

Many books are now being written about the ill-effects of sugar and proposing sugar-free diets. Although this is all music to my ears, there is a tendency to go overboard. Some diets suggest avoiding fruit, high-carbohydrate vegetables and cereals. They advocate a high-protein, high-fat, low-carbohydrate diet that isn't balanced, healthy or sustainable in real life.

If we are not careful, it is easy to become obsessive and wary of eating any food with a natural sugar content. But it is important that we don't throw the baby out with the bathwater. We need carbohydrates in our diet to make serotonin – a mood-enhancing hormone. Cutting out naturally sweet foods and carbohydrates altogether is not good for our mental health and also means that we miss out on foods with a high level of nutrients. In Eastern traditions where food is used as medicine, sweet ingredients are used to balance the flavours of salty, spicy, pungent and bitter. This doesn't necessarily mean adding sugar, but neither does it mean cutting out all foods that are naturally sweet.

Many of the so-called 'superfoods', ones containing the highest level of antioxidants, are fresh and dried fruits and fresh vegetables. Dates, prunes, figs, raisins, cranberries, pomegranates, blueberries and raspberries are among the top 15 antioxidant foods (as tested by the US Department of Agriculture in 2010). These foods also contain fibre that slows their digestion and absorption, thus preventing the pure 'sugar hit' of highly processed sweeteners.

Eating a high-protein diet as part of a low-carbohydrate regime is not good for our health, either. As well as being high in saturated fat, excess protein puts a strain on our kidneys and excess red meat consumption has been linked with cancer. The incidence of kidney stones has almost trebled in the last few years and it is thought to be due to the increase in high-protein diets. These produce acid waste products that our kidneys must try to eliminate.

A BALANCED APPROACH

I have always been anti added sugar ever since I trained as a nutritional therapist and wrote my first book in the 1980s, and I still feel that sugar is a major health issue. It is important, however, that the 'free from added sugar' diet we follow is healthy and easy to maintain. We need to follow an eating plan that fits into our lifestyle rather than a fad diet that works for a few months but doesn't teach us how to eat for life. A common-sense diet means no dieting.

The art of eating healthily is to avoid blood-sugar levels rising or falling too quickly. To do this, it is necessary to avoid added sugars and to make sure that the absorption of food higher in natural sugars and carbohydrates is slowed down during the process of digestion by combining it with fibre, fat or protein from another source. We tend to do this without thinking about it. You're unlikely to eat a plate of rice or a baked potato on its own, for instance.

When it comes to fruit, I have always recommended that two pieces of fresh fruit per day are adequate, and that it's not advisable to drink commercially made fruit juice or smoothies on a regular basis, even though they are seen as healthy. A glass of fruit juice contains the equivalent of four to five pieces of fruit without the body needing to do any work to break them

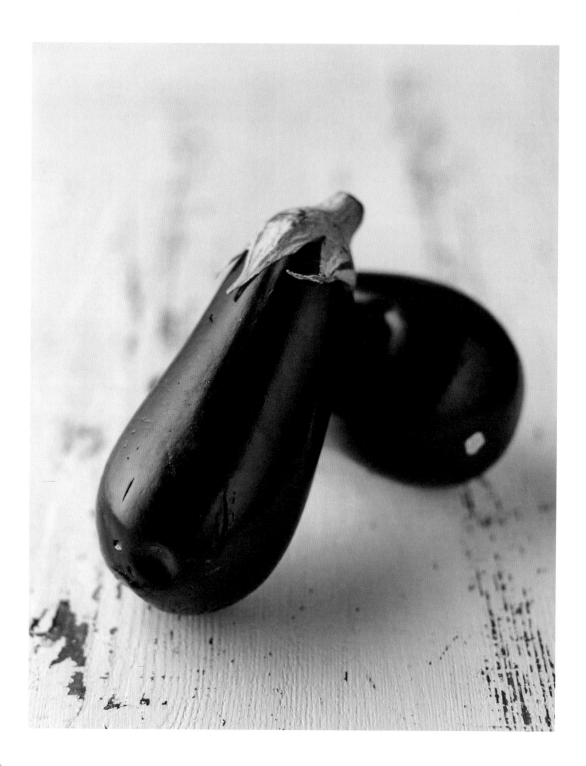

Introduction

down. The fruit in commercial smoothies, although whole, has its fibre broken down, making it easily absorbed. Eating fruit for a snack is still a good idea, but nowadays I often eat them with a few nuts or an oatcake to slow their transit further.

Dried fruit is good for us as it is full of vitamins, minerals and antioxidants, but it needs to be limited in a similar way to fresh fruit. Used sensibly alongside other foods that lower its absorption rate, dried fruit makes a delicious and naturally sweet addition to any diet.

If I was being a purist, then I wouldn't include sweeteners such as honey, blackstrap molasses or pomegranate molasses in this book. But these are major superfoods; eaten as they are in small amounts, and balanced with other slower-release foods, they provide a positive addition to a healthy diet. In other words, let's use common sense along with wholesome healing foods.

Swing High, Swing Low

As well as preventing blood sugar from shooting too high, it is also important to stop it from dipping too low. This happens after eating sugary or over-processed foods when the pancreas has removed this sugar from the bloodstream. But it is also happens if we don't eat the right food at regular intervals. It may sound healthy to under-eat, but this puts pressure on our adrenal glands as they try to support us by mobilising stored sugar. Lots of people burn themselves out this way and probably three-quarters of the population have some level of adrenal exhaustion. You don't ever need to go hungry and you should certainly never feel faint or ill through lack of food.

A friend of mine whose husband was pre-diabetic was finding that his blood sugar was always too high after eating breakfast, even though he was eating a sensible, sugar-free meal. I suggested that she tried giving him a light supper before bedtime of low-glycaemic (see page 16) foods such as

oatcakes and nut butter. Almost instantly, his blood-sugar levels stabilised.

A similar effect has been noticed in tests on diabetics: those who skipped breakfast were found to have higher blood-sugar levels after lunch. If we don't eat sufficient food regularly, the body releases stored sugar in response to this stress – but because it doesn't know if the stress is caused by lack of food or if it needs enough energy to run a marathon, it releases lots of sugar just in case. If we ran the marathon, this sugar would be used for energy but for most individuals the sugar just remains in the bloodstream.

Naturally Sweet

Having read about the harm caused by too much sugar, please rest assured that you can still have sweets and treats. A life of abstinence and denial, as well as being no fun, is not good for us either. On the other hand, the more you consume food in its natural state, the less you need worry about the negative effects of sugar.

In the cakes and puddings section, I avoid added sugar in recipes and use the natural sweetness from fruit with the occasional spoon of blackstrap molasses or honey. The trick is to balance the fast-release foods with slower-release ingredients, and this is one of the reasons I try to include foods such as nuts, seeds, ground almonds, oils and vegetables in these recipes.

It is also not just about what you eat, but when you eat it. A cake or a pudding consumed after a meal containing protein, fat and fibre will have less impact than one eaten in the middle of the afternoon on an empty stomach. If I need something sweet mid-afternoon, I'll tuck into one of my flapjacks or a piece of fruit cake (see pages 218–220 and 214), which I know contain lots of slow-release ingredients. The more 'cakey' cakes such as the Chocolate Cake on page 223 are ideal for special occasions when more of a celebratory centrepiece is needed.

Sugar Substitutes

Now that 'sugar-free' is in vogue, you will start to see lots of recipes in magazines and cookery books claiming to be just that. These are generally using other forms of sugar, such as pure glucose, fructose, agave syrup or maple syrup. In other words, nothing has changed – the recipes still contain a large amount of sugar.

Other recipes contain sugar substitutes such as xylitol and stevia, natural sweeteners manufactured from plants and trees that are not absorbed in the same way as sugar across the intestinal wall. This sounds very positive as they are low calorie and slow release, but the verdict is still out on their safety and health benefits. They can cause bloating, diarrhoea and flatulence, among other side effects.

Some of these side effects could be due to the processing of the products. Stevia in its plant form has been used for centuries as a sweetener, so it would seem harmless enough. But when it is processed as a sugar substitute, is it still metabolised in the same way? Because these sugar substitutes are sweet on the palate, the body assumes it is receiving sugar and primes itself to do so. Glucose is cleared from the bloodstream by the pancreas and blood sugar drops, but no real sugar/glucose is provided for the body to compensate. When this happens, adrenalin and cortisol surge to mobilise sugar from other sources to bring blood-glucose levels back up. The frequent release of the stress hormones (adrenalin and cortisol) is damaging to our adrenal glands and our overall health. The consequences of excess stress hormones include a supressed immune system, increased inflammation and lower thyroid function, to name a few.

The inappropriate use of sugar substitutes (they are often used like for like to replace sugar in recipes) does not stifle an over-sweet tooth and, used in such large quantities, would be very expensive. I don't feel they're needed, as nature has provided us with many wholesome sweeteners that, if used in moderation, will not upset our blood-sugar balance or affect our health. Small amounts of natural sweeteners are more acceptable, especially for candida sufferers who may not cope well with other sweeteners.

Artificial sweeteners such as aspartame and saccharin are often hidden in ready-prepared food, but these are chemically derived and therefore best avoided. Aspartame, in particular, has been linked with neurological problems and gastrointestinal symptoms.

Why One Chocolate is Never Enough

Research is now starting to reveal that sugar has addictive properties as powerful as those of cocaine. Our bodies produce a hormone, leptin, which acts like an appetite thermostat, but we're gradually becoming resistant to this hormone and it is the over-consumption of sugar that is causing this resistance. It means that our appetites don't abate as long as we are eating sugary foods.

Very little attention has been paid so far to our compulsive attitude towards sugar and refined carbohydrates. This is partly because eating sugary foods is socially acceptable – just look at the cupcake craze – and partly because we have been laying the blame for our obesity and health problems upon saturated fat.

Sugar is not just empty calories, as was always thought, but a time bomb waiting to explode. Once you remove sugar from your diet and support your blood-sugar levels with other foods, you will be amazed how much easier it is not to be tempted by sweet things. Often your body is craving them just because your blood-sugar levels are at rock bottom.

Sugar cravings can also be linked to our emotions. We have grown up thinking of a sugar fix as a treat and so when we are depressed, stressed, tired or upset, we turn to sugar to help us feel better. The fact that this is only a temporary fix that makes things worse in the long run is irrelevant at the time.

GLYCAEMIC INDEX

There is much talk about the glycaemic index (GI) of carbohydrates, which relates to the speed at which they are broken down and released as sugar into the bloodstream. Low-GI foods are slow release; high-GI foods are fast release. This is further complicated by the glycaemic-load rating. So, for instance, the carbohydrate in watermelon is deemed fast release, or high GI, yet only 6g of a 100g piece of watermelon is carbohydrate, which is not reflected in the overall GI rating. If you then include the satiety rating, or how long a food will keep you feeling full, then potatoes (which rate high on the glycaemic scale) also rate high on the satiety scale. It is therefore easy to jump to conclusions about certain foods, based on their GI ratings, without seeing the full picture and hence cutting out foods that are highly nutritious.

Slow Release and Fast Release

To simplify all this complicated research, which doesn't always agree on GI ratings, I've created the chart on page 16, which divides foods into my version of slow, medium and fast releasing. I've also included other foods in the list, such as fats and proteins, which wouldn't be in a glycaemic list because they are not carbohydrates. I just want you to get a good idea of the foods that will keep your blood sugar stable.

This doesn't mean that you should just eat foods from the slow-release section, as this would lead to an imbalanced diet. Similarly, if a food is in the fast-release section, it can be eaten but it is best not to eat it on its own. For instance, I never eat rice cakes unless they are combined with a slow-release food such as a pâté or nut butter or used to dip in the yolk of an egg.

DITCH THE DIET

Calorie counting and following crash or highly restricted diets has always seemed such a negative approach to eating, as far as I am concerned, and it's so unnecessary. It's all about what you shouldn't eat rather than what you should. I much prefer to concentrate on eating real and natural food whenever I feel hungry. And provided you eat sufficient of the right kind of food at regular intervals, you will lose any excess weight and feel healthier. The only diet that works is one that you can stick to in the long term, one that allows you to enjoy food and not feel deprived.

When you reduce your intake as part of a diet, your body goes into famine mode. Assuming food must be in short supply, your metabolism slows down to make the best use of the food it is receiving. Then when you start to eat normally again, your body no longer needs the extra and the result is weight gain. The trick is to eat five times a day, and this is a regime I still follow myself. Obviously, you are not going to lose weight if you eat cakes and biscuits five times a day, but provided you eat natural foods, like the ones in these recipes, you can still have treats and lose weight.

Eating regularly helps to keep your blood-sugar and energy levels stable and speeds up your metabolism. It's when your blood sugar dips and soars that you start to gain weight (see pages 8–11). If you eat over-processed or sugary foods (even a white sandwich, some fruit juice and a cereal bar for lunch), your blood sugar peaks and the excess is deposited as fat. If your blood sugar drops too low, then you will crave foods (often sugary) and often end up consuming more than your body needs. I rarely eat sugary foods, especially on their own, though occasionally I am tempted by a scone for afternoon tea when out with friends. But what I find is that, a couple of hours later, I feel desperate for food and need to

SLOW- AND FAST-RELEASE FOODS

Slow-release

Pumpernickel bread
Oatcakes and porridge oats
Buckwheat and quinoa
Beans, pulses and
   houmous
Nuts, seeds and nut
   butters
Oils and natural fats, such
   as olive and coconut
Olives
Sugar-free natural yogurt
Unsweetened soya and
   nut milks
Meat, fish and eggs
Apricots, peaches,
   cherries, raspberries,
   strawberries,
   blueberries, apples,
   plums, grapefruit,
   oranges and pears
Dried apricots
Broccoli, cabbage,
   cauliflower, spinach,
   kale, Brussel sprouts,
   avocados, asparagus,
   celery, courgettes,
   aubergines, cucumbers,
   leeks, onions,
   mushrooms, peppers,
   tomatoes, green beans,
   mangetout, raw carrots,
   salad leaves, radishes
   and fennel

Medium-release

Honey
Wholemeal bread
Brown, basmati and
   Arborio rice
Rice flakes and millet
   flakes
Wholegrain sugar-free
   breakfast cereals
Sugar-free muesli
Cornmeal and popcorn
Gluten-free pasta
   (depending on
   ingredients)
70–90% dark chocolate
Pomegranate and
   blackstrap molasses
Pineapples, kiwi fruit,
   mangos, bananas and
   pawpaws
Dates, sultanas and dried
   cranberries
Sweetcorn, beetroot,
   swedes, boiled
   potatoes, broad
   beans, carrots, peas
   and steamed sweet
   potatoes
Pure fruit juice (depending
   on the fruit)

Fast-release

Sugar
Sweets and chocolates
White bread
White rice
Rice cakes
White rice noodles
Shop-bought biscuits,
   cakes, puddings and
   energy bars
Commercial cereals, such
   as cornflakes, crisped
   rice and puffed rice
Beer, wines and spirits
Fizzy drinks
Sweetened fruit juice
Grapes and melon
Baked and mashed
   potatoes
Parsnips and pumpkins

eat again well before the time I normally have my evening meal. Thus I end up eating more calories than my body needs simply because my blood sugar is on a roller-coaster ride.

You should always aim to eat a good breakfast, lunch and evening meal, with snacks added, depending on where your biggest food gaps are. If you eat breakfast at 7am and lunch at 1pm, then you need a snack mid-morning. If you eat your evening meal early, perhaps with the children, then an early supper may be a more sensible option than a mid-afternoon snack.

Although I recommend eating regularly, when you are busy in the day and need the energy it is also a good idea to fast as long as possible overnight, as this gives the internal organs a rest. I usually don't eat after 7.30pm and don't eat breakfast until 8.30am, so my body has more than a 12-hour rest (see breakfast section for exceptions to this). Just work around your lifestyle following the recipes in this book and start enjoying food as the pleasure that it should be.

Fats

Now that some of the blame for obesity and other health problems has been attributed to sugar, where does that leave fat? First, a fat-free diet is not a good idea, as some fats are essential for our health. The problem is that many of the fats we eat, especially in processed food, are what are known as trans fats. These are fats that have been changed from liquid to solid form to suit the food industry, or ones that have been transformed into trans fats by being overheated during cooking. These are the fats we need to avoid.

Eating fats in the form of food – such as nuts, seeds, olives, avocados, fish and meat – means that we eat fats that are good for us. When heating oils and fats for cooking, we need to use ones that are stable at higher temperatures (see page 20) so that we don't compromise our health. If you follow a diet using the types of recipes in this book, not only will you not be eating too much fat, but you will also be obtaining the essential fats that your body needs.

STOCK UP ON THE STAPLES

Eating healthily when you lead a busy life is not so much about spending time in the kitchen or supermarket, but rather about planning ahead. This first of all involves stocking your kitchen with the basics. Within these recipes I have used a limited selection of ingredients, in order to simplify both the recipes and your store cupboard.

Have a look through the list and jot down any that you don't have with a view to adding them to your store cupboard. You'll reuse them constantly, I promise you, and once they are installed in your kitchen, you will be able to make any of the recipes with the minimum of fuss. Take a look at the food facts (pages 20–23) for more information to help you make the best choices when you buy. Try buying wholefoods in bulk, either online or in wholefood shops. This will save you time as well as money and will ensure that the ingredients are there when you need them. See the list of suppliers at the back of this book (page 286).

Fresh Vegetables and Fruit

In addition to the items in the storecupboard chart on page 19, always have a good selection of fresh vegetables and fruit, preferably stored in the fridge to prevent them from going limp.

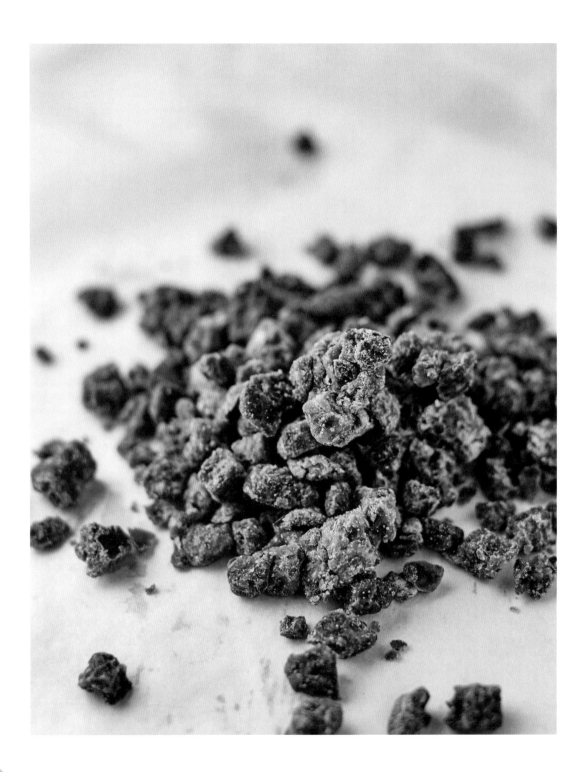

STOCK UP YOUR STORECUPBOARD

GRAINS AND PASTA
Basmati rice
Arborio rice
Brown rice flakes
Millet flakes and grains
Quinoa flakes and grains
Buckwheat flakes and grains
Gluten-free oats
Polenta or medium-ground maize meal
Gluten-free pasta
Flat rice noodles

BAKING
Gluten-free plain flour (see page 22)
Gluten-free baking powder
Bicarbonate of soda
Blackstrap molasses
Honey
Cacao, cocoa or carob powder
70–90% dark chocolate
Vanilla extract
Almond extract
Desiccated coconut
Gelatine

DRIED FRUIT
Apricots, prunes, cranberries, sultanas, dates and cherries
Candied peel and crystallised ginger (optional)
Freeze-dried fruit

OILS AND CONDIMENTS
Olive oil
Coconut butter/oil
Rice bran oil
Sesame oil

Stock cubes
Salt and pepper
Mustard powder
Pomegranate molasses

DRIED HERBS & SPICES
Sage
Basil
Oregano
Rosemary
Thyme
Bay leaves
Fennel seeds
Paprika and sweet smoked paprika
Turmeric
Cumin seeds and ground cumin
Ground coriander
Garam masala
Green cardamom pods
Chilli powder
Chinese five-spice powder
Cinnamon
Mixed spice

TINS AND BOTTLES
Tinned chopped tomatoes
Tomato passata
Sun-dried tomatoes
Tomato purée
Olives
Tinned or bottled beans and pulses (cannellini, chickpeas, butter beans, lentils, red kidney beans)
Tinned or bottled fish (tuna, salmon, sardines, mackerel, anchovies)

Coconut milk
Artichoke hearts

PACKETS
Dried porcini mushrooms
Dried whole brown and split red lentils
Gluten-free oat cakes
Rice cakes

FRIDGE
Dairy-free milk/yogurt
Lemons
Knob of fresh root ginger
Garlic
Chillies
Tamarind concentrate
Chorizo
Sun-blushed tomatoes
Nut butters
Nuts (almonds, ground almonds, cashews, Brazils, hazelnuts, walnuts, pine nuts)
Seeds (chia, pumpkin, sesame, sunflower, linseeds, ground linseed)

FREEZER
Lemon rind/juice
Piece of peeled fresh root ginger
Peas, sweetcorn and baby broad beans
Cooked prawns
Raw tiger prawns
Meat and fish
Chopped herbs
Berries

A FEW FOOD FACTS

MEAT AND FISH

Meat and poultry:
Eat meat less often and in smaller portions so that you can afford better quality. Buy from your local butcher or farmers' market – preferably meat that's organic and/or grass fed. This meat has more good-for-you omega-3 fatty acids and less saturated fat. Search out sausages that are free from preservatives and buy in bulk and store in your freezer.

Fish:
Smaller coldwater fish are a good choice as they contain fewer pollutants, as do wild and organic fish as opposed to farmed. For essential fats go for salmon, trout, mackerel, sardines and herrings – fresh, bottled or tinned.

Chorizo:
Chorizo is available free from preservatives (see the list of suppliers on page 286). I like to cut it into small dice and then freeze it (remove the skin if it seems tough). You can use it straight from frozen, which means it never goes mouldy sitting in the fridge.

OILS, CONDIMENTS AND FLAVOURINGS

Coconut oil:
Often called coconut butter, and in its purest ('virgin') form still tasting of coconut, coconut oil is also available in a purified form, which removes the coconut flavour. This oil, which sets at room temperature, is ideal for heating as it has a high smoke point. It can be used in baking instead of butter or other oils and for spreading on bread or crackers. It is my number one choice for cooking.

Olive oil:
This is ideal for savoury cooking and salad dressings. It has a lower smoke point than coconut oil, so it shouldn't be used for hot frying. Its health benefits have been well documented. Try to buy extra-virgin and organic if possible.

Rice bran oil:
This oil has a light, delicate flavour and a high smoke point, making it ideal to use in baking. It is extracted from the germ of brown rice, so it retains the nutrients from the whole rice grain.

Sesame oil:
This strong, pungent oil is only used in small quantities, but it adds an extra dimension to salads and stir-fries.

Stock:
Negotiating the stock market is a bit of a minefield, but gluten- and yeast-free stock cubes are available. I try to avoid any containing hydrolysed vegetable or animal protein, as this is a very chemical process. The little pots of stock are not hydrogenated, but do all seem to contain yeast and/or dairy. You can also buy fresh stock from the supermarket or make your own (see page 203).

Mustard:
Mustard powder is available wheat-, dairy- and vinegar-free in many supermarkets or wholefood shops. Check the ingredients in ready-made mustards, though, as many contain vinegar or wheat.

Pomegranate molasses:

Made from the concentrated juice of the pomegranate, this has a sour as well as sweet taste and is extremely rich in antioxidants, giving it superfood status. Available from the specialist food section in supermarkets, it's used in small quantities in certain recipes.

Salt:

Use Himalayan or sea salt, both of which contain naturally occurring minerals, rather than table salt, which often contains additives.

Root ginger:

Although I always keep a knob of fresh root ginger in the fridge, I also store a peeled piece in the freezer for emergencies. Ginger can be grated from frozen and this is a good way of keeping it if you don't use it very often.

Sun-dried and sun-blushed tomatoes:

Sun-dried are dense, flattened tomatoes often sold in bottles in oil and sometimes in vinegar. A dried version is the purest form but these need to be reconstituted before use. Sun-blushed and sun-kissed versions are more lightly dried and still retain their tomato shape. They are available in bottles but also in chiller cabinets at the supermarket.

Tomato purée:

I like to buy tomato purée in bottles and decant it into ice-cube trays in the freezer. One cube roughly equals one tablespoon. This saves money and avoids bottles or tubes going off at the back of the fridge.

GRAINS AND PASTA

Rice:

I prefer to use brown basmati rice, as it is so quick and easy to cook (about 25 minutes) and has the lowest GI rating (see page 15) of all the rice products. Brown rice is also available in a flaked form, which is ideal for use in breakfast cereals.

Oats:

Although oats contain a protein similar to gluten, it is the way they are processed that really affects their gluten content. Gluten-free oats (marked on the label) are readily available and easily tolerated by most individuals on a gluten-free diet.

Buckwheat:

Buckwheat has a wonderful, though unusual nutty flavour. It has a low GI rating (see page 15) but, best of all, it only takes only 10 minutes to cook. The trick is to master the cooking technique as it quickly overcooks. I started to get the measure of it when I bought a packet from an East European shop where it comes in perforated packets ready to drop into a pan of boiling water and is unable to disintegrate because of the packet. I have since improvised by cooking it in a metal sieve.

Millet:

Whole millet is cooked in the same way as rice and can be used in any dish where you would normally use rice. It takes approximately 20 minutes to cook. I have used it in its flaked form, especially in the breakfast recipes. It has a distinctive flavour but is the least acidic of all the grains, so is very good for you.

Quinoa:

This tiny South American non-grass grain is higher in protein than other grains, so is a good choice for vegetarians. It is quick and easy to cook, taking only 10 minutes, and can take the place of rice in recipes. It is also available in a flaked form, which I have used in the breakfast recipes.

Gluten-free pasta:

This is now readily available and difficult to distinguish from wheat pasta. as the quality keeps improving. It is increasingly being made from low-GI ingredients such as beans, buckwheat, quinoa and sweet potatoes (see page 15).

DAIRY-FREE MILK, CREAM AND YOGURT

Dairy-free milks:

A wide range of alternative milks is now available in the shops. Labels do need to be read, though, as some milks contain added sweeteners and flavourings. These days I often make my own by blending 1 mug of almonds or desiccated coconut to 6 mugs of water.

Coconut milk and yogurt:

Coconut is available in many different forms for use in cooking. Most of the milks on the market are quite acceptable, though some makes contain more additives than others. Creamed coconut is the purest, but this needs to be reconstituted with water. Coconut yogurt is becoming increasingly available, though it is expensive.

Coconut cream:

Coconut cream, which is used in these recipes, is available in some supermarkets, but it is best produced by pouring the liquid from a tin of coconut milk (not the 'light' version) that has been left in the fridge overnight. I try to always keep a tin in the fridge just in case. If you open the tin at the bottom, it will be easy to pour off the liquid, which can be kept to use in smoothies or soups.

BAKING

Gluten-free flour:

It really is worth making your own flour, as it produces a lighter texture in baked goods than ready-prepared, all-purpose brands. Individual flours are readily available from wholefood shops or internet suppliers. If you buy ready-prepared flour, you may need to adjust the level of liquid in recipes. This is my favourite recipe for gluten-free plain flour.

125g (4½oz) each of brown rice flour and sweet white sorghum flour
175g (6oz) each of cornflour (not cornmeal and preferably yellow unbleached), potato starch and tapioca flour
75g (3oz) buckwheat flour

Make up batches of flour in an airtight container large enough to allow you to shake to mix.

Bicarbonate of soda and gluten-free baking powder:

Used as raising agents in baked goods, these are readily available from the supermarket.

Cacao, cocoa or carob powder:

Cacao powder is the raw, unheated version of cocoa powder and is interchangeable in recipes. Read labels if you have a severe food allergy, as many state that they have been made in factories containing nuts and milk. Carob powder can be used as an alternative to cocoa powder for those who want to avoid stimulants.

Dark chocolate:

This is now on the list of 'good for you' foods, being high in antioxidants, vitamins and minerals – provided the chocolate has over 70% cocoa solids, that is. It does also contain some sugar, but I accept this small amount in recipes (see page 262 for a sugar-free version).

Vanilla and almond extract:

Make sure you buy extract, not essence, as the essence is chemically derived. Most extracts are held in alcohol, but alcohol-free products are available. Vanilla is available in many other forms, the purest being natural vanilla pods (1 pod equals 3 teaspoons of extract). See the back of the book for suppliers of alcohol-free products (page 286).

Gelatine:

The gelatine in my recipes is in sheet form and is very easy to use. Five sheets sets about 570ml (1 pint) of liquid, but this varies with different brands so check the quantities and adjust accordingly. You can use vegetarian gelatine if you prefer.

Honey:

Honey has been used as a sweetener for thousands of years, but it does need to be used in moderation. An occasional teaspoon or tablespoon as part of a recipe is, as far as I am concerned, quite acceptable. Look for mild-tasting varieties that are local, raw and unheated, as these will be the most nutritious. If you prefer not to use honey, try agave syrup instead.

Blackstrap molasses:

When white sugar is refined, it is stripped of all its nutrients. Blackstrap molasses is made up of all the nutrients but does contain a little sugar. It is high in minerals and has a strong, treacle-like taste, so only needs to be used in small amounts.

Stevia:

Sold as 'Truvia' in supermarkets, this herbal sweetener has a low GI rating (see page 15) but it is still a processed food. It is best to use it only in very small amounts when extra sweetness is necessary or if you have a candida problem and cannot tolerate other sweeteners. If you can, buy stevia in leaf form or as ground leaves and infuse in liquid (like making a cup of tea) before adding the liquid to recipes.

FRUIT AND NUTS

Lemon juice and rind:

Lemon juice is available preservative free in bottles, but I often buy six organic lemons and shave off parings with a vegetable peeler to store in the freezer before squeezing the juice and freezing it in ice-cube trays for adding to recipes. Juice has been used in cake recipes to react with the bicarbonate of soda. If you cannot tolerate citrus juice, try using vitamin C powder (see below).

Vitamin C powder:

Vitamin C is available in the baking section in some supermarkets and in wholefood shops. If you are using it instead of citrus fruit, use ¼ teaspoon vitamin C instead of 1 tablespoon of lemon juice.

Dried fruit:

Try to buy dried fruit from wholefood shops to avoid sulphur dioxide, which is used as a preservative, and oils used to prevent the fruit from sticking together.

Freeze-dried fruit:

Useful for adding flavour to foods, especially in place of dried fruit. They are expensive, but you need only a small amount as the flavour is intense. Most supermarkets now stock them.

Nuts and seeds:

I like to buy these in bulk, as they work out much cheaper. I also like to store them in the fridge in glass jars, as nuts and seeds readily go rancid. To toast nuts or seeds, toss in a dry pan over a medium heat – or heat under a medium grill – for a couple of minutes until they start to brown, keeping a close eye on them as they burn easily.

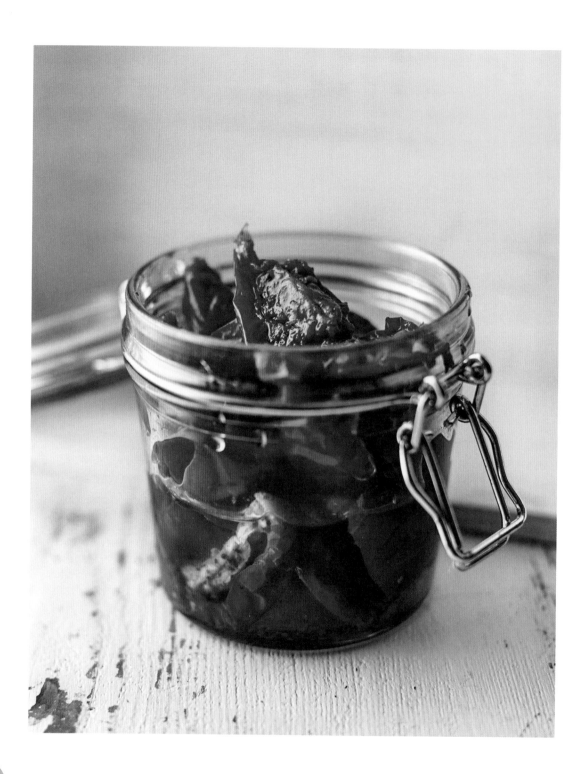

EQUIPMENT

I'm not a great fan of gadgets and I rarely go into a kitchen shop unless I need to replace something. I exist with a pared-down list of what I consider essentials. A mixing bowl isn't essential; a pan will suffice. A wide range of kitchen knives just wouldn't be used. I have a 10cm (4in) paring knife and a 15cm (6in) chopping knife that I also use for carving meat, plus a bread knife. However, I wouldn't be without a knife sharpener, a food processor and a slow cooker. Below is a list of what I consider essential. This doesn't include every piece of kitchen equipment, but those fringe items that make cooking easier.

Pots and pans:
A set of stainless-steel pans, plus a steamer, a flat paella-type pan with a lid and a frying pan; a large casserole dish and a slow cooker.

Baking trays and tins:
2 large baking trays, including a 30cm x 38cm (12in x 15in) tray for tray bakes; a 20cm x 33cm (8in x 13in) brownie tin; a 450g (1lb) loaf tin; a 20cm (8in) deep-sided round cake tin (preferably loose-bottomed); two 23cm (9in) round sandwich tins; a 12-hole muffin tin.

Knives:
Very good-quality kitchen knives and sharpener (see above).

Other basics:
Lemon squeezer, garlic press, small balloon whisk, wooden spoons, spatulas, sieve, pastry brush, wire cooling rack.

Measuring equipment:
Electronic kitchen scales, a set of measuring spoons, a large measuring jug and a small accurate 55ml (2fl oz) measure; kitchen timer.

Food processor:
Makes beating, blending, chopping and grating into a simple process.

Hand-held stick blender:
This is ideal for blending soups and sauces. The one I have also has a useful grinding attachment and a whisk.

A NOTE ON QUANTITIES

Serving quantities:
Many of the recipes in this book serve two, which means that they can easily be doubled if you need to serve four, or halved if you are serving just one person. Where recipes keep or freeze well (casseroles, soups and one-pot dishes) or are meant for entertaining (some puddings), they make enough for four to six servings. It's a good idea to jot down the quantities you need to suit your requirements next to those already given. Don't worry about spoiling the text – this is a book to be used, not a coffee-table decoration!

Spoon measurements:
Teaspoon (tsp) and tablespoon (tbsp) measurements in the recipes have been made using measuring spoons. They are level unless stated otherwise, though 'level' has been added where a more precise measurement is essential, such as in baking.

SNACK HAPPY

Many health and diet books say we shouldn't eat between meals and make us feel guilty for not having the willpower to last out. So why am I including a section on snacking? It's because I disagree. In principle, the liver should mobilise reserves to support our energy needs between meals, but few people these days have a liver that's up to the job. Moreover, few people these days eat sufficiently well at breakfast and lunch to last to the next meal without snacking. Eating snacks helps to keep blood-sugar levels even. If blood sugar dips too low, not only do we feel hungry but we are likely to make poor food choices as we crave sugary foods or ones high in refined carbohydrate. If our blood sugar goes too high, because we have succumbed to the wrong type of snacks, excess sugar is stored as fat and we are heading towards serious health problems. (See pages 8–11 for more about this.) Keeping blood sugar on an even keel by eating the right kind of food at regular intervals means that not only do we have more energy but our internal organs perform more efficiently, too. Energy enables everything to work optimally and as a result we feel good physically, mentally and emotionally.

Don't worry about putting on weight by including snacks, because you won't. In fact, one of the easiest ways to lose weight is to speed up your metabolism by eating five slow-release meals per day. (For more on slow- and fast-release foods, see page 15.) But try not to snack too late (unless you have health problems), as your internal organs will also benefit if you can give them a 12-hour rest overnight.

I have tried in this section to give you lots of ideas for fairly instant everyday snacks – things that you can pick up and eat or put together with very little effort. There are also a few that need to be baked, but these are worth the effort when you just want something different or a special treat. Always plan to have snacks in your eating regime. They are especially important for anyone who works long hours (eating breakfast early and dinner late), for young children and for people with health problems. I never go out without some snack food; sometimes it doesn't get eaten, but usually I'm really glad I had the foresight to bring something with me.

SAVOURY SNACKS

Oatcakes
I love the fact that these come in little cellophane packets. They are so easy to grab and pop in a handbag or briefcase just in case. Gluten-free ones are readily available – look for those made with non-hydrogenated fats. Try oatcakes on their own or with a few almonds and dried apricots or spread with nut butter or pâté (see pages 78–83).

Rice Cakes
I'm not a great fan of rice cakes because they contain carbohydrates that are very quick release. However, they are a useful vehicle and, if eaten with the right food, their GI (see page 15) is lowered. Try them spread with nut butter and mashed banana or topped with sliced avocado and tomato.

Pâté and Crackers
There are lots of pâtés in the lunch section (see pages 78–83) and most take only minutes to make. Serve these with gluten-free crispbreads, oatcakes or try the Artisan Crispbreads on page 232.

Dips and Crudités

Try watering down houmous or pâté (see pages 77–83) so that they become a dipping sauce to go with crudités (such as baby vegetables or ones cut into batons).

Toast

Whenever I make my gluten-free bread (see pages 227–231), I like to freeze some slices ready to pop in the toaster when needed. You can serve toast 'buttered' with coconut oil and topped with avocado, pâté (pages 78–83) or nut butter. (See also the toppings on page 44.) Read labels on commercial gluten-free bread before buying, as many contain sugar and are not very sustaining.

Soup

This is an ideal snack if you know you are going to be eating lunch or dinner late. There are some really speedy versions in the lunch section (pages 50–61), and shop-bought soups – if they're made with 'real' ingredients and no sugar or other additives – can be a good alternative otherwise.

Kale Crisps

See page 270.

Popcorn

Sugar-free popcorn is now available in supermarkets and shops, or make your own following the instructions on the packet. It's very simple.

Platter of Savoury Nibbles

Children love these – it means they don't get overwhelmed by large quantities of just one type of food. Try one when they arrive home from school ravenous. Include foods such as nuts, seeds, olives, slices of chorizo, cherry or sun-dried tomatoes, cubes of cheese (if tolerated), kale crisps (see page 270), oatcakes, avocado and celery.

SWEET SNACKS

Platter of Sweet Nibbles

Include things such as a selection of chopped fresh fruit, a few pieces of dried fruit, nuts, seeds, 70–90% dark chocolate, an oatcake with nut butter or a handful of granola (see page 39).

Box of Nuts and Dried Fruit

I always keep a container of mixed nuts and fruit in the fridge ready to grab if I'm off out for the day. Just make up your own favourite selection. As well as nuts and seeds and dried fruit, you could include coconut flakes, a few banana chips (these do contain some sugar), cacao nibs or a few squares of 70–90% dark chocolate.

Fresh Fruit

Aside from single pieces of fruit like bananas, apples and oranges, you can always chop up fruit to take with you, popping it into a sealed container. This works especially well for young children, who may find fruit easier to eat this way. Nowadays I try to eat something more sustaining with my fruit, such as nuts or yogurt, to prevent my blood sugar from crashing later, and I try to avoid the quick-release fruits (see page 16), such as grapes or melon, between meals.

Yogurt with Fruit

Non-dairy alternatives to standard yogurt are readily available these days, including goat's milk, soya and coconut. I prefer to buy natural yogurt and add my own fruit, as fruit yogurts tend not to contain much fruit but do have a lot of sugar. Try yogurt topped with finely diced fresh fruit, or stewed fruit, with a sprinkle of granola (see page 39).

Stewed Fruit

It's good to have a bowl of stewed fruit in the fridge that you can dip into for snacks as well as serve for puddings or on breakfast cereals. Try adding some granola (see page 39), toasted nuts and seeds, chia seeds or seed mix, dairy-free natural yogurt or Cashew Cream (see page 236) to make it more substantial.

Muesli

I always have a container of homemade muesli (see pages 35–36) in the cupboard and find I use it more for snacks than for breakfast. Served with a little fresh fruit and yogurt or dairy-free milk, it's ideal for a mid-afternoon or supper snack.

Chia Seed Pots

See page 38.

Cakes and Flapjacks

I love to have some ready-baked goods (see pages 211–224) in the freezer for those afternoons when only a cake will do. If you have them stored in individual pieces, then they won't take long to defrost. Try to serve ones made with sustaining ingredients, such as nuts, seeds, fruit and vegetables, for mid-afternoon snacks.

Energy Balls

See page 263.

Ice Lollies

Freeze homemade smoothies (see pages 42–43) in ice-lolly moulds and keep in the freezer ready for hot summer days.

Ice Cream

Have the ingredients for some of the dairy-free ice-cream recipes (see pages 254–256) ready frozen so that on a hot summer afternoon you can quickly blend them to produce a delicious and healthy homemade treat.

DRINKS

Milky Drinks

A milky drink provides a quick and easy but light snack. I sometimes have a soya decaf latte if I'm out and about or meeting friends. At home, you can make your own versions with any of the alternative dairy-free milks now available. Try to avoid milks with added sweeteners and don't expect them to support you for too long. Heat up the milk with added cacao, cocoa or carob powder, chicory, or cinnamon and vanilla extract.

Smoothies

Provided these contain some substance in the form of seed mix, ground almonds, avocado or oil (see page 42), smoothies provide a quick and easy way to snack. They are also a good way to get nourishment into unsuspecting children. (See some of the recipes in the breakfast section, pages 42–43.)

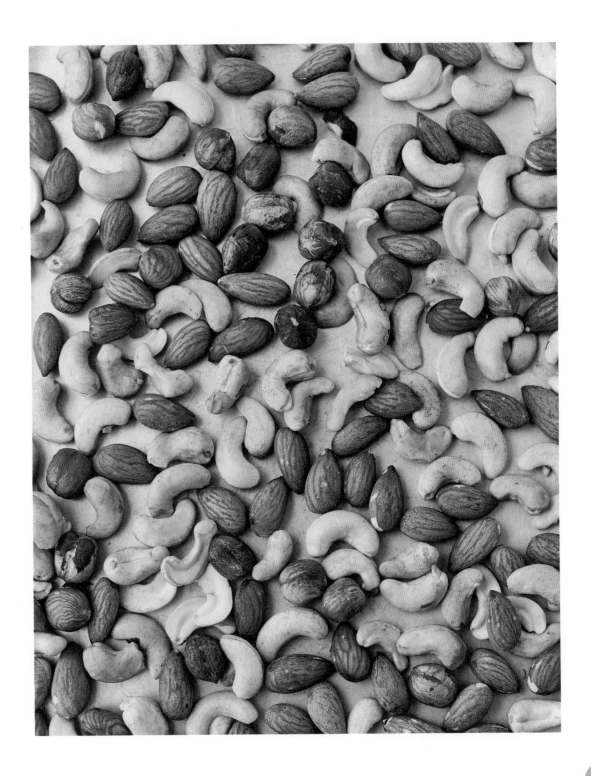

Break
your Fast

We're often told that breakfast is the most important meal of the day, and there's a lot of truth in this. If you split the word up, it says 'break fast' and that's exactly what you're doing. You have fasted overnight, often since early evening, and you now need to break your fast and give your body the fuel it needs in order to function at its best. If you consume unrefined complex carbohydrates and/or fats and protein for this first meal of the day, then your blood sugar will be supported during the morning. You will have more energy and be able to concentrate much better than if you skip breakfast or eat over-processed and sugary breakfast foods. If you don't eat a substantial breakfast, it's all too easy to start snacking on the wrong kind of food mid-morning as your blood sugar dips and you develop cravings.

Some people struggle to eat breakfast, partly because they're not in the habit of having it, but also because their blood sugar may have dropped too low overnight and they actually feel sick at the thought of eating first thing. They often wake with a headache or feeling quite down and out of sorts. When I worked as a nutritional therapist, I used to suggest that these clients ate something slow release (see page 16) for supper, just before bed. I'd recommend oatcakes with nut butter or a bowl of muesli. If this still wasn't sufficient, I'd then suggest they set the alarm for

4am, eat a snack and go back to sleep. Four in the morning is the point at which our blood sugar is at its lowest. It is also the time that people typically wake with panic attacks, an overactive mind, hot flushes or negative thoughts, which can be triggered by low blood sugar. If you have problems and think that your blood sugar may be dipping too much in the night, try supporting it with your diet and see whether things improve.

If you want your children to do well at school and get a good start in life, then it helps to feed them regularly with the right kind of food. When I was in practice as a nutritional therapist, a child would often be brought to see me because of some health problem, and it was lovely to see their surprise and delight when, after adjustments to their diet, their school grades improved and they started to enjoy lessons more because they could concentrate better. We can alleviate so many problems just by eating well. And a good breakfast is the foundation of eating properly each day.

Breakfast Cereal Base Mix

I use a small, straight-sided mug to measure out my cereal and I keep this mug in the cereal container.

Make up a cereal base mix using the cereals you like and what you can tolerate. I like to use a mixture of roughly equal parts of **gluten-free oats, quinoa, millet, brown rice flakes** and **buckwheat flakes**. Store this in a large, resealable container or keep each cereal in an individual jar and choose a different one or a different combination each day. Next you need to work out a portion size depending on your appetite.

Ground Seed Mix

Ground seed mix is now readily available in supermarkets and health-food shops or you can make your own by grinding a mixture of three parts **linseeds** to one part each of **pumpkin, sunflower** and **sesame seeds** and store in a glass jar in the fridge.
This provides the right balance of essential fats.

Power Porridge

Serves 2

Adding ground almonds and fruit to the Breakfast Cereal Base Mix (see page 33), gives a creamier texture. I've used fruit readily available in winter, as this is when I tend to make this porridge; more acidic summer fruits don't work as well, I find. If you cannot tolerate ground almonds, try grinding other nuts, such as cashews or hazelnuts, or use one of the seed mixes now available.

2 mugs Breakfast Cereal Base Mix (see page 33)

1 mug dairy-free milk

2 tbsps sultanas

1 tsp mixed spice

4 mugs boiling water

1 large banana or pear

2 tbsps ground almonds

1. Place the cereal, milk, sultanas and mixed spice in a saucepan and stir to combine.

2. Add the boiling water and mix. Bring to the boil, stirring regularly, then simmer on a low heat for about 5 minutes or until the porridge is smooth and creamy.

3. Peel the banana and cut it into small pieces, or chop up the pear, removing the core, and add to the pan with the ground almonds. Stir to combine and serve immediately.

Variations

For these variations, include the following in place of the sultanas, mixed spice, banana/pear:

Apricot, Cinnamon and Banana: Add 1 teaspoon of ground cinnamon, 2 tablespoons of chopped dried apricots and a sliced banana.

Chocolate, Sultana and Banana: Add 2 teaspoons of cacao, cocoa or carob powder, 2 tablespoons of sultanas and a sliced banana.

Chocolate, Coconut and Pear: Add 2 teaspoons of cacao, cocoa or carob powder, 1 tablespoon of desiccated coconut, 2 tablespoons of sultanas and a diced pear.

Date, Vanilla and Persimmon (Sharon Fruit): Add ½ teaspoon of vanilla extract, 2 tablespoons of chopped dates and a diced persimmon.

Apple, Date and Cinnamon: Add ½ teaspoon of ground cinnamon, 2 tablespoons of chopped dates and a finely sliced apple at the beginning of cooking, so that the apple has time to soften.

Easy Everyday Muesli

Makes 10 mugs

This is best made in bulk and stored in an airtight container so that you can dip in whenever you need a quick breakfast or snack. If you cannot tolerate oats, use 2 mugs each of quinoa, buckwheat and millet flakes. I don't use rice flakes because I want this muesli to be instant and rice flakes benefit from pre-soaking because they are quite hard. You can toast the nuts and sunflower seeds if you want extra crunch (see page 23). Any size of mug will suffice; the bigger the mug, the more cereal you will make.

4 mugs gluten-free oats (mixture of jumbo and porridge)

2 mugs quinoa or buckwheat flakes

1 mug desiccated coconut

½ mug Ground Seed Mix (see page 33)

½ mug sunflower seeds

½ mug chopped walnuts

½ mug chopped almonds

½ mug dried cranberries

½ mug sultanas

1. Mix everything together and store in an airtight container.
2. I like to serve this muesli on a base of grated apple with fresh summer fruit, such as sliced peaches, strawberries or plums, piled on top and moistened with dairy-free milk. A little granola (see page 39) sprinkled on top gives added crunch.

Variations

Try the following combinations of dried fruit and chopped nuts to vary your muesli:

Hazelnuts, almonds and apricots

Cherries, blueberries and cashews

Cranberries, cherries and almonds

Dates, apricots and cashews

Cranberries, dates and walnuts

Slivered almonds, cherries and sultanas

Summer Soaked Muesli

Serves 1

When warmer weather comes along, I swap my porridge for this soaked muesli. It is really substantial, will keep you full for hours and the variations are endless. You can have individual containers with dried fruit and nuts for a help-yourself family affair. You'll find recipes for smoothies later in this chapter (see pages 42–43), but sometimes I use a little shop-bought smoothie in this recipe as it's such a small amount.

¾ mug Breakfast Cereal Base Mix (see page 33)

½ mug dairy-free milk or water

1 tbsp Ground Seed Mix (see page 33) or ground almonds

½ eating apple, finely diced or grated

½ mug fruit smoothie or dairy-free yogurt

1 handful of soft fruit pieces (see topping ideas, right)

1 tbsp dried or freeze-dried fruit (see topping ideas, right)

1–2 tbsps chopped nuts (or see topping ideas, right)

1. Soak the cereal base in the milk or water for at least 15 minutes. You can prepare this ahead and leave to soak overnight to save time in the morning.

2. Add the seed mix or ground almonds and the apple, then pour over the smoothie or yogurt (or a mixture of both).

3. Top with the soft and dried fruit (cut up if large) and the chopped nuts and enjoy!

Topping Ideas

The following combinations of soft and dried fruit and chopped nuts work well:

Peach, dried apricots and almonds

Nectarine, dried cranberries and almonds

Strawberries, crystallised ginger (contains a little sugar) and walnuts

Blueberries, prunes and Brazils

Banana, dried blueberries and cashews

Pineapple, prunes and walnuts

Mango, dried apricots and cashews

Raspberries, dried blueberries and cashews

Plums, sultanas and hazelnuts

Figs, prunes and almonds

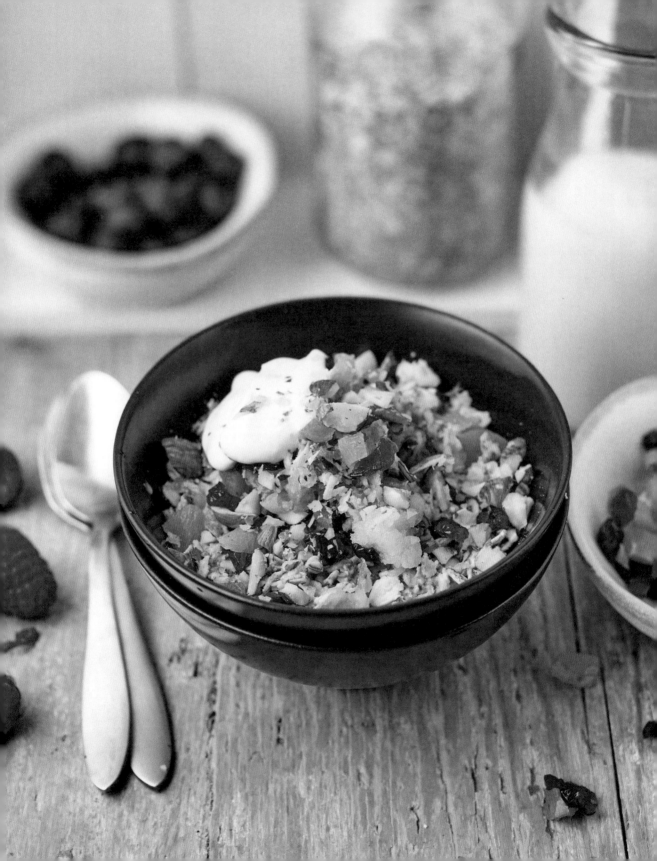

Chia Seed Pots

Serves 2

Soak chia seeds overnight for an easy but decadent breakfast treat. High in anti-inflammatory omega-3s, chia seeds are full of fibre to keep you satisfied for hours. They are also useful for mid-morning or mid-afternoon snacks. The mixture will keep for 2–3 days in the fridge – just dip in whenever you need sustenance or store in little pots ready to take with you when you're on the go.

2 level tbsps chia seeds

170ml (6fl oz) almond or other dairy-free milk (for homemade almond milk, see page 22)

2 tsps honey, mild-tasting runny

½ tsp vanilla extract

To serve

1 ripe banana

1 handful of fresh fruit (such as blueberries, raspberries or chopped peach)

3 tbsps dairy-free yogurt or coconut cream (see page 22)

1 handful of granola (see page 39 – optional)

1. Place the chia seeds and milk in a bowl and whisk to combine. Whisk occasionally over the next 10 minutes until the chia seeds have thickened – this prevents lumps from forming.

2. Mix in the honey and vanilla extract, then place the soaked chia seeds in the fridge to chill and soften for 3–5 hours or preferably overnight.

3. Mash the banana until smooth, then add to the soaked chia seeds. Divide the mixture between two bowls (or pots if transporting) and top with the fresh fruit, yogurt or coconut cream and a scattering of granola just before serving.

Variation

Chocolate Chia Seed Pot: Follow the recipe above but add half a tablespoon of cacao, cocoa or carob powder to the mixture along with the honey and vanilla extract. Top with sliced pear, dairy-free yogurt or coconut cream and some toasted coconut flakes or granola.

Vanilla, Cranberry and Almond Granola

Makes about 700g (1½lb)

Try sprinkling this granola over porridge or muesli to add crunch, or eat as an afternoon snack with diced fresh fruit.

150g (5oz) pitted dates, finely chopped, and 110ml (4fl oz) water (or 1 portion of Date Purée – see page 210)

2 tbsps coconut oil

½ tsp vanilla extract

1 tsp ground cinnamon

50g (2oz) chopped almonds or hazelnuts

50g (2oz) sunflower or pumpkin seeds

25g (1oz) sesame seeds or linseeds

275g (10oz) gluten-free oats or buckwheat flakes

50g (2oz) dried cranberries

25g (1oz) sultanas

1. Preheat the oven to 145°C (125°C fan), gas mark 1½.

2. Place the dates and water in a large saucepan and bring to the boil. Remove from the heat, cover with a lid and leave the dates to soak for about 30 minutes or until they are soft. Once softened, beat the date mixture until smooth or blend in a food processor.

3. Add the coconut oil, vanilla extract and cinnamon and mix in, allowing the coconut oil to melt. (If the dates are cold by this stage, melt the coconut oil in a separate pan before adding.)

4. Add the remaining ingredients and mix well to coat in the date mixture. You can add the dried fruit halfway through cooking in the oven if you prefer it less chewy.

5. Spread the granola on two large baking trays and place on the middle shelf of the oven to bake for 40–45 minutes or until the granola is nicely browned. Mix halfway through cooking as the edges of the mixture will brown first.

6. Remove from the oven and allow it to cool on the trays before storing in an airtight container.

Continued overleaf...

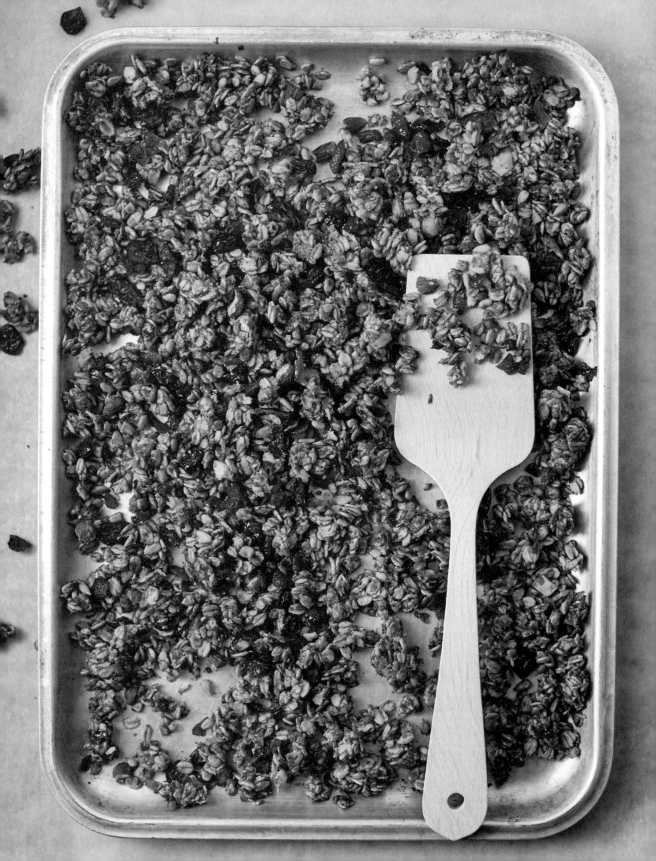

Vanilla, Cranberry and Almond Granola
(continued)

Variations

Double Chocolate and Cherry Granola: A bit indulgent as chocolate does contain a little sugar, but the overall amounts are tiny and this is a real treat when you need something special. Add 1 tablespoon of cacao, cocoa or carob powder to the recipe and substitute dried cherries for the cranberries and sultanas. When the granola has cooled a little, add 50g (2oz) of finely chopped 70–90% dark chocolate and allow it to melt among the clusters.

Marmalade Granola: Using a vegetable peeler, thinly pare the rind of one orange, avoiding the pith as much as possible. Finely slice into 2mm (1/8 in) matchsticks. Place in the pan with the dates and add the juice of two fresh oranges made up to 110ml (4fl oz) with water (if needed) before bringing to the boil and leaving to soften. Omit the ground cinnamon and vanilla extract. Candied peel can be added instead of one of the dried fruits (it does contain a little sugar).

Honey and Ginger Granola: Add 1 tablespoon of mild-tasting runny honey and the squeezed juice of 1 tablespoon of grated fresh root ginger to the date mixture. Miss out the cinnamon and vanilla extract and use cashews or Brazil nuts instead of the hazelnuts or almonds. Crystallised ginger can be used instead of one of the dried fruits (it does contain a little sugar).

Substantial Smoothies

Each serves 2

Because the sugar in a shop-bought smoothie is released too quickly into the bloodstream, I prefer to make my own so that I can offset the fruit with more sustaining ingredients, such as avocado or chia seeds. Smoothies do, however, have their place. They are useful as a starter for breakfast with a second course to follow; to get fruit and vegetables into a reluctant child; or as a mid-afternoon snack. They are also a good first step for people who can't face breakfast and are ideal to feed teenagers who get up late and would otherwise set off for school without anything. If you also have some flapjacks (see pages 218–220) in the freezer, already wrapped, then these can be used as a second course to eat on the journey or on arrival at school or work.

Making a Smoothie

You don't really need a recipe for a smoothie; just make up your own according to what you have available or follow the examples opposite. Always add something substantial to your smoothie, such as nuts, seeds, oats, ground almonds or nut butter. Blitz your ingredients in a blender or food processor until you have a smooth, thick but pourable purée. If you are using grains, whole nuts or seeds, process these first until finely ground before adding the remaining ingredients. Preferably use straight away or store in the fridge for no more than 24 hours.

High-powered Blender

A high-powered blender is a useful piece of equipment for making smoothies as it processes even hard vegetables such as kale or carrots, as well as nuts and seeds, into a smoothie consistency.

Green Smoothie

1 eating apple, chopped

2 kiwi fruits, peeled, or 1
handful of diced pineapple

1 handful of spinach

2 tsps lemon juice

Flesh of ½ avocado

1 mug cold peppermint tea
or 10 fresh mint leaves and
1 mug water

Add all the ingredients to a high-powered blender or food
processor and mix until smooth.

Cooling Summer Smoothie

2 peaches, stoned

2 handfuls of strawberries

4 tsps of chia seeds

1 mug coconut water or
dairy-free milk

Add all the ingredients to a high-powered blender or food
processor and mix until smooth. Drink straight away or the chia
seeds will thicken the mixture.

Comforting Smoothie

1 handful of cashews

1 tbsp of desiccated
coconut

1 banana

1 tbsp of cacao, cocoa or
carob powder

1 mug dairy-free milk

If you are using a food processor, it is best to finely grind the nuts
and coconut before adding the other ingredients and processing
until smooth. If you are using a high-powered blender, add all the
ingredients at the same time.

Berry and Vanilla Smoothie

1 cooked beetroot, chopped

1 handful of mixed berries

2 tbsps of ground almonds

½ tsp of vanilla extract

1 mug cold fruit herbal tea
or dairy-free milk

Add all the ingredients to a high-powered blender or food
processor and mix until smooth.

Gluten-free Toast with Toppings
Each serves 2

Now that I have made successful gluten-free bread (see pages 227–231), I like to keep a loaf sliced in the freezer so that I can dip in whenever I feel like a slice of bread or toast for breakfast. Add coconut oil or a drizzle of olive oil if you cannot tolerate butter for spreading. Try with some of the following toppings and don't forget to include eggs if you don't have a problem with them.

Toppings

Avocado, Olive Oil and Chilli: Chop up the flesh of 1 avocado and place on 2 pieces of toast. Drizzle over a little olive oil and sprinkle with 1 tsp of lemon juice and a pinch of chilli powder or diced fresh chilli.

Smoked Salmon, Avocado and Rocket: Mash the flesh of 1 avocado and spoon onto 2 pieces of toast. Add some strips of smoked salmon, a grind of black pepper, a few rocket leaves and a squeeze of lemon juice.

Sardines, Tomato and Olive Oil: Mash or finely chop 3–4 sardine fillets and use to top 2 pieces of toast. Finely slice a large tomato and add on top. Drizzle over some olive oil and give a grind of black pepper before heating under the grill.

Nut Butter, Banana and Seeds: Spread 4 tablespoons of nut butter of your choice on 2 pieces of toast, then mash a banana and spread on top. Sprinkle over 2 tablespoons of seeds of your choice.

Homemade Baked Beans: Heat through 8 tablespoons of Homemade Baked Beans (see page 144) and use to top 2 pieces of toast.

Mushrooms, Pesto and Mustard: Finely slice 2 handfuls of mushrooms and fry in a little coconut oil or butter with a pinch of dried mustard powder and some salt and pepper. Spread 2 pieces of toast with 2 tablespoons of Pesto Sauce (see page 90) and add the fried mushrooms to serve.

Tray-baked Cooked Breakfast

Serves 2

This healthy cooked breakfast is not only easy to make but there is little washing-up, especially if you line the tray with foil or baking parchment. You could include eggs, scrambled or poached, if these are not a problem, as well as or instead of the smoked salmon. You could serve with Potato Cakes (see page 194), fried leftover potatoes or some gluten-free bread (see pages 227–231), if you prefer.

2 tbsps olive oil

200g (7oz) chestnut mushrooms, halved if large

1 x 250g bunch of asparagus, tailed

1 bunch of cherry tomatoes on the vine (about 12 tomatoes)

4 slices of smoked salmon

Salt and freshly ground black pepper

1. Pre-heat the oven to 200°C (180°C fan), gas mark 6.

2. Place 1 tablespoon of oil and a little salt and pepper in a bowl and add the mushrooms. Toss to coat in the oil, then spread out on a large baking tray. Repeat with the asparagus, laying each spear on the tray with a slight gap between.

3. Add the cherry tomatoes to the tray, then bake in the oven for about 10 minutes or until the mushrooms and asparagus are softening slightly.

4. Serve hot with the smoked salmon.

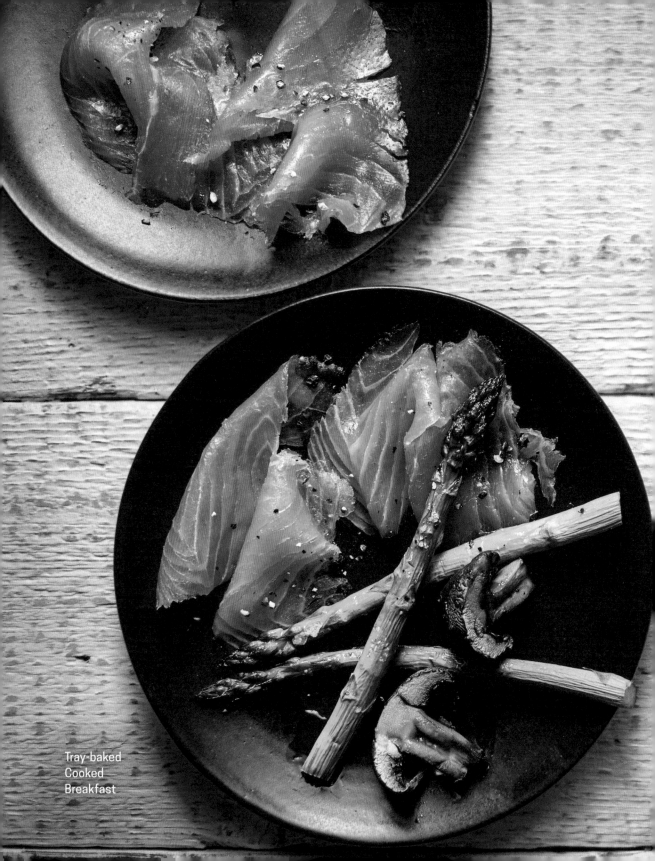

Tray-baked
Cooked
Breakfast

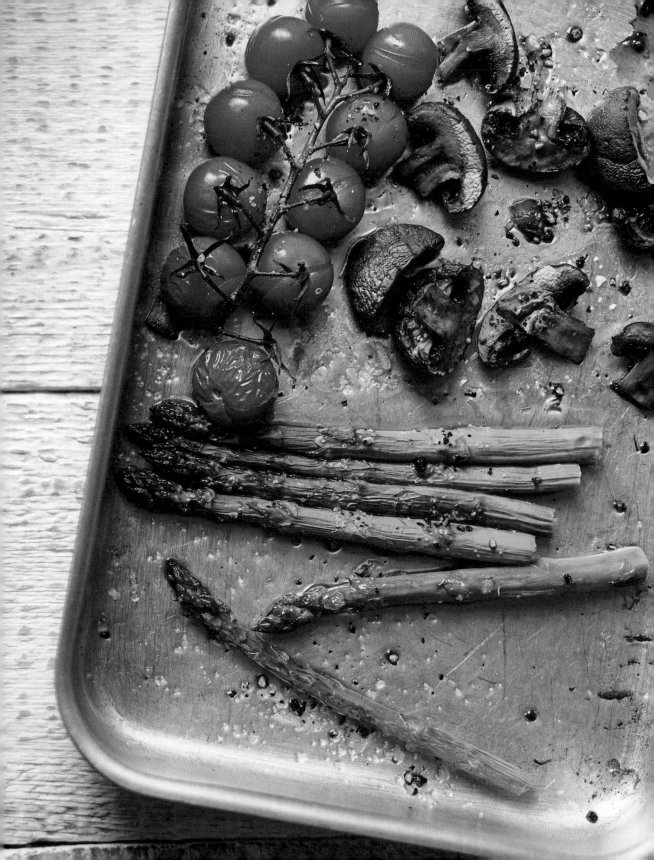

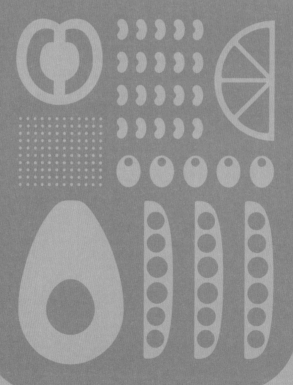

Lunch
on the Go

In this chapter I've included lots of ideas for packed lunches, as few people have the luxury of eating at home. It's also difficult to eat healthily and 'free from' when out and about. Making your own lunches saves money, too, especially if you are assembling a meal from leftovers, whereas the cost of bought-in lunches soon adds up. Bought food, even a ready-prepared salad, is often high in fat and sugar, whereas you can fill your lunchbox with nothing but goodness.

Think about lunches when cooking your evening meal – perhaps cooking some extra chicken, sausages, potatoes, rice or pasta ready to use as a base for next day's lunch. With a little imagination and forward planning, lunch can be a meal to look forward to and needn't take an age to prepare.

The recipes in this chapter are both healthy and substantial. It is so easy to skip lunch or grab something on the run because you're too busy. But if you do, you'll find yourself with an energy or concentration slump mid-afternoon and often with cravings for sweet foods in order to lift your blood sugar and mood. To prevent this, it is important not only to eat the right foods but also to eat regularly and not too late. If you haven't eaten since breakfast, and there's a big gap until lunch, you will still experience a dip even if the food you eat is perfectly balanced nutritionally.

Soups

I'm so pleased with these soups. They are delicious and so quick and easy to make: only 5–10 minutes to prepare and 5–10 minutes to cook. Don't hold me to exact times, but we are talking speedy meals where everything is thrown into a pot and bubbled away. No keeping your eye on a pan of sweating vegetables while you try to do other things. These are soups you can make on a whim when you walk into the kitchen thinking, 'What shall we have for lunch?', or they can be prepared ahead and transported to work in a vacuum flask or resealable container. Most of the soups are blended – using a hand-held stick blender or food processor – and they all freeze well or can be kept for a couple of days in the fridge. The recipes make four average-sized bowls or two large pasta-type bowls. Garnish, if you like, with extra vegetables, chopped herbs, oil or black pepper.

Stock and Stock Cubes

If you have fresh stock, then use it instead of stock cubes – much better and healthier – but I don't expect everyone to make their own. Also, I want these soups to be really quick and easy, and stock cubes (see page 20) fit the bill. I've used chicken or vegetable stock cubes in these recipes. If you'd like to make your own, however, I've included a very simple recipe in the leftovers section (see page 203); alternatively, you can buy fresh, good-quality stock from a supermarket.

Rich Tomato Soup

Serves 2–4

Don't be put off by the thought of anchovies in tomato soup.
The soup won't taste fishy, but you will get an intensely rich flavour.
Because the anchovies are already salty, you won't need to add
any salt to the soup.

1 onion, diced

½ stock cube dissolved in
570ml (1 pint) boiling water

1 tsp dried basil

1 tsp dried oregano

2 x 400g (14oz) tins of
chopped tomatoes

1 x 50g (2oz) tin of
anchovies in oil

Freshly ground black pepper

1. Place the onion, stock and dried herbs in a saucepan, bring to the boil, then reduce the heat and simmer for 5–8 minutes or until the onion is tender.

2. Add the tomatoes and anchovies, including the oil from the tin. Bring back up to a simmer, then blend until smooth. Season with pepper to serve.

Pea and Pesto Soup

Serves 2–4

Dairy-free pesto is readily available in supermarkets, or you could make your own (see page 90). This recipe works well with celery substituted for the leek or onion. Bottled pesto always seems stronger than fresh, almost like creamed basil – hence the variation in quantities.

2 onions, finely diced, or 1 large leek, sliced

1 stock cube dissolved in 1.2 litres (2 pints) boiling water

500g (1lb 2oz) frozen peas

6 tbsps Pesto Sauce (see page 90) or 3 tbsps bottled dairy-free pesto

Salt and freshly ground black pepper

1. Place the onions or leek and the stock in a saucepan, bring to the boil, then reduce the heat and simmer for about 5 minutes or until the vegetables are tender.

2. Add the peas and bring the mixture back up to a simmer. Stir in the pesto to warm through and then blend until smooth. Season to taste with salt and pepper.

Sweet Potato, Carrot and Coriander Soup

Serves 2–4

This gently warming soup is a twist on an old favourite and a great addition to your repertoire. If you don't have a pestle and mortar, just grind the cardamom seeds using the bottom of a glass on a plate.

1 onion or small leek, diced

1 large or 2 medium-sized sweet potatoes, peeled and diced

2 large carrots, sliced

Seeds from 5 cardamom pods, crushed

1 stock cube dissolved in 1.2 litres (2 pints) oiling water

2 tbsps chopped coriander

Salt and freshly ground black pepper

1. Place all the ingredients (except the coriander, salt and pepper) in a saucepan, bring to the boil, then reduce the heat and simmer for 5–8 minutes or until the vegetables are just cooked.

2. Blend until smooth, add the coriander and season to taste with salt and pepper.

Courgette and Broad Bean Soup

Serves 2–4

Every time I make this recipe, I think that there can't possibly be enough ingredients to make a tasty soup, but every time it surprises and delights me. It makes the most delicious, creamy soup, despite the few ingredients. If you are using frozen beans, buy only the baby ones as the others can have tough skins that don't blend very well.

3 large courgettes, sliced

1 stock cube dissolved in 1.2 litres (2 pints) boiling water

450g (1lb) fresh podded broad beans or frozen baby broad beans

Salt and freshly ground black pepper

1. Place all the ingredients (except the salt and pepper) in a saucepan, bring to the boil, then reduce the heat and simmer for 4–5 minutes or until the vegetables are just cooked.

2. Blend the soup until smooth and creamy, and season to taste with salt and pepper.

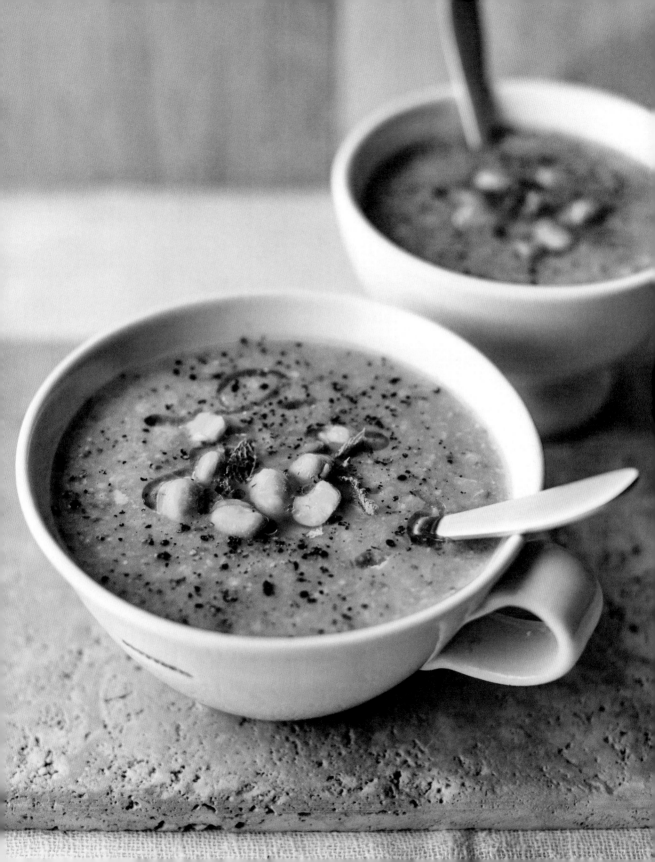

Tomato, Smoked Paprika and Butter Bean Soup

Serves 2–4

This is the soup to make when there is nothing in the fridge but you need sustenance. You will be surprised and delighted with the results.

1 large leek or onion, finely diced

1 tsp sweet smoked paprika

½ stock cube dissolved in 725ml (1¼ pints) boiling water

1 x 400g (14oz) tin of butter beans, drained and rinsed

1 x 400g (14oz) tin of chopped tomatoes

200ml (7fl oz) coconut milk

Salt and freshly ground black pepper

1. Place the leek or onion in a saucepan with the smoked paprika and stock. Bring to the boil, then reduce the heat and simmer for 5–8 minutes or until the vegetables are just cooked.

2. Add the butter beans, chopped tomatoes and coconut milk to the pan and heat through. Blend the soup until smooth and season to taste with salt and pepper.

Creamy Vegetable and Butter Bean Soup

Serves 2–4

Play around with the vegetables in this semi-puréed soup according to what you have available. Parsnip, celeriac, fennel and butternut squash all work well, as long as you have about 700g (1½ lb) of prepared vegetables in total. To make the soup into an even thicker broth, add the rest of the tin of butter beans and a handful of cooked chicken along with the peas.

1 onion, diced

1 leek, sliced

1 large carrot, diced

2–3 sticks of celery, diced

1 potato or sweet potato, peeled and diced

1 stock cube dissolved in 1.2 litres (2 pints) boiling water

½ x 400g (14oz) tin of butter beans, drained and rinsed

1 handful of frozen peas

Salt and freshly ground black pepper

1. Place the fresh vegetables and the stock in a saucepan. Bring to the boil, then reduce the heat and simmer for 5–8 minutes or until the vegetables are just cooked.

2. Blend half of the soup with the butter beans, then return this to the pan (containing the unblended half of the soup), add the peas and heat through. Season to taste with salt and pepper.

Spiced Butternut Squash Soup
Serves 2–4

Sweet potato works equally well instead of butternut squash in this velvety, flavoursome soup. Both sweet potatoes and butternut squash are high in carotenoids, which give their flesh its bright orange colour. These antioxidants have an anti-inflammatory and anti-ageing effect on the body's cells.

1 small butternut squash, peeled, deseeded and diced (about 450g/1lb of flesh)

1 large onion or 1 leek, finely sliced

1 tsp Chinese five-spice powder

1 stock cube dissolved in 1 litre (1¾ pints) boiling water

200ml (7fl oz) coconut milk

Salt and freshly ground black pepper

1. Place the vegetables, spice and stock in a saucepan, bring to the boil, then reduce the heat and simmer for 5–8 minutes or until the vegetables are tender.

2. Add the coconut milk and heat through. Blend the soup until smooth, then season to taste with salt and pepper.

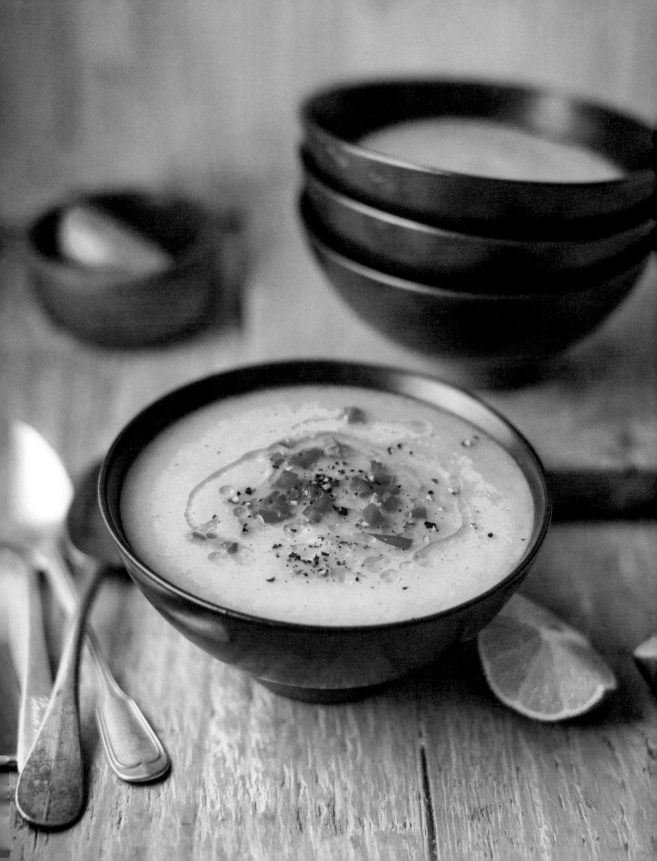

Moroccan Spiced Cauliflower Soup

Serves 2-4

Cauliflower may seem like an unusual ingredient here, but it works really well to produce this subtly spiced, creamy soup. It is made extra creamy with the addition of ground almonds, but miss these out if you cannot tolerate nuts.

½ cauliflower (about 400g/14oz), broken into florets and the stem sliced

1 onion, diced

2.5cm (1in) piece of fresh root ginger, peeled and grated

1 stock cube dissolved in 1.2 litres (2 pints) boiling water

1 tsp ground cinnamon

1 tsp ground cumin

½ tsp garam masala

½ tsp turmeric

Seeds from 10 cardamom pods, crushed

50g (2oz) ground almonds

Salt and lots of freshly ground black pepper

Paprika, for sprinkling

1. Place the vegetables, ginger, stock and spices in a saucepan and bring to the boil. Reduce the heat and simmer for 5–8 minutes or until the vegetables are just cooked.

2. Add the ground almonds and blend the soup until smooth. Season to taste with salt and pepper and add a sprinkling of paprika to serve.

Wild Rocket, Spinach and Watercress Soup

Serves 2–4

For a variation on this soup, use 200g (7oz) of baby spinach leaves instead of the rocket, spinach and watercress and add half a teaspoon of freshly grated nutmeg.

1 large leek, mainly white stem, sliced

1 potato, peeled and diced

1 stock cube dissolved in 1 litre (1¾ pints) boiling water

200ml (7fl oz) coconut milk

1 x 130g (4½oz) packet of mixed wild rocket, spinach and watercress

Salt and freshly ground black pepper

1. Place the leek, potato and stock in a saucepan, bring to the boil, then reduce the heat and simmer for 5–8 minutes or until the vegetables are just cooked.

2. Add the coconut milk, rocket, spinach and watercress and bring back up to a simmer. Cook for a further minute, then blend the soup until smooth. Season to taste with salt and pepper.

Salad Pots

The art of eating a gluten- and yeast-free diet is to think further than just sandwiches and consider the delicious alternatives. My favourite lunch if I'm out and about is a homemade salad pot. As I really want these salad pots to be easy to make, I've sometimes suggested using tinned beans and fish and frozen vegetables. Where cooked ingredients such as meat are called for in a recipe, try to cook these while you have the oven on for your evening meal. Even better, plan your evening meals so that you have leftovers to use the next day. Fresh herbs are usually optional in recipes, even though they make a wonderful addition, as I don't always have them around.

Once you've made your salad, pop it into a sealed container and refrigerate it until needed. If you know your salad pot will not be refrigerated when out and about, think first before including ingredients such as such as prawns or fish. If it's hot and I'm out, I usually include some frozen vegetables such peas or sweetcorn, which will help to keep my salad cool.

These salad pots are also ideal for summer entertaining and picnics as you can make them ahead then serve a selection of them. That's my sort of entertaining – easy but delicious dishes, and everyone will love them. If you are vegetarian, don't dismiss the meat- and fish-based salad pots: by substituting beans, pulses, nuts, tofu or cheese and eggs (if these are tolerated), you have a wealth of pots to choose from.

Salad Pot Base Ingredients

The base for your salad pot can be **cooked rice, millet, quinoa, buckwheat, potatoes, pasta, tinned beans (cannellini, chickpeas or butter beans)** or **lentils,** the quantity depending on your appetite. It is a good idea to dress pasta as soon as it is cooked to stop it from sticking together. If you prefer to avoid too much starch, try a base of **vegetable noodles** (see page 126) – lightly steamed or sautéed – or use **lettuce, rocket, watercress** or **spinach leaves,** but be aware that these will not keep you full for as long. It's best to put salad leaves at the top of your salad pot to prevent them from wilting and mix them in when you are ready to eat.

Salad Dressings

Salad dressings can be found on pages 110–111. I always have a jar of Pomegranate Molasses Dressing (page 110) ready mixed as it is so easy to make and it goes well with all the salad pots.

Curried Cauliflower, Cranberry and Walnut Salad Pot

Serves 2

Cauliflower has grown in popularity in the last few years as people are beginning to realise that it's a powerhouse of nutrients. I love its crunchy texture when eaten raw in a salad and this mildly spicy version combines some lovely flavours and textures.

½ fresh red chilli, deseeded and finely diced (optional)

2 handfuls of frozen peas

2 handfuls of small cauliflower florets

2 tbsps red onion, finely diced

2 parings of lemon rind, finely sliced

2 tbsps dried cranberries or raisins

1 small handful of walnut pieces

2 portions Salad Pot Base (such as cooked rice, millet or buckwheat – see page 62)

6 tbsps Coconut Lime and Chilli Dressing or dressing of your choice (see pages 110–111)

Salt and freshly ground black pepper

1. Combine all the ingredients for the salad in a bowl or pan.

2. Mix in the salad dressing and season with salt and pepper, if needed. Transfer the salad to resealable containers if not eating at home.

Chicken, Sweetcorn and Bacon Salad Pot
Serves 2

This is a delicious and filling lunch that will provide you with sufficient fuel and nutrients to keep you going during a busy afternoon.

2 rashers of crisp cooked bacon, cooled and sliced

½ courgette, grated

1 handful of sweetcorn kernels

1 handful of mangetout or sugar snap peas, sliced

2 spring onions, finely sliced

1 handful of shredded cooked chicken

2 portions of Salad Pot Base (such as cooked rice, buckwheat or diced new potatoes – see page 62)

4–6 tbsps Pomegranate Molasses Dressing or dressing of your choice (see pages 110–111)

Salt and freshly ground black pepper

1. Combine all the salad ingredients in a bowl or pan and mix with the dressing.

2. Season the salad with salt and pepper, if needed, and transfer to resealable containers if not eating at home.

Chicken, Cranberry and Five-spice Salad Pot

Serves 2

I love this salad as it contains some of my favourite ingredients. Chinese five-spice gives a wonderful background flavour and the crunchy cashew nuts contrast beautifully with the tender chicken and tart cranberries.

6 white mushrooms, quartered

4 tbsps Pomegranate Molasses Dressing or dressing of your choice (see pages 110–111)

1 level tsp Chinese five-spice powder

2 spring onions, finely sliced

2 handfuls of shredded cooked chicken

2 tbsps dried cranberries

1 tbsp chopped mint or coriander (optional)

2 portions of Salad Pot Base (such as cooked rice or buckwheat – see page 62)

Salt and freshly ground black pepper

1 handful of cashews, toasted (see page 23), to garnish

1. Marinade the mushrooms in the dressing and five-spice powder while you assemble the remaining ingredients.

2. Toss everything together in a bowl or pan and season to taste with salt and pepper.

3. Transfer the salad to resealable containers if not eating at home. Garnish with the toasted cashew nuts when ready to eat.

Sausage and Lentil Salad Pot

Serves 2

I sometimes use the ready-cooked lentils sold in pouches at the supermarket. Cooked with vegetables and spices, the lentils are very tasty and convenient to use, but check the ingredients in case they include any that you can't eat. Tinned lentils are fine, or you could cook your own dried ones and save money. Ideally, make this when you have leftover cooked sausages.

2 large or 4 small cooked gluten-free sausages, sliced

½ x 400g (14oz) tin of lentils, drained and rinsed, or ½ x 250g (9oz) pouch of ready-cooked lentils

8 sun-blushed tomatoes, diced

2 spring onions, finely sliced

2 sticks of celery, finely diced

4 radishes, finely sliced

1 portion of Salad Pot Base (such as cooked rice or quinoa – see page 62)

4–6 tbsps Pomegranate Molasses Dressing or dressing of your choice (see pages 110–111)

Salt and freshly ground black pepper

1. Combine all the ingredients for the salad in a bowl or pan.

2. Mix with the dressing and season with salt and pepper, if needed. Transfer to resealable containers, if transporting your salad, and look forward to a delicious and filling lunch.

Crayfish and Mango Salad Pot

Serves 2

With its contrasting colours and textures, this salad looks as good as it tastes!

2 handfuls of rocket

1 carrot, grated

½ red pepper, deseeded and diced

Flesh of ½ just-ripe mango, diced

2 tbsps red onion, finely diced

125g (4½oz) cooked crayfish tails or prawns

½ fresh red chilli, deseeded and finely diced (optional)

1 tbsp chopped coriander (optional)

2 portions of Salad Pot Base (such as tinned cannellini beans or cooked pasta – see page 62)

5–6 tbsps Coconut Lime and Chilli Dressing or dressing of your choice (see pages 110–111)

Salt and freshly ground black pepper

1. Keeping the rocket to one side, combine the remaining salad ingredients in a bowl or pan.

2. Mix with the dressing and season with salt and pepper, if needed. Transfer to resealable containers, if transporting your salad, with the rocket piled on top, ready to mix in when you eat.

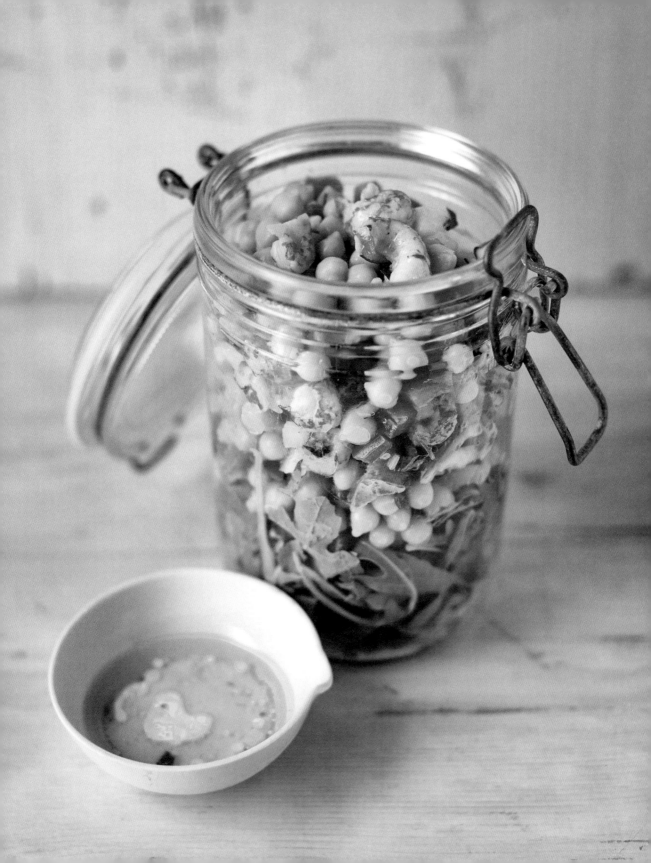

Smoked Trout and Grapefruit Salad Pot

Serves 2

Oily fish such as trout is a good source of omega-3 fatty acids, while grapefruits are high in vitamin C, making this salad highly nutritious as well as very tasty.

1-2 smoked trout fillets, flaked

7cm (3in) piece of cucumber, diced

Diced flesh of 1 grapefruit and grated zest of ½ grapefruit

1 handful of watercress or 5 radishes, sliced

2 portions of Salad Pot Base (such as cooked new potatoes or pasta – see page 62)

4–6 tbsps Pomegranate Molasses Dressing or dressing of your choice (see page 110–111)

Salt and freshly ground black pepper

1. Combine all the salad ingredients in a bowl or pan and toss in the dressing.

2. Season with salt and pepper if needed, then transfer to resealable containers if out and about.

Sardine, Tomato and Spinach Salad Pot
Serves 2

This great lunch will keep your taste buds satisfied at the same time as nourishing your body with essential fats from the sardines, the powerful antioxidant lycopene from the tomatoes and iron from the spinach.

1 handful of cooked green beans, sliced

1 x 120g (4oz) tin of sardines in tomato sauce, roughly chopped

10 cherry tomatoes, halved

10 black olives, pitted and halved

2 portions of Salad Pot Base (such as cooked pasta or tinned chickpeas – see page 62)

4–6 tbsps Pomegranate Molasses Dressing or dressing of your choice (see page 110–111)

1 handful of baby spinach, rocket or watercress

Salt and freshly ground black pepper

2 tbsps pine nuts, toasted (see page 23), to garnish

1. Combine all the salad ingredients except the green leaves and pine nuts in a bowl or pan. Mix with the dressing and season with salt and pepper, if needed.

2. Transfer to resealable containers if taking your salad out, placing the green leaves on top, ready to mix in when you eat. Serve sprinkled with toasted pine nuts.

Tuna, Sweetcorn and Celery Salad Pot

Serves 2

This salad is an old favourite of mine. I love it because it can be made when there are very few fresh salad ingredients left in the fridge, yet the contrasting textures and flavours make a delicious dish.

1 x 200g (7oz) tin of tuna, drained

2 handfuls of sweetcorn kernels

2 sticks of celery, finely diced

½ eating apple, diced

1 small handful of walnut pieces

6 tinned anchovies, finely sliced

2 portions of Salad Pot Base (such as cooked buckwheat or quinoa – see page 62)

4–6 tbsps Pomegranate Molasses Dressing or dressing of your choice (see pages 110–111)

Freshly ground black pepper

1. Combine all the ingredients for the salad in a bowl or pan, mixing them with the dressing.

2. You shouldn't need to season with salt as the anchovies are salty, but add pepper if you like. Transfer the salad to resealable containers if not eating at home.

'Nothing in the Fridge' Salad Pot

Serves 2

This salad pot relies heavily on tinned and frozen ingredients, so is ideal to make when the fridge is empty. It's also a good one to bear in mind if you are going to be in a hot car or temperatures are soaring and you don't have the facilities to refrigerate. The frozen ingredients help to keep it cool but will be defrosted by the time you are ready to eat. I like to add fresh mint to this salad, as I always have some in the garden or freezer and I love the way the flavour permeates the salad after a few hours.

2 handfuls of frozen peas

2 handfuls of frozen sweetcorn kernels

2 handfuls of frozen prawns or 1 x 200g (7oz) tin of tuna, drained

4 tinned anchovies, finely diced, plus 1 tsp anchovy oil reserved from the tin

2 sun-dried tomatoes, finely diced

10 black olives, pitted and halved

1 tbsp chopped mint, fennel or coriander (optional)

2 portions of Salad Pot Base (such as cooked rice, millet or quinoa – see page 62)

4 tbsps Pomegranate Molasses Dressing or dressing of your choice (see pages 110–111)

Freshly ground black pepper

1. Combine all the ingredients for the salad in a bowl or pan and mix with the dressing.

2. You shouldn't need to season with salt as the anchovies are salty, but add pepper if you like. Transfer the salad to resealable containers if out and about.

Mediterranean Salad Pot

Serves 2

It's good to make this salad pot with a quinoa base, for extra protein. Try adding some slices of avocado if you are eating it straight away (avocado browns easily if left too long, even if tossed in lemon juice). Raisins make a good substitute for sun-dried tomatoes.

1 small courgette, thinly sliced

½ small red onion, finely diced

½ red or yellow pepper, deseeded and diced

8 cherry tomatoes, halved

12 black or green olives, pitted and halved

2 sun-dried or 6 sun-blushed tomatoes, diced

1 tbsp chopped basil, mint or coriander (optional)

2 portions of Salad Pot Base (such as cooked quinoa or buckwheat – see page 62)

4–6 tbsps Pomegranate Molasses Dressing or dressing of your choice (see pages 110–111)

Salt and freshly ground black pepper

1. Stir gently to combine all the salad ingredients in a bowl or pan.

2. Mix in the salad dressing and season with salt and pepper if needed. Transfer the salad to resealable containers if not eating at home.

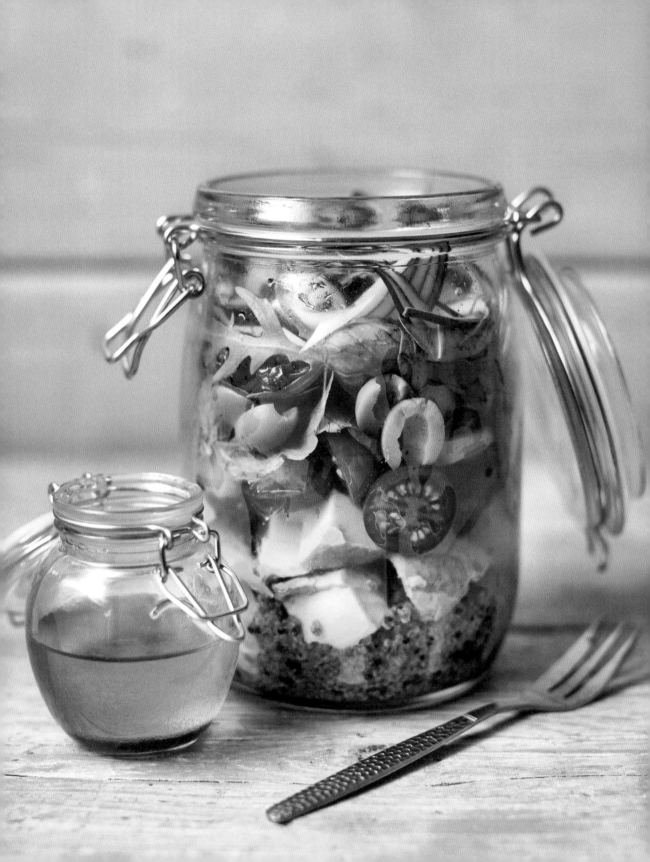

Pâtés and Dips

These simple pâtés and dips are perfect for spreading on crispbreads or gluten-free oatcakes to accompany soups (see pages 50–61). They can also be used for sandwich and baked potato fillings (see pages 85–87) or packed into little pots for eating on the go. Loosened with a little water, they make ideal dips to serve with crudités. They will generally serve four, depending on what you use them for. They also freeze well.

Carriers for Dips

You can use a whole range of 'carriers' for dips, from oatcakes, rice cakes or gluten-free crackers (try the Artisan Crispbreads on page 232) to crudités – fruit and vegetables cut into sticks where appropriate, such as apples, carrots, celery, peppers, cucumber, courgette, baby sweetcorn, sugar snap peas, radishes, green beans, cauliflower and broccoli florets. These are ideal in lunchboxes, or to serve as a second course after a bowl of soup. They are good to keep in the fridge for when children come home from school, or when you return from work ravenous and in need of something to nibble. Use any of the pâtés in this section, adding a little water where necessary to make the pâté into a dip consistency.

Easy Houmous

Serves 4

Although houmous is easy to buy ready made, some brands contain sugar and you will save money by making your own. This recipe uses tinned chickpeas, though you could substitute frozen ready-cooked chickpeas, available from some supermarkets. It also omits the usual tahini paste, which I always find has gone out of date by the time I rescue it from the back of the fridge.

1 x 400g (14oz) tin of chickpeas, drained and rinsed

1 tbsp sesame seeds

1 tsp grated lemon zest and 2 tbsps lemon juice

2 tbsps olive oil

1 tsp sesame oil

1 garlic clove, crushed

2–3 tbsps water

Salt and freshly ground black pepper

1. Place all the ingredients except the water and seasoning in a food processor and blend until smooth.

2. Add sufficient water to soften the mixture if it is too stiff, and season to taste with salt and pepper.

Variation

You can vary your houmous by blending in other ingredients, such as the flesh of 1 small avocado, 4–5 sun-dried tomatoes, 2 roasted red peppers or 2 tablespoons chopped fresh coriander.

Sun-dried Tomato and Mackerel Pâté

Serves 4

Tinned tuna or sardines would make a good substitute for the mackerel in this flavoursome pâté.

1 x 120g (4oz) tin of mackerel fillets, drained

4–6 sun-dried tomatoes

2 tbsps tomato purée

3–4 tbsps water

1. Blend the mackerel, sun-dried tomatoes and tomato purée until smooth in a food processor, or finely chop the sun-dried tomatoes and then mash everything together with a fork. Add sufficient water to loosen the mixture and produce a soft pâté.

Red Lentil and Sweet Potato Pâté

Serves 4

This recipe produces a smooth, golden pâté full of fibre from the lentils and beta-carotene from the sweet potatoes. It also tastes scrummy and is very moreish.

150g (5oz) dried red split lentils, rinsed and drained

1 sweet potato (about 200g/7oz), peeled and cut into large chunks

1 tsp sweet smoked paprika

½ tsp dried thyme

½ stock cube dissolved in 425ml (15fl oz) boiling water

2 tsps pomegranate molasses or lemon juice

Salt and freshly ground black pepper

1. Place the lentils and sweet potato in a saucepan with the smoked paprika, thyme and stock. Bring to the boil, then reduce the heat and cook for about 15 minutes or until the lentils and sweet potato are tender and almost all of the liquid has been absorbed.

2. Blend the mixture in a food processor with the pomegranate molasses or lemon juice until smooth and creamy. Season to taste with salt and pepper.

Artichoke and Olive Pâté

Serves 4

This is such a simple pâté to make, yet it tastes as though you must have spent ages preparing it. Just bask in the praise and don't let on that it was so easy!

8 tinned or bottled artichoke hearts

1 garlic clove, crushed

16 green olives, pitted

4 tinned anchovy fillets in oil, plus 1 tsp oil from the tin

1 tbsp olive oil

Freshly ground black pepper

1. Drain or squeeze the liquid from the artichoke hearts and add them to a food processor with the garlic, olives, anchovies, anchovy oil and olive oil.

2. Blend until smooth and season with black pepper. (You shouldn't need to season with salt as the anchovies are salty.)

Kalamata Olive and Lentil Pâté

Serves 4

Everyone who tastes this asks for the recipe! Based on a traditional Greek recipe, it produces a delicious, piquant and slightly salty pâté.

125g (4 ½ oz) ready-cooked Puy or whole brown lentils (from a tin or pouch)

110g (4 oz) pitted Kalamata olives

1 tsp dried oregano

1 tsp grated lemon zest and 1 tbsp lemon juice

55ml (2fl oz) olive oil

Freshly ground black pepper

1. Place the lentils in a food processor with the olives, oregano, lemon zest and juice, and blend until fairly smooth.

2. With the processor still running, drizzle the olive oil slowly into the mixture via the feeder tube and blend until very smooth. Season with black pepper – you won't need any salt because the olives are quite salty.

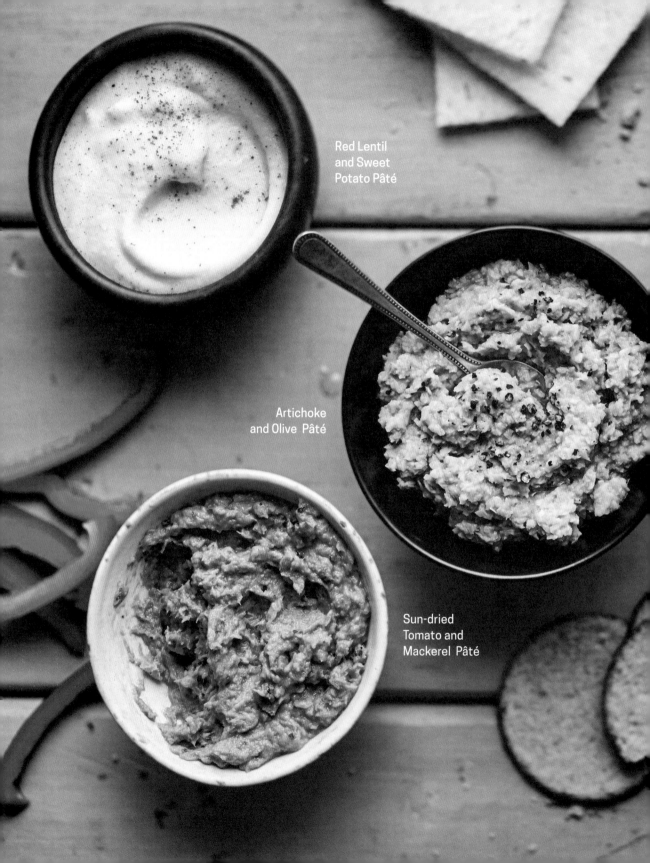

Red Lentil
and Sweet
Potato Pâté

Artichoke
and Olive Pâté

Sun-dried
Tomato and
Mackerel Pâté

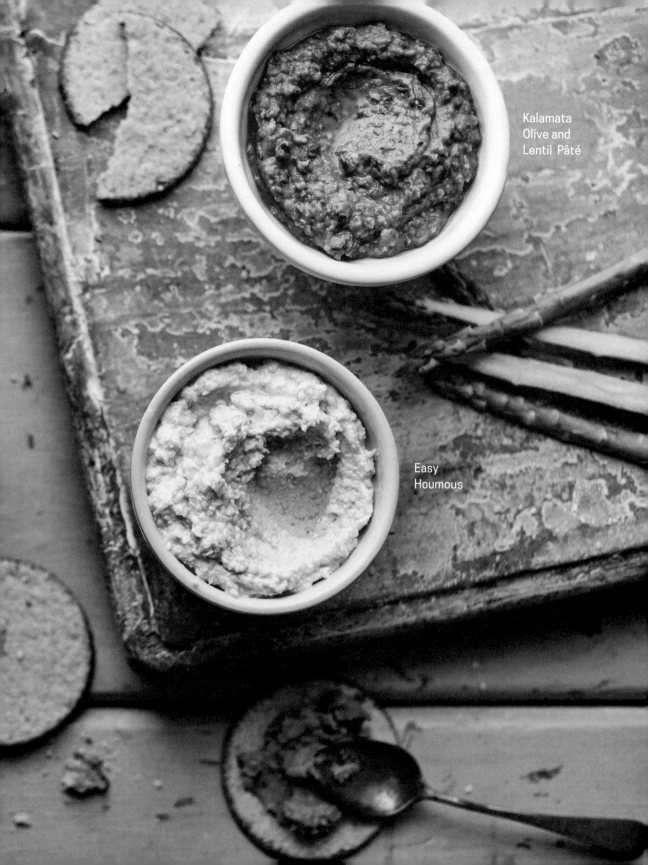

Kalamata
Olive and
Lentil Pâté

Easy
Houmous

Mushroom Pâté

Serves 4

With its intense flavour and deep rich colour, this pâté is delicious served hot or cold.

10g (½oz) dried porcini mushrooms

2 tbsps oil (see page 20)

310g (11oz) field mushrooms, sliced

1 garlic clove, crushed

½ tsp dried thyme

½ tsp dried oregano

2 tbsps ground almonds or 1 slice of gluten-free bread (see pages 227–231)

Salt and freshly ground black pepper

1. Soak the dried porcini mushrooms in sufficient hot water to cover.

2. While the dried mushrooms are soaking, heat the oil in a large frying pan and fry the sliced field mushrooms and garlic over a medium heat for 4–5 minutes or until the mushrooms release their juices.

3. Drain and dice the soaked porcini mushrooms, then roughly chop and add to the pan with the dried herbs. Continue to cook until all the liquid has evaporated – about another 8 minutes.

4. Transfer the mixture to a food processor, along with the ground almonds or slice of bread, and blend until smooth, seasoning to taste with salt and pepper.

Cashew Nut Cheese

Serves 4

Reminiscent of cream cheese, this slightly tart but sweet cashew nut pâté makes a lovely option if you cannot (or choose not to) eat dairy. The cashew nuts have to be soaked well in advance, however, so you need to think ahead when making this dish.

150g (5oz) cashew nuts, soaked in 425ml (15fl oz) water for at least 6 hours

2 garlic cloves, crushed

50g (2oz) coconut oil

2 tbsps lemon juice

55ml (2fl oz) olive oil

55ml (2fl oz) boiling water

1 tbsp chopped coriander, dill or fennel (optional)

Salt and freshly ground black pepper

1. Drain and rinse the soaked cashews and blend in a food processor until finely ground.

2. Add all the remaining ingredients except the herbs and seasoning and process until you have a smooth cheese. Season to taste with salt and pepper and fold in the herbs (if using).

Baked Potatoes and Sweet Potatoes

The thought of a warming baked potato with a delicious filling is something I look forward to in the autumn. Sweet potatoes are ideal as they have a slower absorption rate than standard potatoes, as well as being high in beta-carotene, but you can substitute ordinary potatoes if you prefer. This is a selection of delicious and more unusual fillings. You could also use the pâtés on pages 77–83 as a topping.

Baking a Potato

Baking potatoes is simple. Simply scrub them and pop them in the oven just as they are. You can oil them or wrap them in foil if you want softer skins. Standard potatoes take about 1 hour to cook, and sweet potatoes 30–40 minutes, at 200°C (180°C fan), gas mark 6.

Baked Potato Fillings
Serves 2

Make one of these fillings while your potatoes or sweet potatoes are baking – they are all quick and easy to prepare. When the potatoes are cooked, split them and roughly mash a little of the flesh with a fork so that when you pile over the filling it soaks in.

Lentil and Mushroom

1 tbsp oil

1 garlic clove, crushed

200g (7oz) chestnut mushrooms, sliced

125g (4½oz) ready-cooked lentils (from a tin or pouch)

½ tsp dried thyme

2 tbsps tomato purée

2–3 tbsps water

Salt and freshly ground black pepper

1. Heat the oil in a pan, add the garlic and mushrooms and cook over a medium heat for 4–5 minutes or until they start to soften.

2. Add the lentils, thyme and tomato purée and heat through, mashing a little with your wooden spoon and adding sufficient water, if needed, to loosen the mixture. Season with salt and pepper, pile into the baked potatoes and serve.

Sardine and Tomato

1 x 120g (4½oz) tin of sardines in tomato sauce

2 tbsbs tomato purée

2 large fresh tomatoes, finely diced

1. Roughly chop the sardines, then add the tomato purée and chopped tomatoes and mix to combine.

2. Pile the mixture into the baked potatoes and serve.

Continued overleaf...

Baked Potato Fillings (continued)

Asparagus, Pea and Pesto

6 asparagus spears, cut
into 3cm (1¼in) lengths

4 good handfuls of peas

4 tbsps Pesto Sauce
(see page 90)

2–3 tbsps water

1. Cook the asparagus spears in a small pan of boiling water for
about 2 minutes or until just tender. Remove from the pan with
a slotted spoon and keep warm while you cook the peas.

2. Drain the peas and mash or blend in a food processor with the
pesto and sufficient water to loosen the mixture. Season with
salt and pepper, then pile into the baked potatoes and top with
the asparagus.

Smoked Mackerel, Beetroot and Avocado

Flesh of 1 medium avocado

2 parings of lemon rind,
finely sliced

1 tbsp lemon juice

1 smoked mackerel fillet,
flesh flaked

2 small cooked beetroots
(not in vinegar), finely diced

1 spring onion, finely sliced

2–3 tbsps water

Salt and freshly ground
black pepper

1. Roughly mash the avocado flesh with a fork, then add the
remaining ingredients except the water and seasoning and mix
to combine.

2. Add sufficient water to loosen the mixture and season to
taste with salt and pepper. Pile the mixture into baked
potatoes and serve.

Spinach and Tomato

1 tsp oil

4 good handfuls of baby
spinach leaves

1 garlic clove, crushed

2 large tomatoes, finely
diced

2 sun-dried tomatoes,
finely diced

Salt and freshly ground
black pepper

1. Heat the oil in a pan, add the spinach and garlic and cook over
   a medium heat, stirring, for 2–3 minutes or until the spinach
   is wilted.

2. Add the fresh and sun-dried tomatoes and heat through,
   but don't cook, the tomatoes. Season to taste with salt
   and pepper, pile into the baked potatoes and serve.

Roast Chicken, Avocado and Sweetcorn

Flesh of 1 medium avocado

1 tbsp lemon juice

½ tsp mustard powder
or 1 tsp grainy mustard

2 handfuls cooked,
diced chicken

2 handfuls sweetcorn

Salt and freshly ground
black pepper

1. Roughly mash the avocado flesh with a fork and combine with the
   rest of the ingredients. Add a little water if needed to loosen
   the mixture.

2. Season to taste with salt and pepper, pile the mixture into the
   baked potatoes and serve.

Pasta
and Pizza

Pasta

Everyone loves pasta – so tasty as well as quick and easy to prepare. In fact, you can have most of these dishes on the table in 15–20 minutes.

There is now a wealth of alternative pastas on the market and they really are very good, competing well with standard wheat pasta and increasingly made with low-GI ingredients such as beans, buckwheat and sweet potato. I like pasta spirals because they hold the sauces better, but choose whichever shape you prefer. Follow the directions on the packet for the quantities of pasta to use and cooking times, as these will vary depending on the type of pasta.

You will notice from these recipes that I like to add lots of vegetables to my pasta dishes. I'm a vegetable fiend and I like to try to eat at least five portions a day and preferably more. Research is now suggesting that we should probably be aiming for eight portions of fruit and vegetables a day, so these pasta sauces offer an ideal way to include them.

If you prefer to eat less carbohydrate, then replace the pasta with a similar quantity of vegetable 'noodles' – made using a spiraliser or a julienne peeler – from vegetables such as courgettes, or try cutting leeks or cabbage into ribbons. Steam these lightly or sweat them in a little oil (see page 20), then use them instead of the gluten-free pasta. Just be aware that vegetable pasta will not keep you full for as long.

Pesto Sauce

Serves 2–3

This pesto sauce is used in some of the following pasta recipes, but it can also be used on its own swirled into a bowl of steaming hot pasta. Dairy-free pesto is now readily available, but it is usually stronger-tasting (almost like a creamed basil), so you need to taste the pesto as you add it to recipes and adjust the amount accordingly. You can make pesto using other herbs and it often works out much cheaper. Using half spinach and half basil creates a gentler-flavoured pesto and also cuts the cost. It's easier to make a larger quantity in the food processor, so feel free to increase the quantities in this recipe and freeze some for another day.

40g (1½ oz) pine nuts, cashews or blanched almonds

75g (3oz) fresh basil, coriander, rocket or watercress (with stalks removed)

1 garlic clove, crushed

1 tbsp lemon juice

2 tbsps light oil (such as rice bran)

1 tbsp olive oil

About 30ml (1fl oz) water (or enough to blend to a soft consistency)

Salt and freshly ground black pepper

1. Blitz the nuts in a food processor until finely ground, then add the herbs or green leaves and process again.

2. Add the garlic, lemon juice, oils and water and process to mix before seasoning with salt and pepper to taste. The pesto will keep in the fridge for a few days, but also freezes well if it is not needed straight away.

Pasta with Spinach, Courgette and Bacon

Serves 2

This delicious and filling bowl of pasta will provide you with enough nutrients and energy to keep you going on a busy day. Avocados contain essential fats and even some protein, as well as giving this pasta a lovely creamy texture. Pesto Sauce (see page 90) could be used instead of the avocado in this recipe.

2 portions of gluten-free pasta

2 tsps oil (see page 20)

2–3 rashers of bacon, finely diced

1 garlic clove, crushed

6 spring onions, finely sliced

1 courgette, coarsely grated

2 good handfuls of baby spinach leaves

Flesh of 1 large ripe avocado (about 200g/7oz)

1 tsp pomegranate molasses

1 tbsp lemon juice

Salt and freshly ground black pepper

1. Cook the pasta in a large pan of boiling water according to the packet instructions.

2. Meanwhile, heat the oil in a separate pan and fry the bacon over a medium heat for 4–5 minutes or until it begins to brown, then add the garlic, spring onions, courgette and spinach and continue to cook for another 3–4 minutes or until the vegetables start to soften.

3. Blend the avocado until smooth in a food processor with the pomegranate molasses and lemon juice, or mash together with a fork.

4. Drain the pasta, reserving some of the cooking liquid, and return to the pan. Add the bacon and vegetable mixture, the blended avocado and enough cooking liquid to loosen the mixture. Season to taste with salt and pepper and serve.

Pasta with Asparagus, Peas and Broad Beans

Serves 2

This is a lovely dish to make in the summer when all the vegetables are fresh, but it's also fine to use frozen peas and broad beans. Cooked chicken pieces can be added instead of, or as well as, one of the vegetables.

2 portions of gluten-free pasta

2 handfuls of peas

2 handfuls of baby broad beans

1 handful of asparagus, tailed and cut into short lengths

Flesh of 1 large ripe avocado

4–6 tbsps Pesto Sauce (see page 90) or 2–3 tbsps bottled dairy-free pesto

Salt and freshly ground black pepper

1 handful of cashews, toasted (see page 23), to garnish (optional)

1. Cook the pasta in a large pan of boiling water according to the packet instructions, adding the peas, beans and asparagus to cook in the same pan for the last 3 minutes.

2. Blend the avocado and pesto until smooth and creamy in a food processor, or mash together with a fork.

3. Drain the pasta and vegetables, reserving some of the cooking liquid, and return to the pan. Combine with the avocado sauce, adding enough cooking liquid to loosen the mixture.

4. Season to taste with salt and pepper and serve garnished with the toasted cashews (if using), chopped if you prefer.

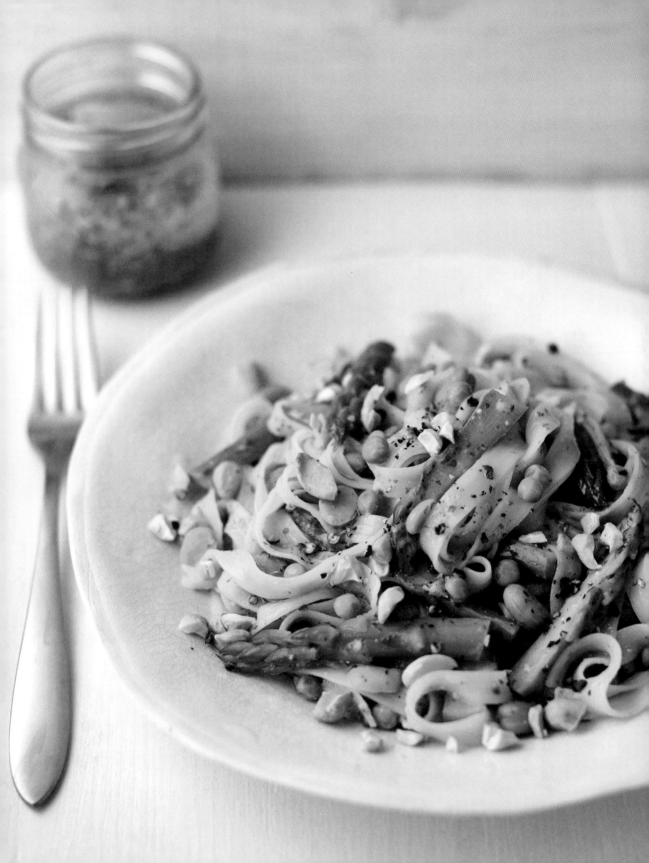

Pasta with Chicken, Mushrooms and Toasted Cashews

Serves 2

You would never think that this dish, with its delicious creamy sauce, is gluten- and dairy-free. Raw diced chicken breast can be used instead of cooked chicken (or omit altogether if you are vegetarian). Just fry the meat for a few minutes before adding the mushrooms.

2 portions of gluten-free pasta

2 sticks of celery, sliced, or 1 handful of sweetcorn kernels

1 handful of broccoli florets or sliced green beans

1 tbsp oil (see page 20)

1 garlic clove, crushed

6 large chestnut mushrooms, sliced

½ tsp dried thyme

¼ stock cube dissolved in 225ml (8fl oz) boiling water

200ml (7fl oz) coconut milk

1 tsp mustard powder or 1 tbsp grainy mustard (see page 20)

2 level tbsps gluten-free plain flour (see page 22)

2 handfuls of shredded cooked chicken

Salt and freshly ground black pepper

1 handful of cashews, toasted (see page 23), to garnish

1. Cook the pasta in a large pan of boiling water according to the packet instructions, adding the celery or sweetcorn and green beans or broccoli to cook in the same pan for the last 5 minutes.

2. Meanwhile, heat the oil in a separate pan, add the garlic, mushrooms and thyme and fry over a medium heat for 4–5 minutes or until the mushrooms have softened.

3. Whisk together the stock, coconut milk, mustard and flour and add to the mushrooms. Bring the mixture to the boil, stirring all the while, then reduce to a simmer and cook for 2 minutes before adding the cooked chicken to heat through.

4. Drain the pasta and vegetables, reserving some of the cooking liquid, and combine with the chicken and mushrooms, adding a little cooking liquid, if needed, to loosen the mixture. Season to taste with salt and pepper and serve garnished with the toasted cashews.

Pasta with Mushrooms, Walnuts and Broccoli

Serves 2

This is a favourite recipe of mine. Despite being vegetarian this pasta dish, with its meaty texture and full-bodied flavour, will not disappoint confirmed carnivores.

1 large carrot, roughly chopped

6 large chestnut mushrooms, roughly chopped

1 handful of walnut pieces

½ tsp fennel seeds

½ tsp dried oregano

1 tbsp oil (see page 20)

2 tbsps tomato purée

150ml (5fl oz) boiling water

2 portions of gluten-free pasta

1 good handful of purple-sprouting broccoli, cut into short lengths, or small broccoli florets

1 good handful of celery or fennel, diced

Salt and freshly ground black pepper

1. Pulse the carrot and mushrooms in a food processor until finely diced, then add the walnuts, fennel seeds and oregano and pulse again, until everything is fairly finely ground but a few walnut pieces are still visible.

2. Heat the oil in a pan and cook the processed mixture over a medium heat for 5 minutes. Add the tomato purée and boiling water and continue to cook while you prepare the pasta.

3. Cook the pasta in a large pan of boiling water according to the packet instructions, adding the broccoli and celery or fennel to cook in the same pan for the last 4 minutes.

4. Drain the pasta and vegetables, reserving some of the cooking liquid, and combine with the carrot and walnut mixture, adding a little cooking liquid, if needed, to loosen the mixture. Season to taste with salt and pepper and serve.

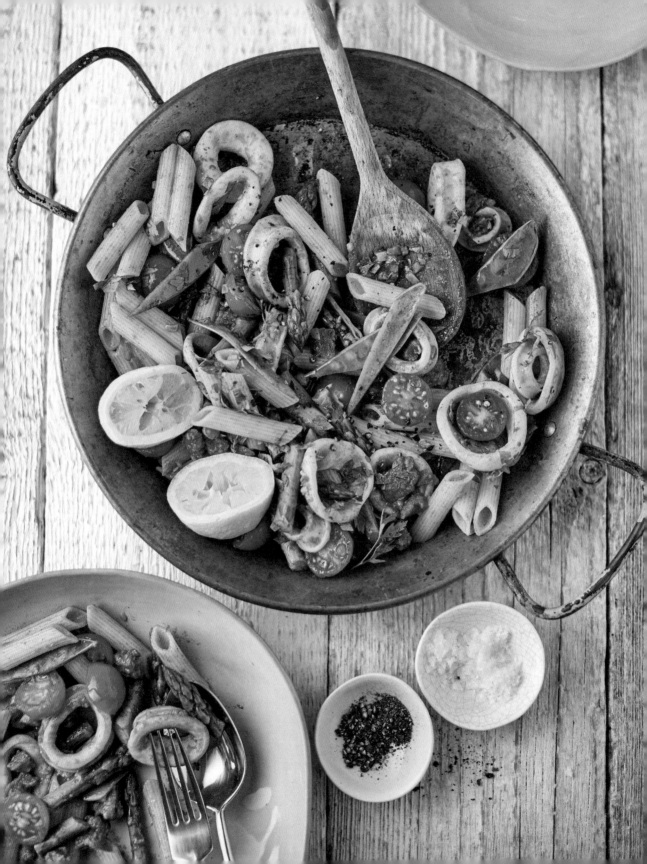

Pasta with Squid and Chorizo

Serves 2

If you keep diced chorizo in the freezer, as well as frozen squid, this recipe will only take minutes to make, yet the combination of colours, textures and flavours puts it in the gourmet class.

2 portions of gluten-free pasta

1 handful of baby sweetcorn, halved lengthways, or asparagus spears, tailed and sliced into 3cm (1¼in) lengths

2 handfuls of mangetout or sugar snap peas

7.5cm (3in) piece of chorizo, finely diced

1 garlic clove, crushed

2 handfuls of fresh or frozen squid, sliced

½ tsp sweet smoked paprika

3 tbsps tomato purée

1 tsp pomegranate molasses or 1 tbsp lemon juice

12 cherry tomatoes, halved

Salt and freshly ground black pepper

1. Cook the pasta in a large pan of boiling water according to the packet instructions, adding the sweetcorn or asparagus and mangetout or sugar snap peas to cook in the same pan for the last 3 minutes.

2. Meanwhile, heat a separate pan and fry the chorizo (no need to add oil) over a medium heat for about 4 minutes or until it begins to brown and release its oil. Add the garlic, squid and smoked paprika and continue to cook for a further 3–5 minutes or until the squid is cooked (this will take slightly longer if using frozen squid), then add the tomato purée, pomegranate molasses or lemon juice, and the cherry tomatoes and just heat through.

3. Drain the pasta and vegetables, reserving some of the cooking liquid, and add to the chorizo mixture. Stir to combine, adding enough of the cooking liquid to loosen the mixture.

4. Season to taste with salt and pepper and serve before the tomatoes lose their shape.

Sardine and Tomato Pasta with Pine Nuts

Serves 2

This is a very good way of getting oily fish into children or even into reluctant adults. The sardines seem to disappear and are hardly noticeable, but the taste is amazing. You could even add an extra tin if you are a sardine fan.

2 portions of gluten-free pasta

1 leek, mainly white stem, thinly sliced

1 handful of green beans, sliced

1 x 120g (4½oz) tin of sardines in tomato sauce, roughly chopped

½ tsp fennel seeds

⅛–¼ tsp chilli powder (optional)

2 tbsps tomato purée

10 cherry tomatoes, halved

10 black or green olives, pitted and halved

2 tbsps sultanas

Salt and freshly ground black pepper

2 tbsps pine nuts, toasted (see page 23), to garnish

1. Cook the pasta in a large pan of boiling water according to the packet instructions, adding the leek and beans to cook in the same pan for the last 5 minutes.

2. Drain the pasta, reserving some of the cooking liquid, and return to the pan. Add the sardines, fennel seeds, chilli powder, tomato purée, tomatoes, olives and sultanas. Stir to combine, adding enough of the cooking liquid to loosen the mixture.

3. Heat through, then season to taste with salt and pepper and serve garnished with the toasted pine nuts.

Pasta with Tuna, Artichokes and Pesto

Serves 2

This quick and easy pasta is one of my lunchtime favourites, as it includes ingredients I usually have to hand. I just swap the vegetables for others, if necessary, and lunch is on the table in minutes.

2 portions of gluten-free pasta

1 small red pepper, deseeded and diced

2 handfuls of small broccoli florets or sliced courgettes

1 x 200g (7oz) tin of tuna in water

5 tinned or bottled artichoke hearts, quartered, or 12 black olives, pitted and halved

6 tbsps Pesto Sauce (see page 90) or 3 tbsps bottled pesto

Salt and freshly ground black pepper

1. Cook the pasta in a large pan of boiling water according to the packet instructions, adding the red pepper and broccoli or courgettes to cook in the same pan for the last 4 minutes.

2. Drain the pasta and vegetables, reserving some of the cooking liquid, and return to the pan. Add the tuna (plus the water in the tin), the artichokes or olives and the pesto. Stir to combine, adding enough of the cooking liquid to loosen the mixture.

3. Heat through, season to taste with salt and pepper, and serve.

Pizza

Just because you don't eat wheat and dairy, it doesn't mean that you can't have a pizza. The pizza base opposite is gluten-free and the topping doesn't have to include cheese. There are some dairy-free cheeses on the market, usually made from soya, but I think I would rather go without. If you can tolerate sheep or goat's cheese, you could use one of these. Because I don't use cheese, I choose to add extra toppings and make sure these contain some tasty ingredients such as sun-blushed tomatoes, anchovies, olives or chorizo. If you have some partly prepared base mixes ready in the freezer (the dry ingredients can be stored, ready weighed, in plastic bags), it means you can have a pizza ready to cook in double-quick time.

Pizza Base

Makes 2 bases

Don't make your pizza bases until you have prepared your toppings and preheated the oven and baking trays. Once you are ready to assemble the pizzas, everything needs to be done quickly as the raising agent in the bases will start to work straight away. To make just one pizza base, simply halve the quantities of the ingredients.

For the wet ingredients

25g (1oz) ground linseed

170ml (6fl oz) boiling water

1 tsp blackstrap molasses

1 tbsp lemon juice or
¼ tsp vitamin C powder
(see page 23)

2 tbsps olive oil, plus extra
for drizzling

30–75ml (1–3fl oz) cold
water

For the dry ingredients

200g (7oz) gluten-free plain
flour (see page 22), plus
extra for dusting

½ level tsp bicarbonate
of soda

1 level tsp gluten-free
baking powder

1 level tsp mustard powder

25g (1oz) gluten-free oats
or buckwheat flakes

½ tsp dried basil

½ tsp dried oregano, plus
extra for sprinkling

1 scant level tsp salt

1. Preheat the oven to 220°C (200°C fan), gas mark 7, and place two baking trays or pizza stones in the oven to heat up.

2. Place the ground linseed and boiling water in a bowl with the molasses, lemon juice or vitamin C powder and the olive oil and leave to soak while you prepare the remaining ingredients.

3. Place two pieces of baking parchment (not greaseproof paper), each about 30cm (12in) square, on a work surface and sprinkle with flour.

4. Sift the flour, bicarbonate of soda, baking powder and mustard powder into a bowl and add the rest of the dry ingredients.

5. Add 30ml (1fl oz) cold water to the soaked linseed and mix well.

6. Combine the soaked linseed with the dry ingredients, mixing quickly and adding more water, if needed, to make a very soft and sticky dough.

7. Split the mixture in two, tipping half onto each piece of baking parchment. Sprinkle the top of each piece of dough with more flour, flatten roughly with the palm of your hand, then roll out into a circle about 4mm (¼in) thick and 28cm (11in) in diameter. I often make two oval bases, as these fit better on my baking trays.

8. Add your choice of toppings (see pages 102–105) and drizzle with oil.

9. Lift each pizza on its piece of baking parchment onto a hot baking tray or pizza stone and bake in the oven for about 15 minutes or until the pizzas are crisping around the edges and the vegetables (if using) have softened. Slide the pizzas off the parchment onto plates and serve.

Pizza Toppings

Your pizza first of all needs a moist layer. I use 2 tablespoons of tomato purée for each pizza, quickly and roughly spread over the surface, but you could use Easy Houmous or Pesto Sauce (see pages 77 and 90) if you can't tolerate tomatoes. Next add some chosen toppings from the list below, putting ingredients that would burn easily, such as spinach or fresh herbs, at the bottom and ones that need to crisp up, such as chorizo, at the top. Choose a good selection from the following, so that your pizza has lots of flavour, or follow the recipes on pages 104–105.

Roasted vegetables: Onion, peppers, aubergine, butternut squash, sweet potatoes or fennel.

Raw vegetables: Use quick-cook vegetables, such as sliced mushrooms, courgette, red pepper, asparagus, thinly sliced red onion and spring onions or baby sweetcorn (halved lengthwise) and cherry tomatoes.

Meat: Choose from ham, bacon or prosciutto (diced) or cooked sausage or chicken (sliced).

Fish: Tuna, sardines or anchovies (tinned or bottled) work well, as do raw prawns, mussels, squid or scallops, and smoked salmon.

Herbs: Place fresh herbs, such as basil, oregano, coriander, fennel or chives, on the base to prevent them from burning or add after cooking. Dried basil, oregano, thyme or fennel can be sprinkled on top before cooking.

Extra flavourings: Olives, pesto, sun-blushed or sun-dried tomatoes, finely sliced garlic and artichoke hearts (tinned or bottled) all give extra flavour. Add spiciness with sliced chorizo (sprinkled on top), finely diced fresh red chilli or peppery rocket leaves (added before other toppings or when the pizza comes out of the oven).

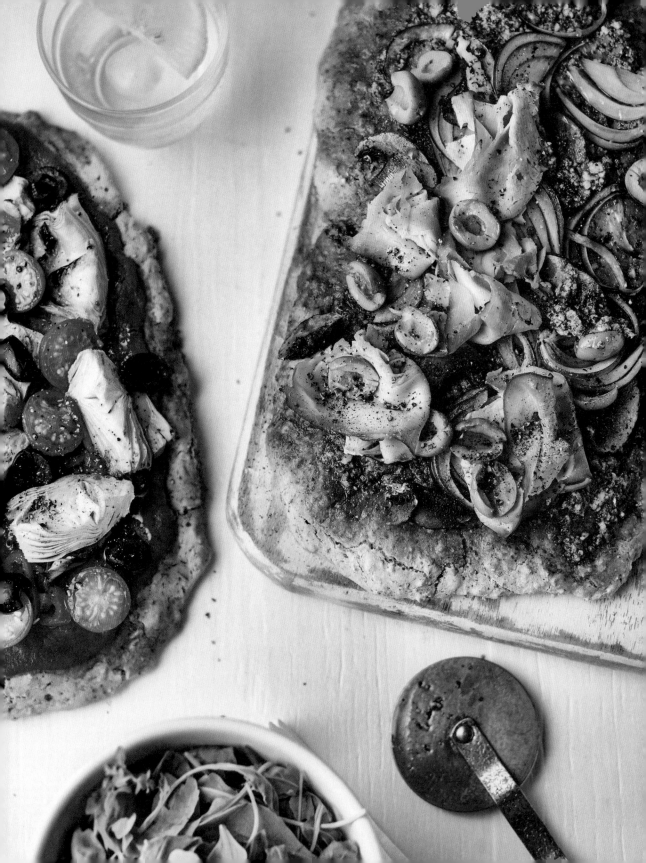

Ham, Mushroom and Pesto

Serves 2

2 handfuls of diced cooked ham

8 chestnut mushrooms, sliced

½ red onion, finely sliced

12 green or black olives, pitted

4 tbsps Pesto Sauce (see page 90)

Olive oil, to drizzle

1. Top your pizza bases with your choice of moist layer (see page 102).

2. Sprinkle the ingredients over, finishing with the pesto, then drizzle with olive oil.

3. Lift each pizza onto a hot baking tray or pizza stone and bake in the oven for about 15 minutes or until the pizzas are crisping around the edges and the vegetables have softened.

4. Slide the pizzas onto plates and serve.

Prawn, Smoked Salmon and Asparagus

Serves 2

8 asparagus spears, tailed, halved lengthways and cut into 3cm (1¼in) lengths

2 handfuls of sweetcorn kernels

4 pieces of smoked salmon, diced

2 handfuls of frozen cooked prawns or fresh uncooked prawns

8 sun-blushed tomatoes, sliced

1 tsp dried oregano

Olive oil, to drizzle

1. Top your pizza bases with your choice of moist layer (see page 102).

2. Sprinkle the ingredients over, then drizzle with olive oil.

3. Lift each pizza onto a hot baking tray or pizza stone and bake in the oven for about 15 minutes or until the pizzas are crisping around the edges and the prawns are cooked through.

4. Slide the pizzas onto plates and serve.

Artichoke, Olive, Chilli and Rocket

Serves 2

4 tinned or bottled
artichoke hearts, cut into
6–8 segments

½ red pepper, deseeded and
finely diced

1 small courgette, very
thinly sliced

12 cherry tomatoes, halved

12 green or black olives,
pitted

½–1 fresh red chilli,
deseeded and very finely
diced

Olive oil, to drizzle

1 handful of rocket leaves,
to serve

1. Top your pizza bases with your choice of moist layer (see page 102).

2. Squeeze any excess liquid from the artichokes, if using tinned ones, then sprinkle all the ingredients except the rocket over the bases. Drizzle with olive oil.

3. Lift each pizza onto a hot baking tray or pizza stone and bake in the oven for about 15 minutes or until the pizzas are crisping around the edges and the vegetables have softened.

4. Top with the rocket, slide the pizzas onto plates and serve.

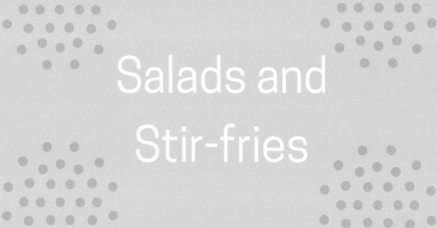

Salads and
Stir-fries

These are meals to make when you don't want to spend time labouring over a hot stove – when the weather is hot or you just want a quick meal. Both salads and stir-fries are very forgiving if you haven't got all the right ingredients. Substitutions are fine – just use whatever you have to hand. It's a great way to use up odds and ends of vegetables left at the bottom of the fridge.

Eating plenty of salads and vegtables is one of the simplest things you can do to attain good health. Full of antioxtidants, vitamins and minerals, salads and vegetables are rich in fibre but low in calories. In areas of the world where people live long, healthy lives, their diets all contain a high percentage of vegetables. Salads and stir-fries offer the perfect opportunity to include lots in your diet.

Substantial Salads

These are not salads to accompany other dishes, but meals in themselves. Served in large individual bowls, they are a feast for the eyes as well as the stomach. You can select from such a wide range of ingredients that salads never need to be boring.

Main meal salads need to be substantial – not just a couple of lettuce leaves and a sliced tomato – otherwise you will be hungry a few hours later and tempted by any snacks available. The salads here consist of a selection of base ingredients made up from the list opposite according to your likes and dislikes and what you have available. Quantities should be ample – the ingredients should cover your bowl or plate and and be piled high to ensure your salad is filling. Then select a hot or cold topping such as chicken, peach and toasted cashews, or roasted sweet potato, red pepper and pine nuts (see the serving suggestions on pages 112–122). Dress your salad with one of the dressings (see pages 110–111), or simply drizzle with good-quality olive oil. You can serve bread or additional potatoes as an extra if you have hearty appetites to satisfy.

Dressings

The dressings on pages 110–111 add an extra dimension to a salad and I am sure you will soon find a favourite. Alternatively, try buying an expensive bottle of olive oil to drizzle over your salad. Olive oils, like wines, vary a lot in flavour, from strong and bitter to light and fruity.

Substantial Salad Base Ingredients

Choose a good selection from the following. See below for an example of the ingredients you might combine to create one base.

Leafy greens: Lettuce, rocket, watercress, spinach, chard, kale, cabbage, mixed salad leaves or Chinese cabbage.

Raw vegetables: Choose a selection from: thinly sliced peppers, celery, fennel, cucumber, red onion, spring onions or radishes; halved cherry tomatoes, baby sweetcorn, mangetout, sugar snap peas or button mushrooms; grated courgettes or carrots; diced avocado or beetroot; broad beans, peas, sweetcorn kernels, cauliflower florets or bean sprouts.

Cooked vegetables: Green beans or asparagus.

Fresh fruit: Diced apple, orange or mango; sliced strawberries or figs; halved grapes.

Dried fruit: Raisins, sultanas or cranberries.

Nuts: Pine nuts, peanuts, cashews, almonds or walnuts.

Seeds: Pumpkin, sunflower or sesame.

Pulses: Cannellini beans, butter beans, red kidney beans, chickpeas or lentils.

Fresh herbs: Basil, fennel, mint, chives or coriander.

Extra flavourings: Olives, sun-dried/sun-blushed tomatoes or artichoke hearts (tinned or bottled).

Sample Substantial Salad Base for Two

4 good handfuls of leafy greens

1 diced stick of celery

7.5cm (3in) piece of cucumber, diced

¼ red onion, sliced

¼ yellow pepper, sliced

8 cherry tomatoes, halved

½ avocado, diced

10 black olives

1 handful of cannellini beans

4–5 strawberries, sliced

Pomegranate Molasses Dressing

Makes 1 jar

This is the easiest, healthiest, tastiest salad dressing ever, and it takes less than five minutes to prepare. You don't even need to be exact about measurements – it will still taste fine. If I had to choose just one, this would be it. You can add other flavourings, if you prefer, such as a teaspoon of honey, mustard powder or fennel seeds.

Pomegranate molasses

Salt and freshly ground black pepper

Olive oil

1. Take a salad dressing jar, or jam jar with a lid, and fill by ⅛ with pomegranate molasses. Add an equal quantity of boiling water and a little salt and pepper. Place the lid on the jar and shake well to combine the ingredients.

2. Open the jar and fill with olive oil, leaving sufficient space at the top to allow the ingredients to mix. Add the lid and shake again to combine, and your dressing is ready. Store at room temperature, rather than in the fridge, to prevent it from solidifying.

Pesto Dressing

Makes about 4 servings

This goes particularly well with vegetarian salads; think roasted vegetables or artichokes and avocado drizzled with pesto dressing.

1 quantity of Pesto Sauce (see page 90) or 4 tbsps bottled pesto

3 tbsps olive oil

3 tbsps water

1. Place all the ingredients in a bowl and whisk to combine. If you are making pesto from scratch (see page 90), then the oil and water can be added to the food processor to combine. Store in the fridge for up to a week or freeze any excess for another day.

Coconut, Lime and Chilli Dressing

Makes about 4 servings

This is the most delicious and easy-to-make salad dressing that will turn any salad into a taste sensation. Why not make up lots and freeze some for another day?

1 tsp grated lime zest

1 tbsp lime juice

1 tsp mild-tasting runny honey (optional)

1 tsp fresh green chilli, deseeded and finely diced

1 tsp ginger juice (squeezed from grated fresh root ginger)

1 tbsp chopped coriander or basil

110ml (4fl oz) coconut cream (see page 22)

Coconut water

Salt and freshly ground black pepper

1. Place all the ingredients except the coconut water and seasoning in a bowl and whisk to combine. Add enough coconut water (from the tin of coconut milk) to produce a runny dressing and season to taste with salt and pepper.

2. Cover and store in the fridge for up to a week or freeze any excess. Remove from the fridge to soften before using and whisk again.

Pear, Walnut and Beetroot Salad

Serves 2

Beetroot is a real superfood that helps the body to detox, while walnuts are full of essential fats. Enjoy them both in this tasty and colourful vegetarian salad.

Dressing of your choice (see pages 110–111)

2 Substantial Salad Bases of your choice (see page 109), including rocket if available

Flesh of 1 large ripe pear, cut into bite-sized chunks

2 cooked beetroots, diced

1 handful of walnut halves

Mint leaves, to garnish (optional)

1. Drizzle the dressing over the salad bases.

2. Scatter over the pear, beetroot and walnuts, and garnish with mint leaves (if using).

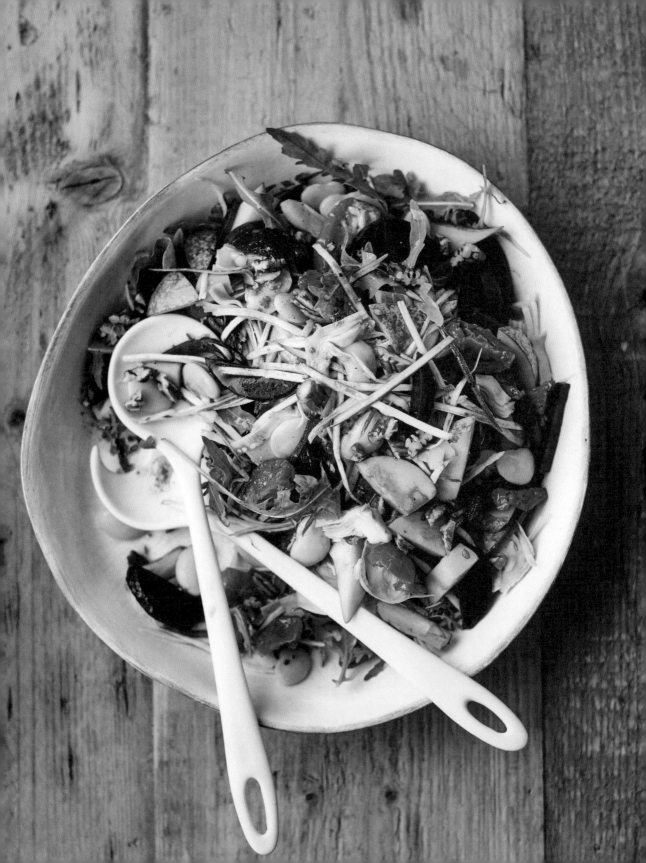

Avocado, Artichoke and Olive Salad

Serves 2

Top your vegetarian salad with these Mediterranean flavours for a nutritious as well as delicious bowl of clean food.

2 substantial salad bases (see page 109)

Salad dressing of your choice (see pages 110–111)

1 large avocado, peeled and flesh diced

4–6 cooked artichoke hearts, cut into wedges

12 black olives, halved

1. Make up the salad bases and drizzle with your chosen dressing.
2. Scatter the avocado, artichoke hearts and olives over the surface and serve.

Sausage, Sun-dried Tomato and Roasted Red Onion Salad

Serves 2

Whenever my oven is on, I try to think of anything else I could cook for meals over the next few days. If you precook the sausage and onion in this recipe, it can be kept in the fridge until needed, then served cold or warmed before adding to the salad.

4 large or 6 medium gluten-free sausages

2 red onions, each cut into 6 wedges

1 tbsp olive oil

2 Substantial Salad Bases of your choice (see page 109)

4 sun-blushed tomatoes, cut into pieces

Pomegranate Molasses Dressing or dressing of your choice (see pages 110–111)

1. Preheat the oven to 200°C (180°C fan), gas mark 6.

2. Prick the sausages and place on a baking tray with the onion wedges, then drizzle the onions with the olive oil. Roast for about 25 minutes or until the sausages and onions are cooked.

3. Top the salad bases with the sun-blushed tomatoes and drizzle with your favourite dressing.

4. Slice the cooked sausages into pieces, scatter on top of the salad with the roasted onions and serve immediately.

Chicken, Peach and Toasted Cashew Nut Salad

Serves 2

This salad looks so inviting with its contrasting colours, textures and flavours. Use mango instead of peach, and toasted pine nuts instead of cashews, for a variation on this recipe.

Coconut, Lime and Chilli Dressing or dressing of your choice (see pages 110–111)

2 Substantial Salad Bases of your choice (see page 109)

2 handfuls of cooked chicken pieces

Flesh of 1 large or 2 small peaches, diced

4 tbsps cashews, toasted (see page 23)

1. Drizzle the dressing over the salad bases.

2. Scatter over the chicken pieces, diced peach and toasted cashews and serve.

Steak and Mushroom Salad

Serves 2

This is a feast of a salad – full of texture and flavour and robust enough to satisfy a hearty appetite.

1 x 225g (8oz) steak (sirloin, rib-eye)

½ tsp mustard powder

2 tsps oil (see page 20)

8 large chestnut mushrooms, sliced

1 garlic clove, crushed

2 Substantial Salad Bases of your choice (see page 109)

Pomegranate Molasses Dressing or dressing of your choice (see pages 110–111)

Salt and freshly ground black pepper

1. Pat the steak dry with kitchen paper and then sprinkle both sides with some salt and pepper and the mustard powder. Heat 1 teaspoon of the oil in a pan and fry the steak on a medium heat for about 3 minutes on each side for medium rare. (Cook it less for rare and more for well done, depending on how you like it and the thickness of your steak.) Remove the steak from the pan and set aside to rest for 5 minutes before slicing thinly.

2. Add the remaining teaspoon of oil to the steak juices in the pan and fry the mushrooms and garlic until they are just cooked but not too soft. Season them with salt and pepper.

3. Drizzle the dressing over the salad bases, then top with the warm mushrooms and sliced steak.

Smoked Mackerel, New Potato and Orange Salad

Serves 2

This is a wonderfully tasty way to get your omega-3 oils from fish, as well as from raw veggies and fresh fruit, in an amazingly appetising dish.

10 new potatoes, cut into bite-sized pieces

Pomegranate Molasses Dressing or dressing of your choice (see pages 110–111)

2 Substantial Salad Bases of your choice (see page 109), including lots of rocket

2 smoked mackerel fillets, flesh flaked

Flesh of 1 orange, diced

1 tsp fennel seeds

1. Cook the potatoes in a large pan of boiling water for about 15 minutes or until just tender, then drain.

2. Drizzle the dressing over the salad bases, then top with the flaked mackerel, diced orange pieces and the hot new potatoes. Scatter with the fennel seeds and serve at once.

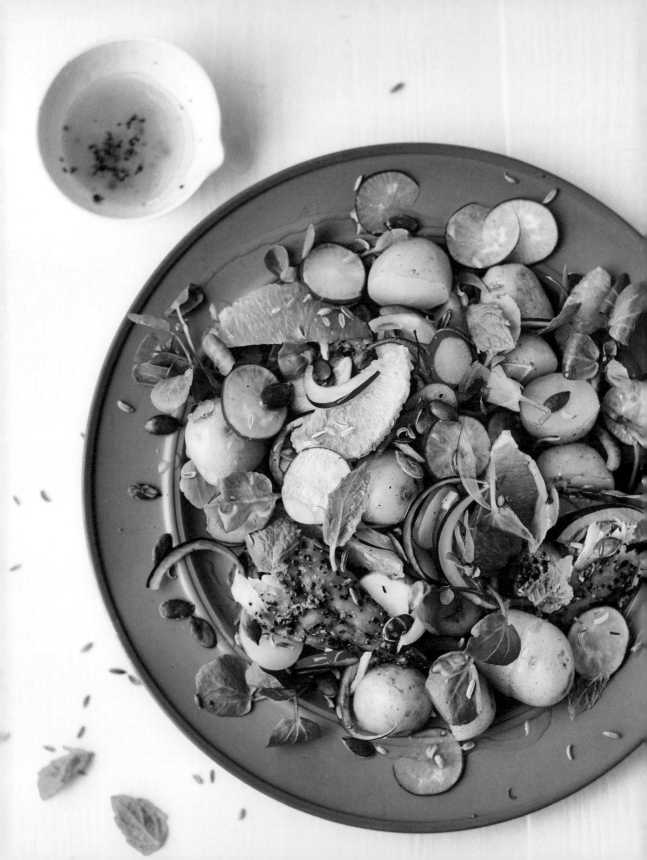

Chorizo, New Potato and Sun-blushed Tomato Salad

Serves 2

This salad is ideal to make when you have leftover cooked new potatoes. For a vegetarian version, swap the chorizo for avocado, artichoke hearts or cubes of feta cheese (if tolerated).

10 cooked new potatoes, sliced into bite-sized pieces

1 tsp oil (see page 20)

7.5cm (3in) piece of chorizo

2 Substantial Salad Bases of your choice (see page 109)

8 sun-blushed tomatoes, cut into pieces

Pomegranate Molasses Dressing or dressing or your choice (see pages 110–111)

1. Fry the potatoes on one side in the oil over a medium heat for 3–4 minutes or until they are lightly browned.

2. Skin the chorizo and, with a sharp knife, cut into quarters lengthways, then cut each quarter into 1cm (½in) pieces. Turn the potatoes over, add the chorizo to the pan and continue to fry for 3–4 minutes or until the chorizo is crispy. Drain the potatoes and chorizo on kitchen paper to remove any excess oil.

3. Top the salad bases with the sun-blushed tomatoes and drizzle over the dressing. Toss over the potatoes and chorizo and serve immediately.

Sweet Potato, Red Pepper and Pine Nut Salad

Serves 2

I like to make really good vegetarian dishes, partly because I love vegetarian food and partly because I feel vegetarians get a poor deal most of the time, especially when eating out.

1 large sweet potato, peeled and cut into bite-sized pieces

2 red peppers, deseeded and quartered

1 tbsp oil (see page 20)

¼ tsp chilli powder

2 Substantial Salad Bases of your choice (see page 109)

Pesto Dressing or dressing of your choice (see pages 110–111)

Salt and freshly ground black pepper

2 tbsps pine nuts, toasted (see page 23), to garnish

1. Preheat the oven to 200°C (180°C fan), gas mark 6.

2. Place the sweet potato and peppers in a bowl or pan with the oil, chilli powder and some salt and pepper. Toss together and then tip into a roasting tin or baking tray. Spread the vegetables in a single layer and roast for about 25 minutes or until just cooked.

3. Drizzle the dressing over the salad bases, scatter over the cooked vegetables and garnish with the toasted pine nuts to serve.

Crab Salad with Mango, Chilli and Lime

Serves 2

I love this dish with its rich coconut dressing and refreshing zingy salad ingredients – it's good to look at as well as tasting heavenly.

Coconut, Lime and Chilli Dressing (see page 111)

2 Substantial Salad Bases of your choice (see page 109)

225g (8oz) white crab meat

Flesh of ½ ripe mango, diced

Flesh of ½ avocado, diced

Coconut flakes, toasted (see page 23), to garnish (optional)

1. Drizzle the dressing over the salad bases.

2. Scatter over the crab meat and diced mango and avocado, and garnish with coconut flakes (if using).

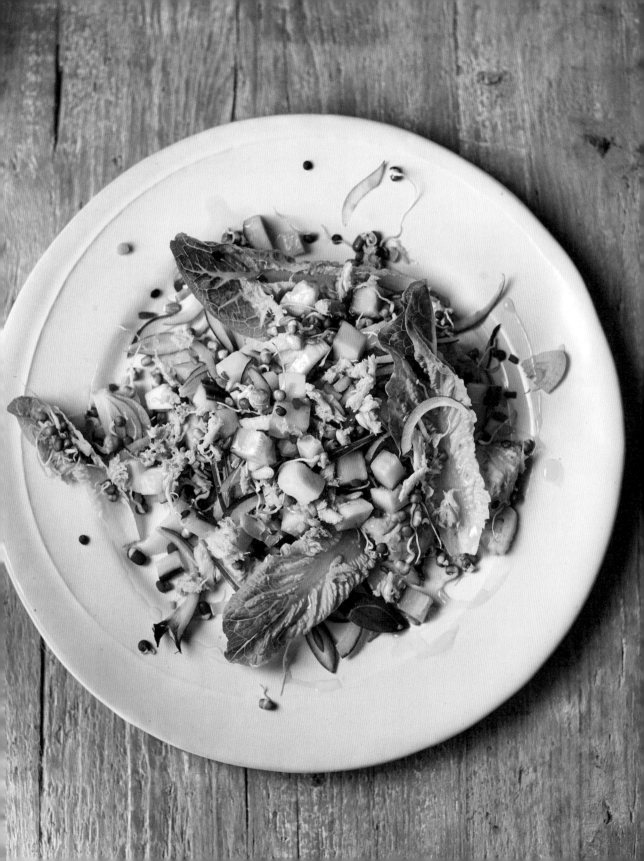

Simple Stir-fries

I love stir-fries – so quick and easy to prepare, yet so healthy. I like to include lots of vegetables in mine, as they provide an easy way to get your 'five a day'. It also means that one portion of meat – say, a chicken breast – is sufficient for two people, making stir-fries very economical. If, however, you prefer more meat and fewer vegetables, or a vegetarian version, just swap things around. Veggie stir-fries benefit from some added protein, such as tofu, nuts, beans and pulses, or eggs (if tolerated), but sometimes it is good just to have vegetables and rice, it's so nourishing and cleansing.

Tamari sauce adds extra flavour but it is made from soya, which may not be tolerated, and because it is fermented is not suitable for those with a yeast intolerance. You also need to check that it is gluten free as some brands are not. Serve stir-fries not only with rice but with cooked millet, buckwheat, quinoa, rice noodles and pasta, or try cauliflower rice or courgette noodles (see page 126). Fresh herbs make a good garnish and add extra flavour.

The art of making a stir-fry is to have all your vegetables still with a bite when you finish cooking. The way you cut up vegetables also has a part to play in how long they take to cook. I use an ordinary non-stick pan, but you could use a wok or even a frying pan. The deeper the sides, the more steam is kept in the pan, so the quicker the ingredients cook. I add to this effect by adding stock during the cooking, which also helps to prevent the vegetables from sticking and burning. I prefer not to cook in smoking fat, as is the norm for stir-fry recipes, as this produces free radicals that are harmful to the body. I stir-fry with a mixture of olive oil and coconut oil.

How to Stir-fry

1. Prepare and chop all the ingredients. Once you start to cook, the point is speed.

2. Heat the pan over a medium/high heat, then add the oil and a moment later start adding the vegetables, ginger, garlic and chilli (if using). Add the thickest and hardest vegetables first, such as onions, carrot and broccoli.

3. Be quick and definite about tossing the ingredients in the oil with a wooden spoon. As soon as the oil starts to disappear, add a couple of tablespoons of stock. Keep adding more stock throughout and keep stirring.

4. Adding the meat will depend on what it is and how it is cut. Generally, it won't take as long as the thicker vegetables, so now is often a good time to add.

5. Add the softer vegetables, such as spinach and mangetout, but don't overcook so they keep a bit of crunch. Bean sprouts will only take a few seconds.

6. See individual recipes (pages 126–135) for when to add the rest of the stock and the remaining ingredients.

Cauliflower Rice and Courgette Noodles

These are all the rage among low-carbohydrate dieters as an alternative to rice or noodles as a base for your stir-fry, but they are also useful for gluten-free meals. Just be careful because they are not as filling as other bases, so they can leave you hungry between meals – especially if your stir-fry doesn't include protein.

Cauliflower Rice

1. Break the cauliflower into even-sized florets – allowing a good handful of florets per person – and remove any leaves and thick stem.

2. Using a food processor, pulse the cauliflower into rice-sized pieces. It's best to chop in batches if you are making more than one portion, to prevent it from turning to mush. You can also grate the cauliflower using a box grater, but watch your fingers and use a larger section of cauliflower.

3. Sweat the cauliflower rice in a dry pan over a medium heat for 3–4 minutes or until it is just starting to soften but still retains a bite. Season with salt and pepper and serve.

Courgette Noodles

1. Allow 1–1½ courgettes per person. Using a spiraliser or julienne peeler, cut the courgette lengthwise into thin strips.

2. Sweat the courgette noodles in a dry pan over a medium heat for 3–4 minutes or until they are just starting to soften but still retain a bite. Season with salt and pepper and serve.

Asparagus, Leek and Almond Stir-fry

Serves 2

This is a favourite recipe of mine, full of wonderful ingredients all held together in a rich, creamy sauce. Asparagus is a great diuretic and can help to banish any heavy puffy feelings, while the almonds, as well as adding protein, are a powerhouse of nutrients, rich in essential fats and minerals.

1 tbsp oil (see page 20)

1 leek, mainly white stem, thinly sliced

1 courgette, sliced

1 x 250g (9oz) bunch of asparagus, tailed and cut into 2.5cm (1in) lengths

10 chestnut mushrooms, halved or quartered

1 tsp grated fresh root ginger

1 garlic clove, crushed

1 tsp dried rosemary

½ tsp dried thyme

¼ stock cube dissolved in 150ml (5fl oz) boiling water

8 tbsps ground almonds

200ml (7fl oz) coconut milk

Salt and freshly ground black pepper

2 tbsps slivered almonds, toasted (see page 23), to garnish

1. Heat a pan or wok over a medium/high heat, then add the oil, followed by the vegetables, ginger, garlic and herbs (see 'How to Stir-fry' on page 125).

2. Toss the ingredients together in the oil; when the oil is absorbed and the pan begins to look dry, add a couple of tablespoons of the stock. Cook for 5–8 minutes, stirring all the time and adding stock at regular intervals, until the vegetables are almost cooked but still retain a little bite.

3. Add the remaining stock, ground almonds and coconut milk, bring to the boil and simmer for 1 minute.

4. Season with salt and pepper and serve garnished with toasted almonds.

Cardamom and Lemon Chicken Stir-fry
Serves 2

This is such a simple yet effective dish, with a lovely combination of flavours. Lemon and ginger really complement the chicken, while the cardamom and Chinese five-spice add an extra dimension. Vary the vegetables according to what you have available.

2 tsps oil (see page 20)

1 tsp sesame oil

1 leek, mainly white stem, thinly sliced

1 sweet potato, peeled and diced

2 handfuls of sugar snap peas

2.5cm (1in) piece of fresh root ginger, peeled and finely diced

1 garlic clove, crushed

1 large skinless chicken breast, sliced into thin strips

Seeds from 6 cardamom pods, crushed

1 tsp Chinese five-spice powder

6 parings of lemon rind, finely sliced

¼ stock cube dissolved in 225ml (8fl oz) boiling water

1 rounded tsp gluten-free plain flour (see page 22)

1 tbsp gluten-free tamari (optional)

Salt and freshly ground black pepper

1. Heat a pan or wok over a medium/high heat, then add the oils, followed by the vegetables, ginger, garlic, chicken, cardamom, Chinese five spice and lemon rind (see 'How to Stir-fry' on page 125).

2. Toss the ingredients together in the oil; when the oil is absorbed and the pan begins to look dry, add a couple of tablespoons of the stock. Cook for 5–8 minutes, stirring all the time and adding stock at regular intervals, until the vegetables are just over half cooked.

3. Whisk the flour with the remaining stock and add to the pan. Bring the mixture to the boil and simmer for 1–2 minutes or until the vegetables and chicken are cooked but the vegetables still retain some bite. Add a little water if the mixture is too thick.

4. Add the tamari (if using) and season to taste with salt and pepper before serving.

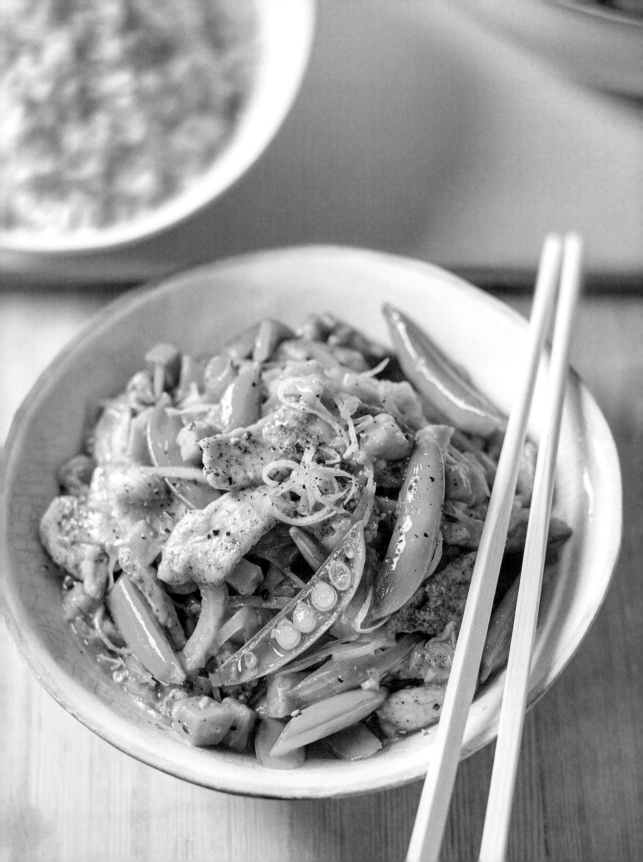

Paprika Pork and Red Pepper Stir-fry

Serves 2

I love the fact that stir-fries are so colourful as well as appetising. Add to that the rich scent of smoked paprika and vegetables cooking and you have a feast for the senses – a dish that tastes as good as it looks and smells. For a sweet-and-sour version of this recipe, add a small handful of fresh or tinned (in fruit juice) chopped pineapple.

2 tsps sesame oil

1 carrot, cut into matchsticks

1 onion, diced

1 red pepper, deseeded and cut into chunks

2.5cm (1in) piece of fresh root ginger, peeled and finely sliced

1 garlic clove, crushed

200g (7oz) pork fillet, cut into thin strips

¼ stock cube dissolved in 225ml (8fl oz) boiling water

1 tsp sweet smoked paprika

1 tbsp pomegranate molasses (optional)

2 tbsps tomato purée

1 rounded tsp gluten-free plain flour (see page 22)

Salt and freshly ground black pepper

chopped coriander, to garnish (optional)

1. Heat a pan or wok over a medium/high heat, then add the oil, followed by the vegetables, ginger, garlic and pork (see 'How to Stir-fry' on page 125).

2. Toss the ingredients together in the oil; when the oil is absorbed and the pan begins to look dry, add a couple of tablespoons of the stock. Cook for 5–8 minutes, stirring all the time and adding stock at regular intervals, until the vegetables are just over half cooked.

3. Add the smoked paprika, pomegranate molasses (if using) and tomato purée and stir to combine.

4. Whisk the flour in the remaining stock and add to the pan. Bring the mixture to the boil and simmer for 1–2 minutes or until the vegetables and meat are cooked but the vegetables still retain some bite. Add a little water if the mixture is too thick.

5. Season to taste with salt and pepper and serve garnished with the fresh coriander.

Chilli Beef Stir-fry

Serves 2

This quick and easy stir-fry ticks all the boxes. It's ready in no time, made with nourishing ingredients and full of contrasting flavours, colours and textures. Vary the vegetables according to what you have available and enjoy this delicious, clean-tasting dish.

1 tsp oil (see page 20)

1 tsp sesame oil

1 onion, diced

2 handfuls of small broccoli florets

2 sticks of celery, thinly sliced

1 green pepper, deseeded and cut into chunks

2.5cm (1in) piece of fresh root ginger, peeled and finely sliced

1 garlic clove, crushed

½–1 fresh red chilli, deseeded and finely diced

200g (7oz) steak (such as rump), finely sliced

¼ stock cube dissolved in 225ml (8fl oz) boiling water

1 tsp mustard powder or 1 tbsp grainy mustard (see page 20)

1 rounded tsp gluten-free plain flour (see page 22)

1 tbsp gluten-free tamari (optional)

Salt and freshly ground black pepper

1. Heat a pan or wok over a medium/high heat, then add the oils, followed by the vegetables, ginger, garlic, chilli and steak (see 'How to Stir-fry' on page 125).

2. Toss the ingredients together in the oil; when the oil is absorbed and the pan begins to look dry, add a couple of tablespoons of the stock. Cook for 5–8 minutes, stirring all the time and adding stock at regular intervals, until the vegetables are just over half cooked.

3. Whisk the mustard and flour in the remaining stock and add to the pan. Bring the mixture to the boil and simmer for 1–2 minutes or until the vegetables and meat are just cooked but the vegetables still retain some bite. Add a little water if the mixture is too thick.

4. Add the tamari (if using) and season to taste with salt and pepper before serving.

Chorizo and Summer Vegetable Stir-fry

Serves 2

For a vegetarian version, omit the chorizo and add toasted cashews before serving. You can also add a teaspoon of sweet smoked paprika and two tablespoons of tomato purée to make up for the chorizo.

1 tbsp oil (see page 20)

1 small onion, diced

8 green beans, sliced

½ red pepper, deseeded and cut into chunks

2 carrots, cut into matchsticks

1 courgette, diced

½ x 250g (9oz) bunch of asparagus, tailed and sliced into 3cm (1¼in) lengths

1 tsp grated fresh root ginger

1 garlic clove, crushed

½–1 fresh red chilli, deseeded and finely diced

1 tsp fennel seeds

10cm (4in) piece of chorizo, finely diced

¼ stock cube dissolved in 225ml (8fl oz) boiling water

1 rounded tsp gluten-free plain flour (see page 22)

1 tbsp gluten-free tamari (optional)

Salt and black pepper

Chopped coriander, to garnish (optional)

1. Heat a pan or wok over a medium/high heat, then add the oil, followed by the vegetables, ginger, garlic, chilli, fennel seeds and chorizo (see 'How to Stir-fry' on page 125).

2. Toss the ingredients together in the oil; when the oil is absorbed and the pan begins to look dry, add a couple of tablespoons of the stock. Cook for 5–8 minutes, stirring all the time and adding stock at regular intervals, until the vegetables are just over half cooked.

3. Whisk the flour with the remaining stock and add to the pan. Bring the mixture to the boil and simmer for 1–2 minutes or until the vegetables are cooked but retain some bite. Add a little water if the mixture is too thick.

4. Add the tamari (if using). Season to taste with salt and pepper and serve garnished with coriander.

Variations

Try other summer vegetables in this recipe, such as broad beans, mangetout, sugar snap peas, fresh sweetcorn and chard. The recipe also works well in winter with more robust vegetables such as parsnips, celery, cauliflower, butternut squash and broccoli.

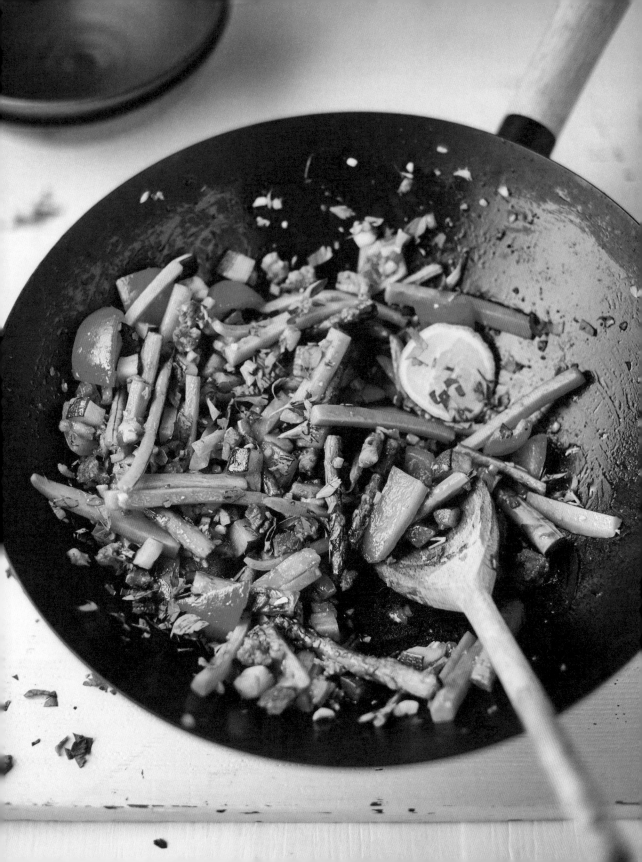

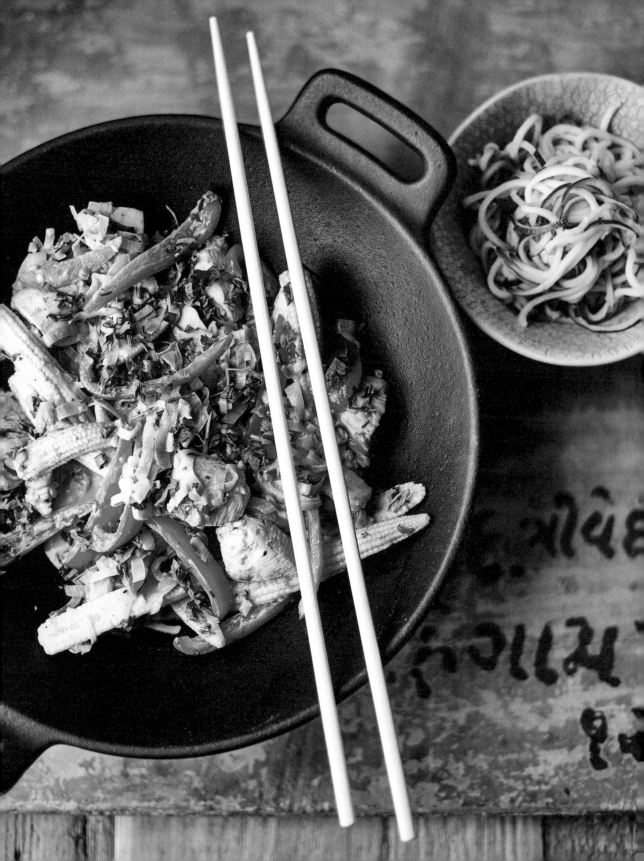

Chicken Tikka Stir-fry

Serves 2

This dish is a healthy version of a classic favourite. It's full of flavour and colour and the ingredients are all held together in a creamy coconut sauce. Omit the chicken and you still have a flavoursome sauce for vegetarians to add their own twist.

1 tbsp oil (see page 20)

1 onion or the white part of a leek, sliced

1 red pepper, deseeded and cut into chunks

1 handful of baby sweetcorn, halved

2.5cm (1in) piece of fresh root ginger, peeled and finely diced

1 garlic clove, crushed

½–1 fresh red chilli, deseeded and finely diced

2 small skinless chicken breasts, thinly sliced

¼ stock cube dissolved in 110ml (4fl oz) boiling water

1 tsp paprika

½ tsp turmeric

2 tsps garam masala

2 tbsps tomato purée

200ml (7fl oz) coconut milk

Salt and freshly ground black pepper

1. Heat a pan or wok over a medium/high heat, then add the oil, followed by the vegetables, ginger, garlic, chilli and chicken (see 'How to Stir-fry' on page 125).

2. Toss the ingredients together in the oil; when the oil is absorbed and the pan begins to look dry, add a couple of tablespoons of the stock. Cook for 5–8 minutes, stirring all the time and adding stock at regular intervals, until the vegetables are just over half cooked.

3. Add the spices and stir-fry for another minute, then add the rest of the stock along with the tomato purée and coconut milk.

4. Bring the mixture to the boil and simmer for 1–2 minutes or until the vegetables and chicken are cooked but the vegetables still retain some bite.

5. Season with salt and pepper and serve.

One-pot Wonders

Create comfort in a pot with these filling, one-pot meals where all your ingredients can be tossed into a single pan or casserole and left to bubble away together, allowing the flavours to mingle.

One-pot cooking is a great way to feed family and friends without the the hassle of having lots of utensils and pans to wash up after the meal. These 'pop it in a pan' dishes are also ideal for students, campers, or anyone with limited cooking facilities.

Don't underestimate the variety of one-pot cooking – there are delicious risottos, chillies and ragouts that can be cooked on top of the stove, as well as warming winter casseroles and stews that can be quickly popped in the oven or slow cooker and left to their own devices while you get on with other things. What's not to love about one-pot cooking?

Speedy Risotto

Risotto is something I have tended to avoid over the years, because the traditional recipe has you standing over the stove ladling hot stock into the pan at regular intervals. But then I tried an experiment: I put all the stock in at the beginning, covered the pot with a tight-fitting lid and cooked it for 20 minutes. The result was a delicious risotto without any hassle. Use fresh stock if you have it – it will make an even better risotto (see page 203).

Arborio Rice and Slower-Release Grains

I have used Arborio rice in these recipes, but if you want your risotto to be slower release (see page 15), use brown rice or buckwheat instead. You will have to check the quantities and timings the first time, as they absorb the stock at different rates. Buckwheat is really speedy, taking 12–15 minutes to cook, but you need more buckwheat (375g/13oz) and less stock (725ml/1¼ pints). The brown basmati rice I used took 30 minutes to cook using the same amount of stock as for Arborio rice.

Cooking Risotto

Keep your eye on the risotto the first time you cook it, as the exact timing will depend on your pan (I use a flat-based, paella-type pan, but you could use a large frying pan with a lid), how well your lid fits and the heat from your cooker. You could cover the top of the pan with foil before putting the lid on if the lid doesn't fit tightly enough.

Speedy Mushroom Risotto
Serves 2–4

This healthy take on a traditional favourite is so full of creamy flavour you'll find it hard to believe that it's dairy-free. You can swap the onions in the dish for leeks, if you prefer.

10g (½oz) dried porcini mushrooms

1 tbsp oil (see page 20)

2 onions, diced

2 garlic cloves, crushed

250g (9oz) chestnut mushrooms, sliced

310g (11oz) Arborio rice

1 stock cube

1 tsp dried thyme

1 tsp dried sage

1 tsp mustard powder or 1 tbsp grainy mustard (see page 20)

Grated zest of 1 lemon

1 tbsp chopped parsley (optional)

6 tbsps coconut cream (see page 22)

A good squeeze of lemon juice

Salt and freshly ground black pepper

1. Place the porcini mushrooms in enough boiling water to cover and leave to soak while you prepare the other ingredients.

2. Heat the oil in a flat-bottomed, paella-type pan or a large frying pan, and sweat the onions and garlic over a medium heat for about 5 minutes or until they start to soften, then add the chestnut mushrooms and continue to sweat for another 3–4 minutes or until they are starting to soften. Add the rice and toss to coat in the oil and juices.

3. Remove the porcini from the soaking liquid (saving the liquid), and squeeze out any excess moisture. Finely chop the porcini and add to the vegetables and rice in the pan.

4. Pour the porcini soaking liquid into a measuring jug – avoiding the last few dregs as they can be gritty. Add the stock cube and top the liquid up to 1 litre (1¾ pints) with boiling water. Stir to combine and add to the rice and vegetables, along with the thyme, sage, mustard and grated lemon zest.

5. Bring the risotto to the boil, turn the heat to medium/low and cover with a tight-fitting lid. Leave to bubble away gently for about 20 minutes or until the rice is soft.

6. Add the parsley (if using), coconut cream and lemon juice, season to taste with salt and pepper and serve.

Speedy Vegetable Paella
Serves 2–4

This is a veggie delight that even confirmed meat eaters will love. You can also change the vegetables for variations on a theme: try broccoli, mushrooms, sweet potatoes or sugar snap peas.

1 tbsp oil (see page 20)

1 onion, diced

1 garlic clove, crushed

½–1 fresh red chilli, deseeded and finely diced (optional)

2 tbsps tomato purée

2 tsps sweet smoked paprika

½ tsp turmeric

½ tsp dried oregano

310g (11oz) Arborio rice

1 stock cube dissolved in 1 litre (1¾ pints) boiling water

1 red or yellow pepper, deseeded and diced

2 medium courgettes, sliced

2 handfuls of frozen peas

1 handful of sweetcorn

4 sun-dried tomatoes, finely diced

12 black or green olives, pitted and halved

Salt and freshly ground black pepper

Lemon wedges, to serve (optional)

1. Heat the oil in a flat-bottomed, paella-type pan or a large frying pan, and sweat the onion, garlic and chilli (if using) over a medium heat for 5 minutes or until they begin to soften.

2. Add the tomato purée, paprika, turmeric, oregano and rice and toss until the rice is coated in the oil and flavourings.

3. Pour in the stock and bring the mixture to the boil. Turn the heat down to medium/low and cover with a tight-fitting lid.

4. Leave to bubble away gently for about 8 minutes, then mix in the pepper, courgettes, peas, sweetcorn, sun-dried tomatoes and olives. Bring back to a simmer, then cover again with the lid and continue to cook for a further 12 minutes or until the rice and vegetables are tender.

5. Season to taste with salt and pepper and serve with lemon wedges, if you like.

Variation
You could turn this into a more traditional paella by adding the diced meat from two chicken thighs with the rice and a handful of raw king prawns when you add the vegetables.

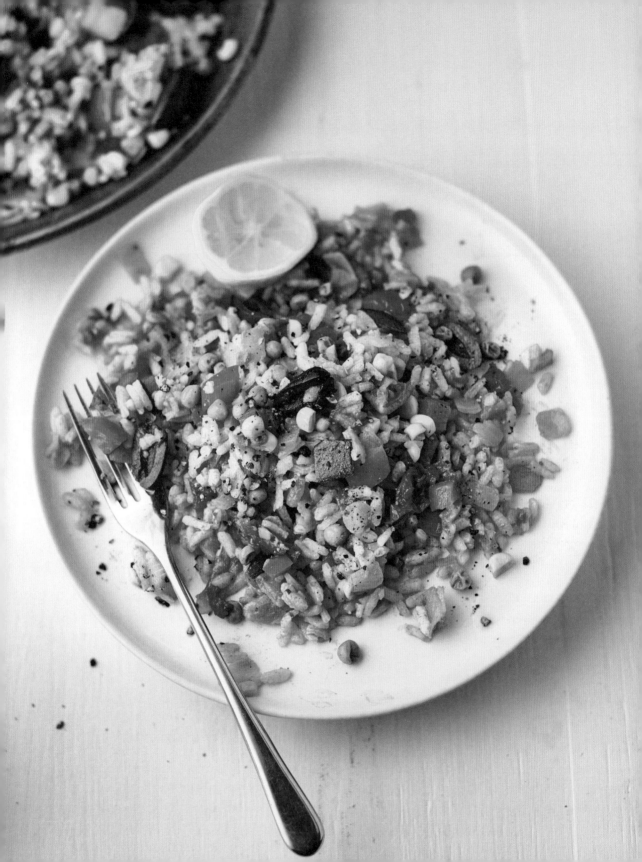

Speedy King Prawn and Smoked Salmon Risotto

Serves 2–4

High in nutrients, this fantastic seafood dish is full of flavour and so versatile. You could serve it for a summer lunch with a crunchy green salad or tuck into a warming bowl on a cold winter's night. It's easy to make and there is very little washing up!

1 tbsp oil (see page 20)

1 large onion, diced

1 garlic clove, crushed

½–1 fresh red chilli, deseeded and finely diced (optional)

310g (11oz) Arborio rice

1 stock cube dissolved in 1 litre (1¾ pints) boiling water

2 handfuls of frozen peas

1 red or yellow pepper, deseeded and diced

1 small courgette, sliced

4 parings of lemon rind, finely sliced

4 slices of smoked salmon, diced

110g (4oz) raw king prawns

1 tbsp chopped parsley, mint or coriander (optional)

A good squeeze of lemon juice

Salt and freshly ground black pepper

1. Heat the oil in a flat-bottomed, paella-type pan or a large frying pan, and sweat the onion, garlic and chilli over a medium heat for 5 minutes or until the onion starts to soften.

2. Add the rice and toss to coat in the oil and juices.

3. Pour in the stock and bring the mixture to the boil, then reduce the heat to medium/low and cover with a tight-fitting lid.

4. Leave to bubble away gently for 10 minutes, then add the peas, pepper, courgette, lemon rind, smoked salmon and king prawns and stir to combine. Bring back to a simmer, cover with the lid and continue to cook for another 10 minutes or until the rice, prawns and vegetables are cooked.

5. Add the herbs (if using), a good squeeze of lemon juice and some salt and pepper to taste before serving.

Ragouts and Chillies

The following one-pot dishes all involve a selection of ingredients bubbling away in a pan until the flavours have mingled and a rich, tasty sauce is formed. Only a minimal amount of preparation is needed. These are the sort of dishes that I like to double up and freeze so that I have emergency stores for when I need a quick meal or I feel like a day off cooking, though they already serve between four and six people. They work particularly well in a slow cooker as you can forget them completely, with no need to give even an occasional stir. (See page 151 for more on slow cooking.) They lend themselves to numerous accompaniments, too – from rice, quinoa, buckwheat and pasta to baked potatoes or mash. So long as you have something that combines well with the rich sauce, anything goes. If you can't eat tomatoes – and all of these dishes contain them – try using carrot juice instead.

Homemade Baked Beans

Serves 4

If you love shop-bought baked beans but don't like all the sugar or sugar substitutes they contain, then try these. They are really scrummy. Baked beans have never been a favourite of mine, yet I love this version. Haricot beans are traditionally used for this dish, but the ones I tried fell apart in the sauce, so I now use firmer ones such as cannellini or borlotti.

2 tsps oil (see page 20)

2 onions, diced

2 garlic cloves, crushed

4 rashers of smoked bacon, diced (optional)

2 tsps sweet smoked paprika

2 tsps mustard powder

2 tsps pomegranate molasses

2 tsps blackstrap molasses

2 x 400g (14oz) tins of chopped tomatoes

4 tbsps tomato purée

2 x 400g (14oz) tins of borlotti, cannellini or haricot beans, drained and rinsed

Salt and freshly ground black pepper

1. Heat the oil in a large pan and sweat the onion, garlic and bacon (if using) over a medium heat for 5 minutes or until the onion starts to soften. Add the paprika, mustard and pomegranate and blackstrap molasses and mix in.

2. Tip in the tinned tomatoes, tomato purée and beans and bring the mixture to the boil. Reduce the heat to medium/low and simmer, covered with a lid, for 30 minutes.

3. Season to taste with salt and pepper and serve.

Turkey and Mushroom Ragout

Serves 4–6

Use chicken instead of turkey, if you prefer, and don't be afraid of swapping vegetables for what you have available. The flavour is in the sauce, and you never know – you may invent a family favourite.

700g (1½lb) lean turkey, finely diced

1 large onion, finely diced

2 garlic cloves, crushed

3 sticks of celery, finely diced

2 carrots, finely diced

150g (5oz) button mushrooms, sliced

150g (5oz) field mushrooms, finely diced

2 tsps dried rosemary

1 bay leaf

1 x 690ml (1 pint 7fl oz) jar of tomato passata

½ stock cube dissolved in 275ml (½ pint) boiling water (150ml/5fl oz if slow cooking)

Salt and freshly ground black pepper

1. Place all the ingredients (except the salt and pepper) in a large pan or slow cooker, using the stock to rinse out the passata jar. Stir everything together to combine.

2. Bring to the boil, stirring occasionally, then reduce the heat, cover loosely with a lid and simmer on a low heat for 30 minutes or slow-cook for 6–8 hours.

3. Season to taste with salt and pepper, remove the bay leaf and serve.

Chunky Beef Chilli

Serves 4–6

To save time cutting stewing steak into fine dice, ask your butcher to put the meat through a large-holed mincer twice. The chocolate adds an authentic and interesting flavour to this chilli, but it can be left out.

700g (1½lb) lean stewing steak, cut into fine dice across the grain

1 large onion, diced

1 large red pepper, deseeded and diced

2 garlic cloves, crushed

1 tbsp grated fresh root ginger

1 x 400g (14oz) tin of chopped tomatoes

6 tbsps tomato purée

1 tsp ground cumin

1 tsp ground coriander

¼–½ tsp chilli powder

¼ stock cube dissolved in 150ml (5fl oz) boiling water (omit the water if slow-cooking)

1 x 400g (14oz) tin of red kidney beans, drained and rinsed

150g (5oz) sweetcorn kernels

25g (1oz) 90–100% dark chocolate, diced (optional)

Salt and freshly ground black pepper

1. Place the meat in a pan or slow cooker, along with the onion, red pepper, garlic, ginger, tinned tomatoes, tomato purée, spices and stock (crumble over the stock cube if slow-cooking).

2. If cooking on the hob, bring the mixture to the boil, stirring occasionally, then lower the heat, cover with a lid and simmer very gently for 1 hour. Add the beans, sweetcorn and chocolate and cook for a further 30 minutes or until the meat is tender. Alternatively, place all the remaining ingredients in the slow cooker and cook for 6–8 hours.

3. Season to taste with salt and pepper and serve.

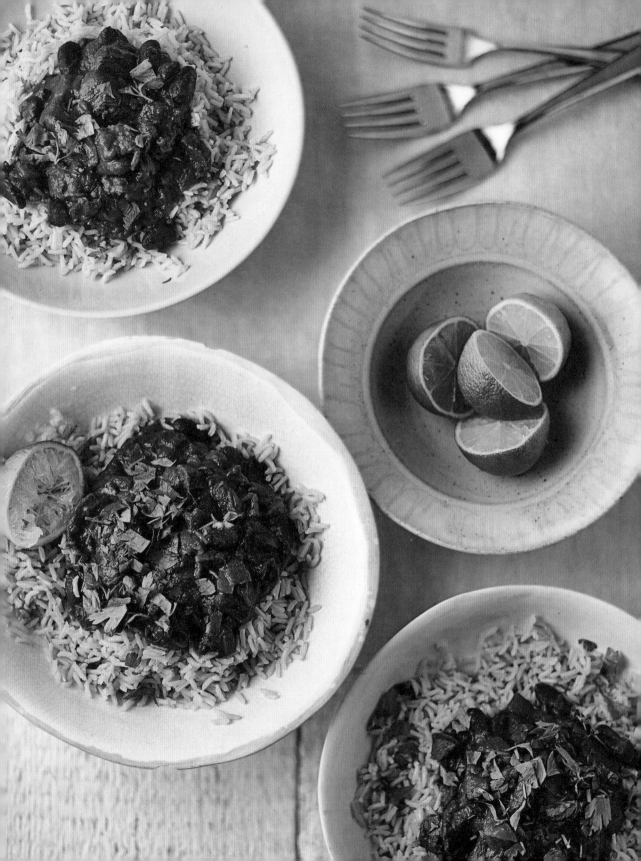

Sausage Ragout

Serves 4

Children will love this dish and will also love helping to make it. My grandchildren enjoy helping with the preparation, especially squeezing the meat out of the sausages.

1 tbsp oil (see page 20)

1 large onion, diced

1 large carrot, finely diced

2 sticks of celery, finely diced

1 garlic clove, crushed

8 gluten-free sausages, skins removed

1 x 400g (14oz) tin of chopped tomatoes

½ stock cube dissolved in 275ml (½ pint) boiling water

2 tbsps tomato purée

Salt and freshly ground black pepper

1. Heat the oil in a pan and sweat the onion, carrot, celery and garlic over a medium heat for 5 minutes or until they start to soften.

2. Stir in the sausage meat, breaking it up into small pieces, and cook for another 5 minutes.

3. Add the chopped tomatoes, stock and tomato purée. Bring the mixture to the boil, then reduce the heat to medium/low, cover with a lid and simmer for about 25 minutes or until you have a thick sauce.

4. Season to taste with salt and pepper and serve.

Butternut and Red Kidney Bean Chilli

Serves 4

This is a tasty vegetarian version of a classic chilli. I love vegetarian food and will often choose it instead of meat or fish, especially if it's as healthy and delicious as this.

1 tbsp oil (see page 20)

1 onion, cut into small wedges

2 garlic cloves, crushed

2 sticks of celery, diced

200g (7oz) chestnut mushrooms, halved if large

½ butternut squash, peeled, deseeded and cut into bite-sized chunks

1 red pepper, deseeded and cut into bite-sized chunks

1 tsp ground cumin

1 tsp ground coriander

½ tsp ground cinnamon

1 tsp sweet smoked paprika

¼–½ tsp chilli powder

2 x 400g (14oz) tins of chopped tomatoes

½ stock cube dissolved in 55ml (2fl oz) boiling water

3 tbsps tomato purée

1 x 400g (14oz) tin of red kidney beans, drained and rinsed

150g (5oz) sweetcorn kernels

2 tbsps chopped coriander (optional)

Salt and freshly ground black pepper

1. Heat the oil in a large pan and sweat the onion, garlic and celery over a medium heat for 5 minutes or until they start to soften, then add the mushrooms and sweat for another 3–4 minutes.

2. Add the butternut squash, red pepper and spices and sweat for 3–4 minutes, then add the chopped tomatoes, stock, tomato purée, red kidney beans and sweetcorn.

3. Gently bring the mixture to the boil, then lower the heat, cover with a lid and simmer for 30–40 minutes, stirring occasionally, or until the vegetables are just cooked.

4. Add the chopped coriander (if using) and season to taste with salt and pepper. Serve with rice, quinoa, buckwheat, polenta or pasta.

Casseroles and Stews

Most recipes for stews and casseroles suggest you fry the meat in batches until brown and sweat the vegetables before you put the ingredients together. The recipes in this section omit this time-consuming stage, but you won't even notice because there are enough flavoursome ingredients to compensate for the lack of frying. Casseroles and stews therefore become healthier and easier to prepare as everything is just thrown into the pot and bubbled away. If you have a timer on your cooker, or have a slow cooker, then spend just 15–20 minutes preparing your dish before you go out in the morning and come home to the welcome smell of dinner cooking itself. This is what I call hassle-free cooking – ideal for busy lives and perfect for easy entertaining.

The stews in this section are complete meals in themselves and need no accompaniment. As well as meat and/or vegetables, they also contain potatoes or dumplings and in my house are served in a deep bowl, garnished with a little parsley if available. Casseroles, on the other hand, need a side dish of at least some potatoes or cooked grains and preferably some extra vegetables or a salad. If I am using the oven, I often put jacket potatoes to cook alongside, leaving me free until the last minute when I rustle up a salad or cook some fresh vegetables. If you have leftover cooked potatoes, you could make your casserole into a hotpot (see page 192) or add the dumplings from the Vegetable Casserole (page 161) and cook uncovered to make your casserole into a cobbler.

Slow Cooking

Slow cookers not only save you money, as less energy is used to heat them, but they are also so easy to use. They are very forgiving as far as timing is concerned. You can be late home and dinner will still be bubbling away but not dried up as it would in a conventional cooker. I find I need to reduce the liquid in recipes, because so little evaporation takes place. However, timing does vary depending on the make. Mine works well left on auto all day, for instance, which means it alternates high and low temperatures, whereas my son's needs to be on low. Follow the manufacturer's instructions for settings and timings.

If you decide to invest in a slow cooker, buy a large one and cook in bulk. This means you can freeze the surplus and have some nights off cooking. It's just as easy to prepare a casserole for eight as it is for four. I always put meat at the bottom to prevent it from drying out, especially chicken joints. I also remove the skin from chicken as it is not going to brown in the slow cooker and this reduces the amount of fat floating on the surface. The strange thing about slow cookers is that meat cooks more quickly than vegetables, so these need to be cut into fairly small pieces. If you want larger vegetable pieces, then part-cook them first by sweating them in some oil or steaming them.

Chicken and Chinese Five-spice Casserole

Serves 4

This is a favourite recipe of mine – chicken in a mild and delicately flavoured creamy sauce. It's one I often turn to when friends are coming to supper and I want a dish that I know they will love but is easy for me to prepare.

4 chicken thighs, skinned if preferred

2 medium-sized sweet potatoes, peeled and diced

2 medium onions, diced

1 garlic clove, crushed

2.5cm (1in) piece of fresh root ginger, peeled and grated

2 level tbsps gluten-free plain flour (see page 22)

½ stock cube dissolved in 425ml (15fl oz) boiling water (150ml/5fl oz if slow cooking)

⅛–¼ tsp chilli powder (optional)

1 tsp dried oregano

½ tsp dried thyme

1 tsp paprika

1 tsp Chinese five-spice powder

2 tbsps tomato purée (optional)

200ml (7fl oz) coconut milk

4 good handfuls of baby spinach leaves

Salt and black pepper

1. Preheat the oven to 180°C (160°C fan), gas mark 4.

2. Place the chicken in a casserole dish or slow cooker and add the sweet potatoes, onions, garlic, ginger and gluten-free flour. Toss the ingredients to coat them in the flour, then push the chicken joints to the base of the casserole if they are skinned or if you are using a slow cooker.

3. Combine the remaining ingredients (except the spinach and salt and pepper) and pour over the chicken and vegetables.

4. Cover the casserole with a lid and cook on the middle shelf of the oven for about 2 hours, or slow cook for 6–8 hours (check your slow-cooker manual for timing).

5. Fifteen minutes before the end of cooking, toss in the spinach. There may seem a lot, but it will soon wilt down and become part of the sauce.

6. Season with salt and pepper, if needed, and serve.

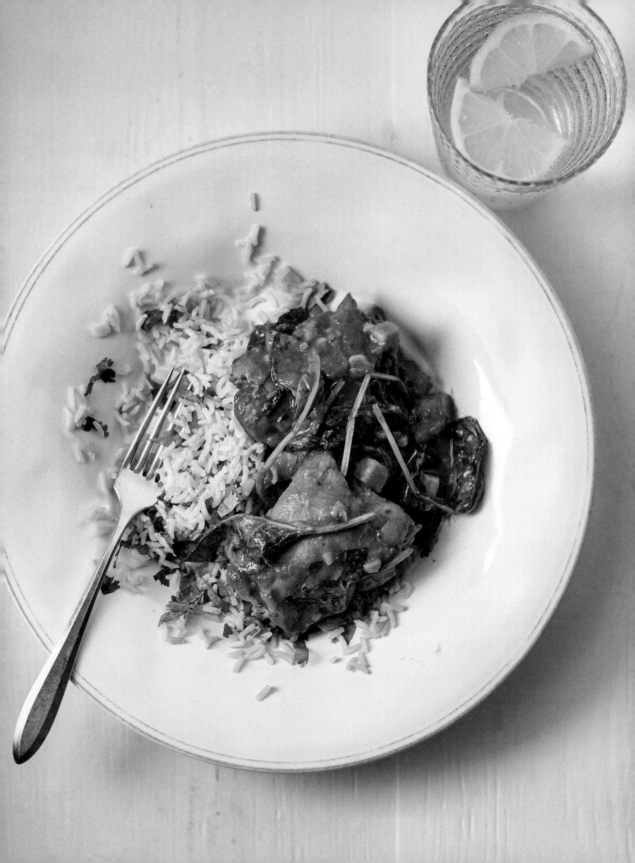

Chicken Casserole with Chorizo and Olives

Serves 4

Don't be put off by the sound of anchovies in a chicken casserole. They melt down and deepen the flavour without making the dish at all fishy; just bear in mind that you probably won't need to add salt as seasoning. If you prefer to remove as much fat as possible, then fry the chorizo in a separate pan for a few minutes and drain on kitchen paper before adding. You could substitute finely diced smoky bacon for the chorizo.

4 chicken thighs, skinned if preferred

10cm (4in) piece of chorizo, finely diced

1 x 50g (2oz) tin of anchovies, finely sliced

2 medium onions, diced

2 sticks of celery, sliced

1 red pepper, deseeded and diced

16 black or green olives

2 garlic cloves, crushed

2 level tbsps gluten-free plain flour (see page 22)

1 bay leaf

½ tsp dried thyme

2 x 400g (14oz) tins of chopped tomatoes

2 tsps pomegranate molasses mixed with 225ml (8fl oz) boiling water (55ml/2fl oz if slow cooking)

¼ tsp ground black pepper

1. Preheat the oven to 180°C (160°C fan), gas mark 4.

2. Place the chicken and chorizo in a casserole dish or slow cooker with the anchovies, onions, celery, red pepper, olives, garlic and gluten-free flour. Toss the ingredients to coat in the flour and then push the chicken joints to the base of the container if they are skinned or if you are using a slow cooker. Push the bay leaf down the side of the dish.

3. Mix together the remaining ingredients and pour over the chicken and vegetables. Cover the casserole with a lid and cook on the middle shelf of the oven for about 2 hours, or slow cook for 6–8 hours (check your slow-cooker manual for timing).

4. Remove the bay leaf and serve.

Lamb or Venison Casserole with Orange and Ginger

Serves 4

This full-bodied traditional casserole is delicately flavoured with orange and ginger, which complement the richness of the meat. Perfect winter comfort food, it's equally good served to guests for entertaining.

700g (1½lb) lean stewing lamb or venison, diced

2 onions, cut into wedges

2 garlic cloves, crushed

2 carrots, cut into chunks

2 sticks of celery, sliced

4 tsps finely grated fresh root ginger

Grated zest and juice of 2 oranges

2 level tbsps gluten-free plain flour (see page 22)

1 x 400g (14oz) tin of chopped tomatoes

2 tbsps tomato purée

1 tsp turmeric

2 tsps paprika

Salt and freshly ground black pepper

1. Preheat the oven to 180°C (160°C fan), gas mark 4.

2. Place the meat in a casserole dish or slow cooker with the onions, garlic, carrots, celery, ginger, grated orange zest and gluten-free flour and toss to coat the ingredients in the flour.

3. Mix the orange juice with the tinned tomatoes and make up to 725ml (1¼ pints) with water, or if slow cooking just mix together the juice and tinned tomatoes. Add the tomato purée, turmeric and paprika and stir to combine.

4. Pour the liquid into the casserole dish or slow cooker and mix well. Cover the dish with a lid and cook on the middle shelf of the oven for 2 hours, or slow cook for 6–8 hours (check your slow-cooker manual for timing).

5. Season to taste with salt and pepper and serve.

Pork Casserole with Pineapple and Peppers

Serves 4

This sweet-and-sour mix of pork and vegetables is gently simmered with an aromatic blend of fruit and spices to produce a succulent casserole.

700g (1½lb) pork fillet, diced

1 large onion, diced

1 red pepper and ½ yellow pepper, deseeded and sliced

1 garlic clove, crushed

½–1 fresh red chilli, deseeded and finely diced

1 tsp Chinese five-spice powder

1 tsp paprika

2 level tbsps gluten-free plain flour (see page 22)

1 x 225g (8oz) tin of pineapple chunks in fruit juice, drained

Grated zest of ½ orange and juice of 1 orange

1 x 400g (14oz) tin of chopped tomatoes

½ stock cube dissolved in ½ pint (275 ml) boiling water (55ml/2fl oz if slow cooking)

1 tsp pomegranate molasses

2 tbsps tomato purée

Salt and freshly ground black pepper

1. Preheat the oven to 180°C (160°C fan), gas mark 4.

2. Place the meat in a casserole dish or slow cooker with the onion, peppers, garlic, chilli, spices and gluten-free flour and toss to coat the ingredients in the flour.

3. Add the pineapple chunks, orange zest and juice and the chopped tomatoes.

4. Mix the stock with the pomegranate molasses and tomato purée and pour into the casserole dish or slow cooker. Stir to combine the ingredients.

5. Cover with a lid and cook on the middle shelf of the oven for about 2 hours, or slow cook for 6–8 hours (check your slow-cooker manual for timing).

6. Season to taste with salt and pepper and serve.

Variation

You can use chicken or duck instead of pork, or try butter beans or tofu (if tolerated) for a vegetarian version.

Creamy Butter Bean, Spinach and Sweetcorn Casserole

Serves 4

My husband, who isn't too keen on vegetarian fare in general, just loves this casserole. It's also delicious served as an accompaniment to meat dishes – try it with sausages or roast chicken.

1 x 400g (14oz) tin of butter beans, drained and rinsed

150g (5oz) red split lentils, rinsed

4 carrots, cut into chunks

225g (8oz) sweetcorn kernels

5 parings of lemon rind, finely sliced

1 stock cube dissolved in 1 pint (570 ml) boiling water (425ml/15fl oz if slow cooking)

2 tsps grated fresh root ginger

1 garlic clove, peeled

1 level tsp ground coriander

1 level tsp ground cumin

2 tsps garam masala

½ tsp turmeric

200ml (7fl oz) coconut milk

16 smallish cauliflower florets

1 x 200g (7oz) packet of baby spinach leaves

Salt and freshly ground black pepper

1. Preheat the oven to 180°C (160°C fan), gas mark 4.

2. Place the butter beans and lentils in a casserole dish or slow cooker with the carrots, sweetcorn and lemon rind.

3. Mix the stock with the ginger, garlic, spices and coconut milk and pour into the dish, then stir to combine.

4. Cover with a lid and cook on the middle shelf of the oven for 1–1¼ hours or until the lentils are just starting to disintegrate. Add the cauliflower and spinach and cook for a further 30–40 minutes or until the cauliflower is just cooked.

5. Season to taste with salt and pepper and serve.

Variation

Creamy Tofu, Spinach and Sweetcorn Casserole: Make the casserole as above, but omit the butter beans. To prepare the tofu, wrap a 200g (7oz) block of tofu in a clean tea towel and place a plate on top with a heavy weight on it. Leave for 30 minutes to remove any excess moisture. Mix 2 tablespoons of lemon juice with the juice from a crushed clove of garlic and from a 2.5cm (1in) piece of grated fresh root ginger, seasoning with salt and pepper. Cut the tofu into bite-sized pieces and fry in 1 teaspoon of oil (see page 20), adding the lemon mixture a tablespoon at a time and allowing it to be absorbed between additions. Keep turning the tofu until it is browned on each side and the juice has all been used. Add to the casserole, along with the spinach, for the last 30minutes of cooking.

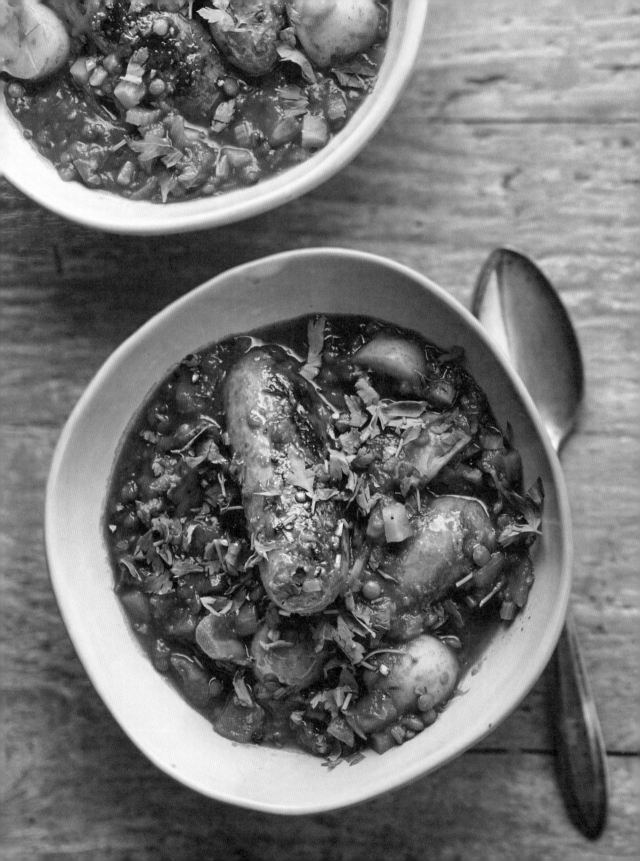

Sausage, Lentil and New Potato Stew
Serves 4

Gluten-free sausages are now readily available in butchers and at the supermarket, while preservative-free ones can be found in some outlets. If you are slow cooking but prefer your sausages browned, fry them for a few minutes before adding them to the cooker. You can also try sweet potato instead of carrots, fennel instead of celery and sweetcorn instead of mushrooms.

150g (5oz) whole brown lentils, rinsed

12 large gluten-free sausages, pricked

4 sticks of celery, sliced

2 leeks or onions, sliced

8 large mushrooms, quartered

2 carrots, diced

10 new potatoes (unpeeled), halved

2 garlic cloves, crushed

1 tsp dried rosemary

1 tsp dried thyme

4 sun-dried tomatoes, finely diced

2 x 400g (14oz) tins of chopped tomatoes

1 stock cube dissolved in 725ml (1¼ pints) boiling water (425ml/15fl oz if slow cooking)

2 bay leaves

Salt and freshly ground black pepper

1. Preheat the oven to 180°C (160°C fan), gas mark 4.

2. Place the lentils in the casserole dish and add the sausages now if slow cooking.

3. Add the vegetables, garlic, herbs and sun-dried tomatoes, then pour over the tinned tomatoes and stock. Tuck the bay leaves down the sides of the dish and place the sausages on top if cooking in the oven.

4. Cover with a lid and cook on the middle shelf of the oven for about 2 hours, or slow cook for 6–8 hours (check your slow-cooker manual for timing).

5. Remove the bay leaves, season to taste with salt and pepper and serve.

Pork, Chorizo and Chickpea Stew

Serves 4

This is a great everyday stew that avoids being ordinary by the addition of some spicy chorizo. If you prefer to reduce the amount of fat in the dish, fry the chorizo in a separate pan for a few minutes to release the oil, then drain on kitchen paper before adding to the stew.

450g (1lb) pork fillet, diced

450g (1lb) new potatoes (unpeeled), halved if large

1 onion, diced

1 carrot, diced

3 sticks of celery, sliced

1 green and 1 red pepper, deseeded and diced

1 x 400g (14oz) tin of chickpeas, drained and rinsed

10cm (4in) piece of chorizo, finely sliced

½ tsp dried thyme

1 tsp dried rosemary

2 level tbsps gluten-free plain flour (see page 22)

1 tbsp pomegranate molasses (optional)

1 tbsp tomato purée

1 stock cube dissolved in 1.2 litres (2 pints) boiling water (860ml/1½ pints if slow cooking)

1 x 400g (14oz) tin of chopped tomatoes

2 bay leaves

Salt and black pepper

1. Preheat the oven to 180°C (160°C fan), gas mark 4.

2. Place the pork and vegetables in a casserole dish or slow cooker with the chickpeas, chorizo, herbs and gluten-free flour and toss to coat the ingredients in the flour.

3. Mix the pomegranate molasses and tomato purée with the stock and pour into the casserole dish or slow cooker along with the tinned tomatoes. Stir to combine, then tuck the bay leaves down the sides of the dish.

4. Cover with a lid and cook on the middle shelf of the oven for about 2 hours, or slow cook for 6–8 hours (check your slow-cooker manual for timing).

5. Remove the bay leaves, season to taste with salt and pepper and serve.

Vegetable Casserole with Herb Dumplings

Serves 4

This is a really tasty vegetarian casserole that can also be served as an accompaniment to meat dishes. It is best cooked in the oven, rather than a slow cooker, as the vegetables need to be chunkier than in a meat casserole and would take too long to cook.

1.4kg (3lb) selection of trimmed/peeled vegetables cut into bite-sized pieces (choose from onions, leeks, carrots, butternut squash, sweet potatoes, celery, fennel, parsnips, swede, mushrooms, peppers)

2 cloves garlic, crushed

½ tsp dried thyme

2 tsps dried oregano

2 tsps paprika

4cm (1½in) piece of fresh root ginger, peeled and finely diced

1 x 400g (14oz) tin of butter beans, drained and rinsed

2 x 690ml (1 pint 7fl oz) jars of tomato passata

150ml (5fl oz) water

Salt and freshly ground black pepper

1. Preheat the oven to 180°C (160°C fan), gas mark 4.

2. Place all the casserole ingredients (except the salt and pepper) in a large casserole dish and mix to combine, using the water to wash out the passata jars.

3. Cover with a lid and cook on the middle shelf of the oven for about 1¾ hours.

4. Meanwhile, make the dumplings. Sift the flour, bicarbonate of soda and baking powder into a bowl and rub in the butter or coconut oil using your fingertips (you can mix the flour and fat in a food processor if you prefer). Add the rest of the dry ingredients and mix to combine.

5. Mix the lemon juice or vitamin C powder with 170ml (6fl oz) of water and add to the dry ingredients. Mix quickly to combine, adding more water if needed, to make a very soft, sticky dough.

Continued overleaf...

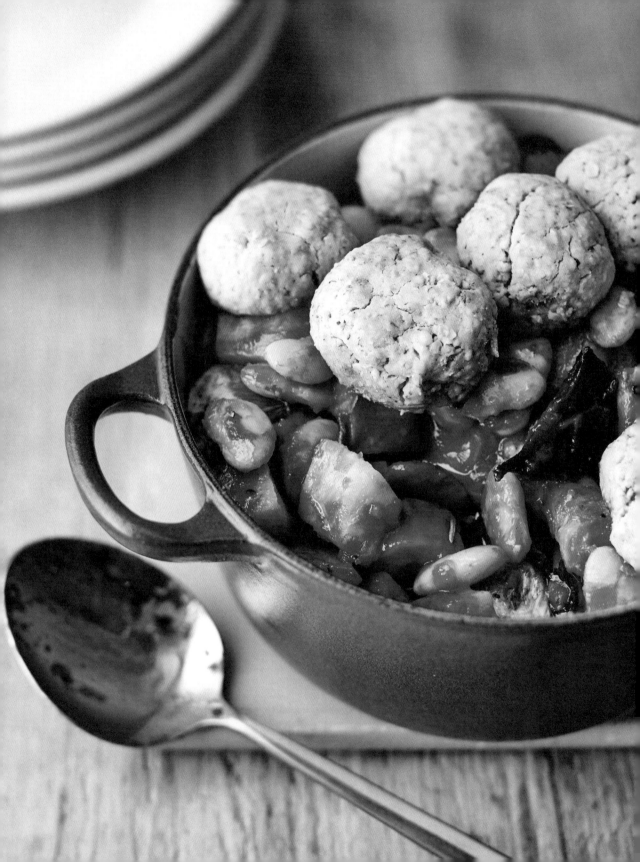

Vegetable Casserole with Herb Dumplings
(continued)

For the dumplings

200g (7oz) gluten-free plain flour (see page 22)

½ level tsp bicarbonate of soda

½ level tsp gluten-free baking powder

75g (3oz) chilled butter (not dairy-free) or coconut oil

110g (4oz) gluten-free oats

1 level tsp mustard powder

½ tsp dried thyme

½ tsp dried oregano

¼ tsp salt

¼ tsp freshly ground black pepper

1 tbsp lemon juice or ¼ tsp vitamin C powder (see page 23)

170–225ml (6–8fl oz) water

6. Remove the casserole dish from the oven and season to taste with salt and pepper. Place rough tablespoons of the dough on top of the casserole – the mixture should make about eight dumplings. (You can roll the dough into balls using floured hands, if you prefer, though this isn't necessary.)

7. Return the dish to the oven, covered, for another 30 minutes or until the dumplings are risen and soft.

Roasts and Tray Bakes

In this section I've tried to create oven meals that are not only easy to prepare but easy to cook, too. With roast joints this means slower cooking, as it's not possible to quickly cook a roast unless you are prepared to hover near the oven to check the juices aren't burning around the edges. Tray bakes are much quicker to cook than roasts and, although you need to keep an eye on them, the bulk of the meal is cooking on the tray so you can get on with other jobs.

When I was growing up, Sunday lunch was always a roast and Monday and even Tuesday meals involved using up the leftovers. I find I'm now going back to this way of eating as there is nothing better than coming home to a second-day roast knowing that very little preparation will be needed. You'll find lots of suggestions for using leftover meat in the 'Love your Leftovers' chapter. You can otherwise freeze leftovers for another day or slice to use in sandwiches. It works out much cheaper to produce your own meat for sandwiches, salads and lunches than buying it sliced from the supermarket or butcher. And it's much nicer.

My Sunday roast is accompanied by roast vegetables and/ or potatoes as well lots of freshly cooked vegetables. This is not only healthier, as meat should be eaten in moderation, but more economical, too, as it helps to eek out an expensive joint. Bear in mind, also, that you'll save money on fuel if you fill the oven while it's on – so why not add other dishes to cook at the same time?

Foolproof Slow Roasts

The meat in these recipes is cooked in a small amount of liquid that combines with any juices produced by the meat as it roasts. The trick is to not let this liquid evaporate or you will have no gravy and lots of washing up as the juices caramelise and burn – a problem I find with most roast recipes. Therefore, rather than putting the meat in a large roasting tin, I cook it in a smaller, higher-sided container covered loosely with foil or a lid. I like to use a large casserole dish, which prevents too much evaporation. If you have to cook in a roasting tin, you will need to add more liquid initially; the amount will depend on the size of your tin. Try an extra 55ml (2fl oz), but keep your eye on the level of liquid until you have worked out the right amount for your container – too much and the meat will steam rather than roast. You may also find that the meat takes a little longer to cook in a more open container.

If you prepare some fresh vegetables at the same time and pop some foil-wrapped baking potatoes in the oven with the meat, then you can have time out while the meal cooks. All you then need to do is quickly cook the fresh vegetables and thicken the gravy and your roast is ready to serve.

On pages 171–172 you'll find some vegetarian roasts that I created in order to have a main vegetarian option to put in the oven along with a joint of meat, though they can of course be cooked on their own for meat-free meals. They are really quick and easy to prepare and the timings are the same as for a joint, so you don't need to keep an eye on them. The Roast Stuffed Butternut Squash could, however, be used as a vegetable accompaniment to roast meat. It's really delicious and I'm sure the meat eaters will love it, too.

Removing the Fat from Cooking Juices

An easy and efficient way to do this is to add a handful of ice cubes to the juices. These quickly cool the liquid and the fat then sticks to the cubes, which can be lifted out with a slotted spoon.

Easy Slow-roast Lamb with Rosemary and Thyme

Serves 6–8

It's not always easy to fit a leg of lamb into a casserole dish, as the bone can get in the way. Look out for short fat joints, large half legs (I used a 1.25kg/2lb 12oz half leg and the timings worked out the same as for a whole leg) or boned joints. If you buy your meat from a butcher, ask them to remove the end of the bone.

1 x 1.75–2kg (4lb–4lb 6oz) leg of lamb

1 tsp butter or oil (see page 20), melted if needed

¼ tsp paprika

55ml (2fl oz) water

½ tsp dried thyme

½ tsp dried rosemary

4 level tsps gluten-free plain flour (see page 22)

½ stock cube dissolved in 275ml (½ pint) boiling water

Salt and freshly ground black pepper

1. Preheat the oven to 170°C (150°C fan), gas mark 3½.

2. Dry the leg of lamb with kitchen paper and place it in the casserole dish or roasting tin (see 'Foolproof Slow Roasts' on page 166). Using your fingers, rub the butter or oil into the skin, along with the paprika and some salt and pepper.

3. Add the water and herbs to the dish or tin, cover with a lid or foil and cook on the middle shelf of the oven for 1½ hours for lamb that's still pink in the middle, 1¾ hours for medium-cooked lamb and 2 hours for well done. Remove the lid or foil for the last 30 minutes if you want a browner roast.

4. Remove the lamb from the dish or tin and skim any fat from the juices using a spoon (or see tip on page 167). Whisk the flour and stock together and add this to the juices. Bring the mixture to the boil, stirring constantly and adding some vegetable cooking water if the gravy is too thick. Season, if needed, before serving.

Variations

Easy Slow-roast Lemon and Garlic Leg of Lamb: Replace the rosemary and thyme with 2 crushed garlic cloves and the grated zest and juice of ½ lemon.

Easy Slow-roast Beef: Follow the recipe for slow roast lamb – for a joint of beef of the same weight, the timings are identical. Just swap the thyme and rosemary for your favourite ingredients. You could try ½ teaspoon of mustard powder rubbed into the skin along with the oil, paprika and seasoning.

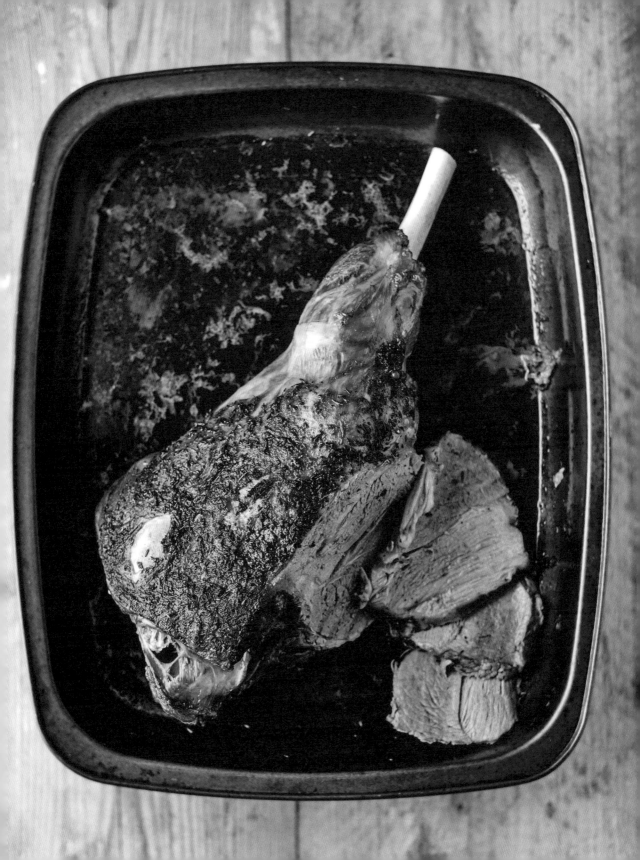

Easy Slow-roast Lemon and Thyme Chicken

Serves 4–6

Everyone loves roast chicken and they'll love this one, too. It works equally well in a slow cooker left on high for about 4 hours or low for up to 8 (check your manual as timings vary). I often put this dish and some foil-wrapped potatoes in the oven with the timer on if I'm out and about, so that I can come home to a ready-cooked meal.

1 x 1.6–1.8kg (3½–4lb) chicken (add an extra 20 minutes' cooking time for every extra 200g/7oz over 1.8kg/4lb)

1 tsp butter or oil (see page 20), melted if needed

½ tsp mild-tasting runny honey

¼ tsp paprika

Juice of ½ lemon

55ml (2fl oz) water

½ tsp dried thyme

4 level tsps gluten-free plain flour (see page 22)

½ stock cube dissolved in 275ml (½ pint) boiling water

Salt and freshly ground black pepper

1. Preheat the oven to 170°C (150°C fan), gas mark 3½.

2. Dry the chicken with kitchen paper and place in a casserole dish or roasting tin (see 'Foolproof Slow Roasts' on page 166). Mix the butter or oil with the honey, paprika and some salt and pepper and rub it into the chicken skin with your fingers.

3. Squeeze over the lemon juice and put the lemon half inside the cavity of the chicken. Add the water and thyme to the casserole dish or roasting tin, cover loosely with a lid or foil and cook on the middle shelf of the oven for 2 hours or until the juices run clear when you insert a knife between the leg and the main body of the chicken. Remove the lid or foil from the dish or tin for the last 30 minutes if the chicken is not browning sufficiently.

4. Remove the chicken from the dish or tin and skim any fat from the juices using a spoon (or see tip on page 167). Whisk the flour with the stock and add this to the juices. Bring the mixture to the boil, stirring constantly and adding some vegetable cooking water if the gravy is too thick. Season with salt and pepper, if needed, before serving.

Variations

Easy Slow-roast Sage and Onion Chicken: Replace the lemon and thyme with an onion, cut into quarters, and ½ teaspoon dried sage.

Easy Slow-roast Garlic and Rosemary Chicken: Replace the lemon and thyme with 8 unpeeled garlic cloves and a bay leaf. Serve the garlic with the roast.

Roast Stuffed Butternut Squash

Serves 2

For this recipe you'll need to choose your butternut squash with care, as they vary a lot in shape and size. You need a medium-sized one with a bulbous end, which is going to be stuffed, and a stalk end that would make a suitable lid.

1 butternut squash

½ stick of celery, finely diced

¼ red pepper, deseeded and finely diced

3 tbsps uncooked quinoa or buckwheat grains

4 sun-blushed tomatoes, finely diced

1 tbsp sultanas

2 parings of orange rind, finely sliced

½ tsp sweet smoked paprika

¼ tsp Chinese five-spice powder

6 tbsps water

Salt and freshly ground black pepper

1. Preheat the oven to 170°C (150°C fan), gas mark 3½.

2. Cut the bulbous end from the squash at the point where it becomes elongated. Using a metal spoon, make a hole in the flesh and scoop out the seeds and any fibrous threads from inside the squash.

3. Combine all the stuffing ingredients except the water, season with salt and pepper and place inside the squash, pressing the mixture down firmly so that it is tightly packed.

4. Pour the water over the stuffing ingredients, then make a lid by cutting a piece off the stalk end of the butternut squash but retaining the stalk as a knob.

5. Wrap the stuffed squash in foil and place on a baking tray in the oven to cook for about 2 hours or until the squash feels soft when you give it a press. Served cut into wedges, it is really good accompanied by the Apricot and Tomato Sauce (see page 173).

Cashew and Ginger Roast

Serves 4–6

This roast is a veggie delight, especially if served with the Apricot and Tomato Sauce opposite. If you are using it as a vegetarian option, cooked alongside a meat roast, you will probably have some left over for lunches or to freeze for another day. Perfect!

Oil, for greasing

1 small onion, roughly chopped

1 stick of celery, roughly chopped

1 large sweet potato, roughly chopped

2 garlic cloves, crushed

5cm (2in) piece of fresh root ginger, peeled and grated

2 handfuls of cashews, cut into 3–4 pieces

1 tsp fennel seeds

8 tbsps uncooked quinoa or buckwheat grains

4 tbsps ground almonds

1 x 400g (14oz) tin of butter beans, drained and rinsed

½ stock cube dissolved in 275ml (½ pint) boiling water

Salt and freshly ground black pepper

450g (1lb) loaf tin

1. Preheat the oven to 170°C (150°C fan), gas mark 3½, then grease the tin with a little oil and line with baking parchment.

2. Cut up the onion, celery and sweet potato separately in a food processor until each is finely diced. Place these in a bowl with the garlic, ginger, cashews, fennel seeds and quinoa or buckwheat.

4. Blend the ground almonds, butter beans and stock until smooth in the food processor, then combine the two sets of ingredients and season with salt and pepper. You won't need much salt if you're using a stock cube.

5. Place the mixture in the prepared loaf tin and cover with foil. Bake in the oven for about 2 hours or until browning on top and crisping around the edges. Invert the tin onto a plate, remove the lining paper and serve the nut roast cut into slices with Apricot and Tomato Sauce (see page 173) spooned over.

Apricot and Tomato Sauce

Serves 4

The deliciously tangy flavour of this sauce provides the perfect accompaniment for either the Cashew and Ginger Roast (opposite) or the Roast Stuffed Butternut Squash (see page 171). It is very easy to make and could be served with other dishes, such as plain cooked chicken or fish.

1 onion, diced

75g (3oz) dried apricots, diced

1 x 400g (14oz) tin of chopped tomatoes

275ml (½ pint) water

Grated zest and juice of 1 orange

Salt and freshly ground black pepper

1. Place all the ingredients (except the salt and pepper) in a pan and bring to the boil. Reduce the heat to low, cover with a lid and simmer for 8–10 minutes or until the apricots and onions are soft.

2. Blend until smooth in a food processor, seasoning to taste with salt and pepper and adding a little extra water if the sauce is too thick.

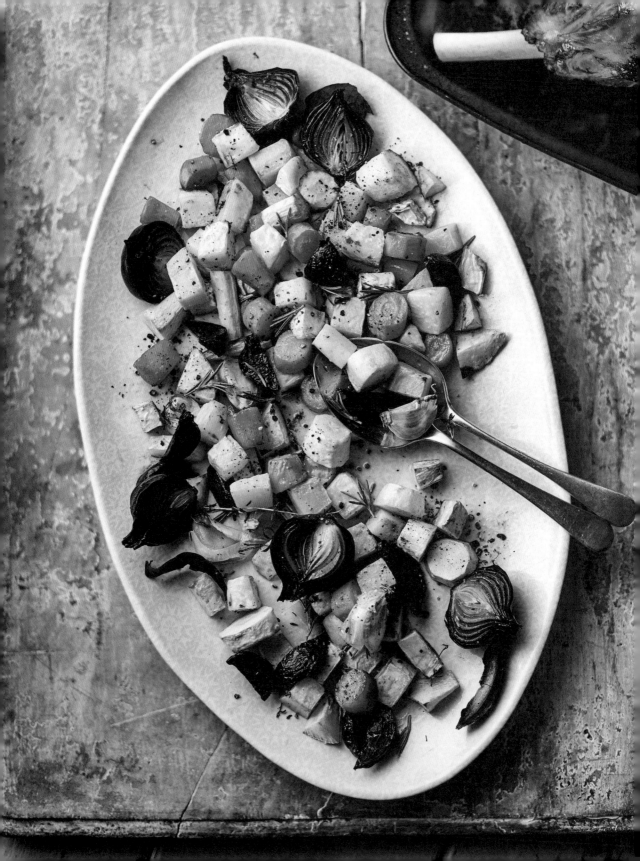

Easy-cook Roast Vegetables

Serves 4–6

These vegetables won't spoil if they are left in the oven for 2 hours with your roast, but you can get away with less cooking time if you are cooking them separately – 1–1½ hours, depending on the size you cut the vegetables. If you have ready-made Pomegranate Molasses Dressing (see page 110), you can use 3 tablespoons of this instead of the oil and lemon juice in the dressing below.

For the vegetables

Select 900g/2lb from the following:

Small white or red onions, halved if needed

Sweet potatoes or butternut squash, cut into large chunks

Carrots, cut into chunks

Parsnips, cut into wedges

Beetroots, cut into thin wedges

Jerusalem artichokes, halved if needed

Swede, cut into small dice

Celeriac, cut into chunks

Garlic cloves, added whole

For the dressing

2 tbsps olive oil

1 tbsp lemon juice

½ tsp mustard powder

1 tsp dried rosemary

½ tsp dried thyme

Salt and freshly ground black pepper

1. Preheat the oven to 170°C (150°C fan), gas mark 3½.

2. Cut a piece of foil two and a half times bigger than your roasting tin. Lay the foil with the centre in the middle of the tin.

3. Make the dressing by whisking together the oil, lemon juice, mustard powder and herbs and seasoning with salt and pepper.

4. Place your choice of prepared vegetables on the foil, pour over the dressing and gently toss to coat the vegetables, taking care not to rip the foil. Alternatively, toss together in a separate pan and transfer to the foil-lined tin; I like to toss beetroot separately to prevent it from colouring the other vegetables.

5. Fold over the foil to make a parcel, turning the edges over a few times to seal. Cook in the oven for 1–2 hours (see above).

Speedy-bake Roast Vegetables

Serves 4–6

These quick-cook roast vegetables are ideal if you are short of oven space, as they can be made while your roast is resting and you are preparing the gravy. They can also be used for vegetarian meals.

For the vegetables

Select 900g/2lb from the following:

Courgettes, sliced

Peppers, diced

Asparagus spears

Whole mushrooms

Red onions, cut into thin wedges

Whole cherry tomatoes

Sweet potato or celeriac, cut into small dice

Baby sweetcorn

Cauliflower florets

Sticks of celery, sliced

Green beans, sliced

For the dressing

2 tbsps olive oil

1 tbsp lemon juice

½ tsp mustard powder

1 tsp dried rosemary

½ tsp dried thyme

Salt and freshly ground black pepper

1. Preheat the oven to 170°C (150°C fan), gas mark 3½, and line a roasting tin with foil or baking parchment, if you wish.

2. Make the dressing by whisking together the oil, lemon juice, mustard powder and herbs and seasoning with salt and pepper.

3. Place your choice of vegetables in the roasting tin, add the dressing and gently toss to coat the vegetables.

4. Roast for 20–30 minutes or until all the vegetables are just cooked, checking halfway through cooking and moving any that are browning too quickly to the centre of the tray.

Potatoes to Accompany Roasts

Baked potatoes are ideal to serve with roasts if you want to avoid having to keep an eye on them while they're cooking. Wrapped in foil, they can happily stay in the oven, undisturbed, for the duration of the cooking. However, what makes a roast meal special are roast potatoes – winter comfort food at its best. Roasted in minimum fat, they still taste delicious, so you don't need to feel guilty about having them!

Really Easy Roast Potatoes

1. Cut peeled potatoes into roast-sized chunks, dry on kitchen paper and toss in 2 teaspoons of oil and a little salt per portion (I use a mixture of coconut and olive oil). I like to use a bowl or pan for this and a large spoon to toss as it's easier and quicker to coat each potato in oil, but you can toss them in the roasting tin.

2. Lay the potatoes in a roasting tin or baking tray, allowing a small gap between each potato. Cooked with your roast, at 170°C (150°C fan), gas mark 3½, they will take about 1 hour to cook and will need turning halfway through.

Extra-crunchy Roast Potatoes

1. Cut peeled potatoes into roast-sized chunks and boil or steam for 5 minutes.

2. Drain, if needed, then shake the potatoes in the pan to roughen the edges. This is what gives the potatoes their crispy outsides and works best with floury potatoes such as King Edwards or Maris Piper.

3. Follow the recipe above, but add 1 tablespoon of oil per portion.

Tray Bakes

The trick with tray baking is to ensure that the vegetables and meat or fish all cook in the same amount of time. This can be achieved through your choice of vegetables or by cutting the vegetables into larger or smaller chunks. Vegetables such as courgettes, peppers, mushrooms and tomatoes cook quickly and are ideal to accompany fish. Potatoes, carrots and parsnips take much longer to cook, but this can be speeded up if you cut them into smaller pieces.

It's really worth mastering the art of tray bakes, as you are cooking a whole meal in one tray – indeed, if you line the tray with baking parchment or foil, you won't even have much washing up. You can also prepare tray bakes ahead of time, ready to pop in the oven when you want to eat. You may decide to serve your tray bake with a salad or some green vegetables, which will need preparing closer to the time, but otherwise you are free to get on with other jobs while dinner cooks. If a tray bake doesn't include potatoes, I often put small potatoes or sweet potatoes in the oven, wrapped in foil, before I start preparing the tray bake so that they will be ready when the dish is cooked.

In all these recipes, the vegetables are tossed in oil and I tend to use a large bowl or pan for this as it makes the process quick and easy. You can toss them in the baking tray, but you will need to be careful that you don't rip the foil or parchment or end up with them on the floor. Your tray needs to easily hold all the ingredients so that they are not too packed together, otherwise they won't brown. Use two smaller trays if you don't have one large one.

There are some fish tray bakes on pages 187–188. Because fish doesn't take long to cook, any vegetables included in the tray bake need to cook quickly, too. This can be achieved either by selecting softer vegetables (such as mushrooms or tomatoes) or by cutting firmer vegetables into smaller pieces. To test if fish is cooked, cut through the fish at its thickest point – it should just have turned from translucent to opaque to be at its best.

Even if you don't eat meat or fish, don't overlook the tray bakes in this chapter. Simply replace the meat or fish with vegetarian alternatives, such as vegetarian sausages, chunks of halloumi or feta cheese, or cubes of tofu tossed in a mixture of oil and smoked paprika or Chinese five-spice powder. Alternatively, add some beans, nuts or seeds near the end of cooking, or try the recipe on page 184.

Spicy Roast Chicken Tray Bake

Serves 2

I love this dish of moist chicken and tender vegetables gently spiced with Eastern flavours. Add more chilli, if you like the extra heat, and serve the tray bake with some rice or quinoa or a salad.

2 tbsps oil (see page 20), melted if needed

1 garlic clove, crushed

1 tsp grated lemon zest and 2 tbsps lemon juice

2 tsps ground cumin

1 tsp garam masala

Seeds from 8 cardamom pods, crushed

⅛–¼ tsp chilli powder

2 carrots or 1 sweet potato, peeled and cut into batons

¼ celeriac or 1 red pepper, cut into chunks

1 onion, cut into 8 wedges

2 large sticks of celery or ½ fennel bulb, sliced

6 large chestnut mushrooms

4 chicken thighs, skinned if preferred

Salt and freshly ground black pepper

1. Preheat the oven to 200°C (180°C fan), gas mark 6, and line the baking tray with foil or baking parchment, if you wish.

2. Place the oil, garlic, lemon zest and juice in a large bowl or pan with the spices and some salt and pepper. Stir to combine and add the vegetables, tossing to coat in the oil mixture, then lift them out with a slotted spoon and spread them evenly on the prepared baking tray.

3. Coat the chicken in any remaining oil mixture and place it among the vegetables. Bake on the middle shelf of the oven for about 40 minutes or until the meat and vegetables are cooked. Check halfway through cooking and move any vegetables that are browning too quickly to the centre of the tray.

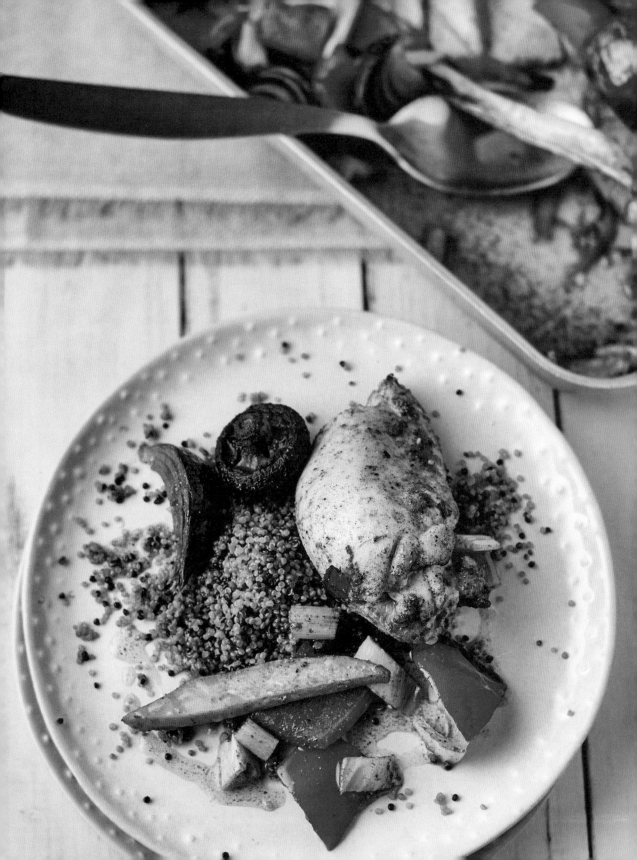

Tray-baked Pork with Apples, Ginger and Parsnips

Serves 2

This is a superb supper dish – quick and easy to make and so delicious. The recipe works best with eating apples that are quite tart, but if you are using baking apples, which disintegrate when cooked, they are best added halfway through cooking.

2 tbsps oil (see page 20), melted if needed

Juice from 1 tbsp grated fresh root ginger

1 tsp mild-tasting runny honey (optional)

1 garlic clove, crushed

2 tsps dried sage

½ tsp dried thyme

1 red onion, cut into 8 wedges

1 parsnip, cut into batons

1 carrot, cut into thin batons

8 small new potatoes (unpeeled), cut into slices 1cm (½in) wide

1 large eating or small baking apple (unpeeled), cored and cut into wedges

2 thick pork chops, excess fat removed

Salt and freshly ground black pepper

1. Preheat the oven to 200°C (180°C fan), gas mark 6, and line the baking tray with foil or baking parchment, if you wish.

2. Place the oil and ginger juice in a large bowl or pan with the honey (if using), garlic, herbs and some salt and pepper. Stir to combine and add the vegetables and apple wedges. Toss to coat in the oil mixture, then lift them out with a slotted spoon and spread them evenly on the prepared baking tray.

3. Rub the pork chops in the remaining oil mixture, then lay them among the vegetables and apple. Bake on the middle shelf of the oven for 30–40 minutes or until the vegetables and meat are cooked. Check halfway through cooking and move any vegetables that are browning too quickly to the centre of the tray.

4. Serve with some fresh green vegetables or a salad, if desired.

Sausage and Red Onion Tray Bake
Serves 2

Sausages work well in tray bakes and they're always popular. This is a warm and comforting dish that I love to serve tipped into large pasta bowls. Sausages are readily available gluten free and even additive free if you do a little searching.

2 tbsp oil (see page 20), melted if needed

1 tsp sweet smoked paprika

½ tsp dried oregano

½ tsp fennel seeds

⅛–¼ tsp chilli powder (optional)

2 red onions, each cut into 8 wedges

2 carrots or 1 sweet potato, peeled and cut into batons

1 red pepper, deseeded and cut into chunks

2 potatoes, peeled and cut into small chunks (dry with kitchen paper)

6 large gluten-free sausages

Salt and freshly ground black pepper

1. Preheat the oven to 200°C (180°C fan), gas mark 6, and line the baking tray with foil or baking parchment, if you wish.

2. Place the oil and paprika in large bowl or pan with the oregano, fennel seeds, chilli powder and some salt and pepper, and mix to combine. Add the onions, carrots or sweet potato, red pepper and potatoes and toss to coat them in the oil mixture, then lift them out with a slotted spoon and spread them evenly on the prepared baking tray.

3. Prick the sausages and rub them with any remaining oil before laying them among the vegetables.

4. Bake on the middle shelf of the oven for 30–40 minutes or until the meat and vegetables are cooked. Check halfway through cooking to turn the sausages over and move any vegetables that are browning too quickly to the centre of the tray.

5. Serve with a fresh green vegetable or salad, if desired.

Ratatouille Tray Bake with Red Kidney Beans and Pine Nuts

Serves 2

This is a tasty, veggie tray bake version of classic ratatouille. Try it served with pasta or pop some small potatoes or sweet potatoes in to bake when you put the oven on.

2 tbsps oil (see page 20), melted if needed

2 tbsps Pesto Sauce (see page 90) or tomato purée

2 garlic cloves, crushed

1 tsp dried basil

½ tsp dried oregano

1 red onion, peeled and cut into 8 wedges

½ aubergine (halved lengthways), cut into slices 1cm (½in) wide

1 large courgette, cut into chunks

1 red pepper, deseeded and cut into chunks

½ fennel bulb, thinly sliced, or 2 sticks of celery, sliced

12 cherry tomatoes

½ x 400g (14oz) tin of red kidney beans, drained and rinsed

10 black olives, pitted and halved

2 tbsps pine nuts

Salt and freshly ground black pepper

1. Preheat the oven to 200°C (180°C fan), gas mark 6, and line the baking tray with foil or baking parchment, if you wish.

2. Place the oil, pesto or tomato purée, garlic, herbs and some salt and pepper in a large bowl or pan and mix to combine. Add the onion, aubergine, courgette, red pepper and fennel or celery and toss to coat in the oil mixture before lifting them out with a slotted spoon and spreading them evenly on the baking tray.

3. Bake on the middle shelf of the oven for 30–40 minutes or until the vegetables are cooked. Check halfway through cooking and move any vegetables that are browning too quickly to the centre of the tray.

4. Add the tomatoes, kidney beans, olives and pine nuts 10 minutes before the end of cooking to heat through and to allow the pine nuts to brown slightly.

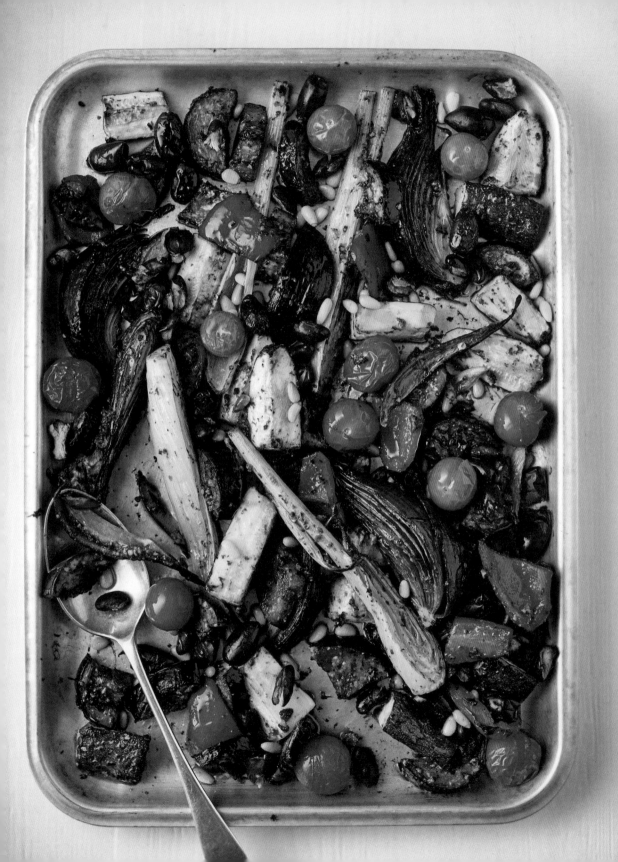

Lemon and Rosemary Lamb Tray Bake
Serves 2

Lemon and rosemary love lamb – they are the perfect partners. Use fresh rosemary, if available, but double the quantity of the dried herb. If you prefer your lamb cooked rare, then add it to the vegetables partway through cooking.

2 tbsps oil (see page 20), melted if needed

1 tsp dried rosemary

10 new potatoes (unpeeled), sliced

1 carrot, cut into batons

1 parsnip, cut into small wedges

1 onion, cut into 8 wedges

1 sweet potato, peeled and cut into cubes

2 thick lamb steaks or 4 lamb cutlets, trimmed of excess fat

1 lemon, thinly sliced and pips removed

Salt and freshly ground black pepper

1 tbsp chopped fresh mint, to garnish (optional)

1. Preheat the oven to 200°C (180°C fan), gas mark 6, and line the baking tray with foil or baking parchment, if you wish.

2. Place the oil, rosemary and some salt and pepper in a large bowl or pan and add the vegetables. Toss to coat in the oil, then lift them out with a slotted spoon and spread them evenly on the prepared baking tray.

3. Rub the lamb steaks in the remaining oil mixture and add them to the tray with the lemon slices, laying them among the vegetables. Bake on the middle shelf of the oven for 30–40 minutes or until the vegetables and lamb are cooked. Check halfway through cooking and move any vegetables that are browning too quickly to the centre of the tray.

4. Garnish with fresh mint (if using) and serve with fresh green vegetables or a salad, if desired.

Monkfish and Parma Ham Tray Bake
Serves 2

This is a fantastic seafood dish that will wow your friends if you invite them to supper. Grainy mustard also works well in this recipe, but it does contain vinegar. It has a mild flavour, so use a level tablespoon instead of the single teaspoon of mustard powder.

2 tbsps oil (see page 20), melted if needed

1 tsp sesame oil

1 tsp grated lemon zest and 2 tbsps lemon juice

1 tsp mustard powder

8 chestnut mushrooms

1 small sweet potato, peeled and cut into 1cm (½in) dice

1 courgette, sliced

8 asparagus spears, tailed and cut into short pieces

12 cherry tomatoes

350g (12oz) monkfish, cut into 8 even-sized chunks

8 slices of Parma-type ham

Salt and freshly ground black pepper

1. Preheat the oven to 200°C (180°C fan), gas mark 6, and line the baking tray with foil or baking parchment, if you wish.

2. Place the oils, lemon zest and juice, mustard powder and some salt and pepper in a large bowl or pan and mix to combine. Add the vegetables and toss to coat in the oil mixture, then lift them out with a slotted spoon and spread them evenly on the prepared baking tray.

3. Coat the fish pieces in any remaining oil and wrap each chunk in a slice of ham before placing it in among the vegetables.

4. Bake on the middle shelf of the oven for about 15 minutes or until the fish and vegetables are cooked.

5. Serve with new potatoes or a green salad, if desired.

Salmon and Prawn Tray Bake
Serves 2

This is a great recipe for packing in the omega-3 oils, which most people are lacking in their diet. As well as being healthy, this dish both looks good and is full of flavour.

6 anchovy fillets, finely diced, and 2 tbsps oil from the tin

1 tbsp lemon juice

½ fresh red chilli, deseeded and finely diced (optional)

1 handful of fine green beans, trimmed and sliced

8 baby sweetcorn

12 sugar snap peas

1 courgette, sliced

2 salmon fillets

6 raw king prawns

½ lemon, halved lengthways and finely sliced

1. Preheat the oven to 200°C (180°C fan), gas mark 6, and line the baking tray with foil or baking parchment, if you wish.

2. Place the anchovies and oil in a large bowl or pan with the lemon juice and chilli (if using) and mix to combine. Add the vegetables and toss to coat in the oil mixture before lifting them out with a slotted spoon and spreading them evenly on the prepared baking tray.

3. Coat the salmon pieces and prawns in any remaining oil mixture and place among the vegetables on the tray. Lay two lemon slices on top of the salmon pieces and place the rest among the vegetables.

4. Bake on the middle shelf of the oven for about 15 minutes or until the fish and vegetables are cooked.

5. Serve with new potatoes or a fresh green salad, if desired.

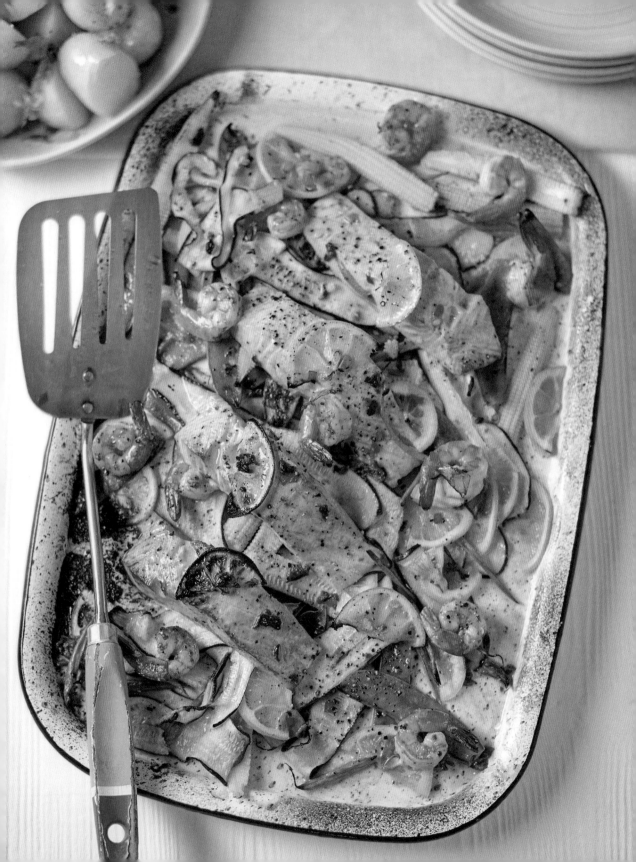

Love your
Leftovers

Not only do I love leftovers, I deliberately cook extra to ensure there will be some. Days when the fridge is full of good things to eat with little preparation needed feel like a holiday to me. I know it would be ideal to have every meal freshly prepared, but we don't live in an ideal world and we have busy lives. Having leftovers means speedy meals made from home-cooked ingredients, without having to resort to convenience food or takeaways.

Using leftovers also opens up a different kind of cooking. I certainly couldn't be bothered to cook and mash potatoes as well as other vegetables, then fry them to make a bubble and squeak. But if you have leftover mash and vegetables, this is an ideal and delicious way to use them up. Using leftovers also saves money, as you waste less, and keeps you slimmer. Rather than forcing down the last of the lamb joint on a Sunday, I scrimp as much as possible to create a Monday supper such as meat and potato hash (see page 194).

Leftover Potatoes

You can never have too much leftover potato or sweet potato, either mashed, boiled or baked. Formed in a cake, if mashed, or cut into cubes if boiled and fried in a little oil, they are the perfect accompaniment to a main dish and ideal to go with leftover roast meat. Another idea is to cut boiled potatoes into small dice, toss them in oil, season with salt and pepper and used as a topping to make a casserole into a hotpot. Diced new potatoes are especially good in a stir-fry instead of grains.

With the addition of a few extra ingredients, your leftovers can be made into a full meal such as Bubble and Squeak (see page 195). Think of crisply fried potatoes mixed with anything from black pudding and bacon to mushrooms and cabbage. Or you could use leftover mash to make Fish Cakes (see page 196) or a Fish Pie (see page 199). Preferably don't store leftover cooked potatoes for more than 24 hours, as they never taste as good if they are kept longer.

Leftover Grains

Whenever I cook rice millet, buckwheat or quinoa I always cook extra for the following day. They are useful to add to a salad pot (see pages 62–74) for lunch and ideal to make into a pilaf (see page 199) or to accompany other meals. If you have leftover grains but not quite enough for a meal, then cook a few rice noodles (these only take a few minutes) and add them to your grains. The combination works well. If I have leftover grains but know I won't be using them, I freeze them in small containers for emergency meals (rice is best not kept for more than 24 hours in the fridge).

Leftover Meat

If I have leftover meat from a roast I try to save some gravy so that I can have a second-night roast, perhaps with some fresh vegetables or Bubble and Squeak if I have leftover vegetables too. Leftover lamb or beef are ideal to make into a One-pan Meat and Potato Hotpot (see page 202) or Shepherd's or Cottage Pie (see page 200). Leftover chicken is so versatile – it is more economical to cook a whole chicken than to buy separate breasts and thighs. After serving roast chicken I remove any remaining meat from the carcass and save it to use in meals over the following days; or I cut the chicken into small pieces and store it in the freezer. A handful of ready-cooked chicken can be added to soups and salads or used in sandwiches and stir-fries. An added bonus is the leftover carcass, which makes wonderful stock (see page 203).

Potato Cakes

Serves 2

These are ideal to make with leftover mashed potato. Adjust the ingredients to make use of one leftover portion or several. Freeze them once cold if you won't be eating them in the next 24 hours.

2 portions of leftover mashed potato (about 350g/12oz)

3 level tbsps gluten-free flour (see page 22)

Oil (see page 20) for frying

1. Combine the mashed potato with the flour, using your hands if necessary to mix really well.

2. With floured hands form the mixture into four cakes, about 1cm (½in) thick and 8cm (3in) in diameter.

3. When ready to serve, fry the cakes (defrosted first, if frozen) in a little oil over a medium heat for 3–4 minutes on each side or until they are golden brown.

4. I love to serve them hot (preferably spread with butter) to accompany a bowl of soup or instead of bread at a weekend breakfast (see page 45).

Potato Hash

Serves 2

Hashes are similar to Bubble and Squeak (see opposite) but use diced potatoes. At least half the ingredients should be potatoes, but after that use your imagination and your leftovers to create your own favourite versions.

2 good-sized portions of leftover boiled or baked potatoes (about 450g/1lb), cut into pieces

Your choice of flavourings (see page 195 for suggestions)

Oil (see page 20) for frying

1. Heat a tablespoon of oil in a large frying pan over a medium heat, then add the potatoes and fry for about 5–8 minutes or until they start to brown a little.

2. Add your flavourings, then continue to stir and fry until everything is cooked or heated through. You may need to add a little more oil depending on the additional ingredients.

3. Serve immediately with the addition of something like Homemade Baked Beans (see page 144) or a fried egg (if tolerated) if you want to stretch your hash still further.

Bubble and Squeak

Serves 2

Bubble and squeak is traditionally a mixture of potato and leftover vegetables, with at least half the mixture being potato. However, there are many variations on this theme and below are some suggestions for additions to your mash. Some of my favourites include tuna, olive and tomato; leek and bacon or chorizo and mushroom. Bubble and squeak can be fried as little cakes or as one large, frying-pan-sized cake, depending on how much potato you have left.

2 good-sized portions of leftover mashed potato (about 450g/1lb)

Your choice of flavourings

Oil (see page 20) for frying

Flavourings

Use a combination of 2–3 of the following (the combined amount should be no more about half that of the mashed potato):

Fish: Smoked mackerel or salmon; tinned sardines, salmon, tuna.

Vegetables: Leftover cooked vegetables; sweetcorn, spring onions; fried mushrooms, leeks, courgettes.

Meat: Cooked ham, bacon, chorizo, sausage.

Extra flavourings: Olives, sun-dried tomatoes; fresh or dried herbs; diced fresh chilli; crushed garlic.

1. Use your hands or a potato masher to break up the leftover mashed potato, as it always solidifies on cooling. Add your choice of flavourings from the list below and mix to combine.

2. To make small cakes, form into rounds about 2cm (¾in) thick with your hands, then fry in a little oil over a medium heat for 3–4 minutes on each side or until browned all over.

3. To make a large bubble and squeak, place the whole mixture in a heated oiled frying pan (preferably non-stick) and press it down to form a large cake. Cook over a medium heat until the underside is golden brown or until the cake moves when you shake the pan.

4. Slip the whole cake out of the pan onto a large plate and drizzle with a little oil. Invert the pan over the bubble and squeak on the plate, then tip everything the right way up so that the bubble and squeak is now in the pan, with the uncooked side at the bottom. Fry gently until the underside is brown and serve cut into wedges.

Salmon Fishcakes

Makes 4–6 fishcakes

Fishcakes are so delicious and always go down well – even children like eating fish prepared this way. Vary the recipe by adding your own favourite types of fish. It could be smoked salmon and prawns, lightly cooked fresh fish, such as smoked haddock or cod, or other tinned fish, like mackerel or sardines.

1 x 215g (7½oz) tin of salmon, deboned but including juices from the tin

4 tinned or bottled anchovy fillets, finely diced

2 tbsps tomato purée (optional)

1 tsp mustard powder

½ tsp grated lemon zest (optional)

2 tbsps chopped parsley (optional)

3 spring onions, finely sliced

2 good-sized portions of leftover mashed potato (about 450g/1lb)

Gluten-free plain flour (see page 22), for dusting

2 tbsps oil (see page 20), for frying

Salt and freshly ground black pepper

1. Combine the salmon and anchovies with the tomato purée, mustard powder, lemon zest, parsley and spring onions.

2. Break up the potato using your hands or a potato masher and mix with the other ingredients, adding enough of the juices from the salmon to make a soft consistency. Season, if needed, with salt and pepper.

3. With floured hands, divide the mixture into 4–6 portions and then flatten into cakes about 2cm (¾in) thick.

4. Heat half the oil in a large frying pan and fry the fishcakes over a medium heat for 3–4 minutes or until golden brown. Turn the cakes over and fry in the remaining oil (if needed) until the second side is cooked.

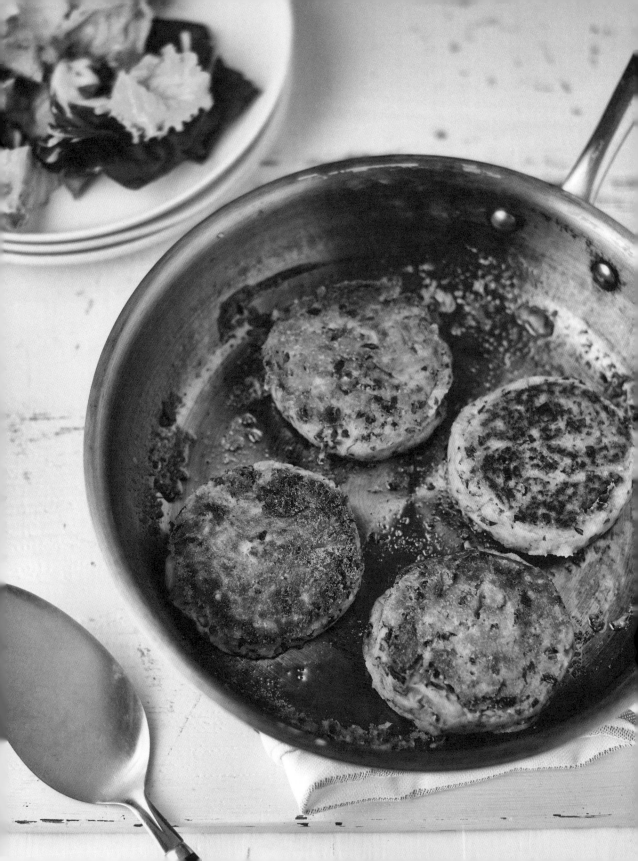

Spiced Vegetable Pilaf

Serves 2

A traditional pilaf is made from rice cooked from scratch with spices, but the dish lends itself to leftovers. As well as cooked grains such as rice, quinoa, buckwheat or millet, you can throw in leftover meat, such as chicken and ham, and use up vegetables such as carrots, parsnip, cauliflower, butternut squash and cabbage. I use a large, deep-sided saucepan with a lid, as this cooks the vegetables quickly, but you could use a lidded frying pan.

1 tbsp oil (see page 20)

2 portion selection of finely sliced stir-fry vegetables (about 450g/1lb after peeling)

2.5cm (1in) piece of fresh root ginger, finely sliced

1 garlic clove, crushed

¼ stock cube dissolved in 150ml (5fl oz) boiling water

1 tsp ground coriander

¼ tsp ground cinnamon

Seeds of 6 cardamom pods, crushed

2 tbsps raisins

2 portions of cooked grains (such as rice, buckwheat, quinoa or millet)

Squeeze of lemon juice

Salt and freshly ground black pepper

Slivered almonds or pine nuts, toasted (see page 23), to serve

1. Heat your pan over a high heat, then add the oil, followed by the prepared vegetables, ginger and garlic. Toss everything together in the oil and lower the heat to medium.

2. Stirring constantly and regularly, add a few tablespoons of stock as the pan begins to dry out, in order to prevent the vegetables from sticking or burning. Add the spices after 3–4 minutes and continue to stir-fry.

3. When the vegetables are almost cooked (after 8–10 minutes), add the remaining stock and the raisins. Stir to combine, then add the cooked grains and cover the pan with a lid. Do not stir, but allow the rice to heat through for a couple of minutes over a medium/low heat from the steam produced by the hot stock.

4. Stir to combine, season to taste with salt and pepper and a squeeze of lemon and serve scattered with the toasted nuts.

Variation:

Chorizo, Chickpea and Smoked Paprika Pilaf: This is ideal to make if you don't have enough rice as the chickpeas bulk up the dish, making it substantial. Follow the above recipe, substituting 1 teaspoon smoked paprika and ½ teaspoon turmeric for the spices and raisins. Add ½ tin of drained and rinsed chickpeas with the rice or other cooked grains and serve scattered with a handful of finely diced and lightly fried chorizo.

Fish Pie

Serves 2

I love fish pie, but it always seems such a chore to make as there are so many processes involved; this one is a cinch, however. If you use one of the ready-frozen fish pie mixes (they usually contain salmon, white fish and smoked haddock) and leftover mashed potato, your pie will be in the oven in less than 15 minutes. (There's no need to defrost the pie mix first – or any of the other frozen ingredients.) Not only that, but it is dairy free and delicious.

275g (10oz) frozen fish pie mix

8 frozen raw king prawns

1 carrot, coarsely grated

1 sweet potato, peeled and coarsely grated

1 handful of frozen peas

1 handful of frozen sweetcorn kernels

1 level tbsp gluten-free plain flour (see page 22)

1 tbsp chopped parsley

2 good-sized portions of leftover mashed potatoes (about 450g/1lb)

Oil (see page 20), for drizzling

Salt and freshly ground black pepper

15cm x 25cm (6in x 10in) gratin dish

1. Preheat the oven to 200°C (180°C fan), gas mark 6.

2. Place the frozen fish pie mix and prawns in a bowl with the vegetables, flour and parsley, season with salt and pepper and mix well together.

3. Transfer to the gratin dish and spread the mashed potatoes on top. (I use my hands or a potato masher to break up cold mash, as it always sets quite solid.)

4. Drizzle the surface with oil and bake in the oven for 30–40 minutes or until the surface of the pie is golden and the fish and prawns are cooked. Serve with a fresh green salad.

Cottage or Shepherd's Pie with Sweet Potato Mash

Serves 2

This dish is ideal to make with leftover meat, but if you also have leftover mashed potato, use it instead of the sweet potatoes or try a combination of both. The recipe makes two good-sized portions, but could easily be stretched to three if served with a salad.

550g (1lb 3oz) sweet potatoes, peeled and cut into chunks

1 tbsp oil (see page 20), plus extra for drizzling

1 medium leek, finely sliced

1 small parsnip or ¼ celeriac, grated

½ tsp dried rosemary

¼ tsp dried thyme

Leftover gravy made up to 370ml (13fl oz) with stock or water

1 tbsp tomato purée

1 level tsp mustard powder

1 level tbsp gluten-free plain flour (see page 22)

1 handful of frozen peas

1 handful of sweetcorn

200–250g (7–9oz) leftover roast beef or lamb, diced

Salt and freshly ground black pepper

15cm x 25cm (6in x 10in) gratin dish

1. Steam or boil the sweet potatoes until just cooked and soft (10–15 minutes).

2. Meanwhile, heat the oil in a pan over a medium/low heat and sweat the leek for about 5 minutes, then add the parsnip or celeriac with the rosemary and thyme and continue to sweat for another 3–4 minutes or until the vegetables start to soften.

3. Whisk the gravy with the tomato purée, mustard powder and flour and add to the pan with the peas, sweetcorn and diced meat. Bring this mixture to the boil, then reduce the heat to low and simmer for 2 minutes or until all the vegetables are cooked. Season to taste with salt and pepper and pour into the gratin dish.

4. Using a potato masher, mash the cooked sweet potatoes until smooth and creamy and season to taste with salt and pepper (you can add a knob of butter, if you like, though it isn't necessary). Pile the sweet potato evenly on top of the vegetables and meat and fluff the surface with a fork. Drizzle with a little oil and then heat under a medium grill for about 10 minutes or until browning on top.

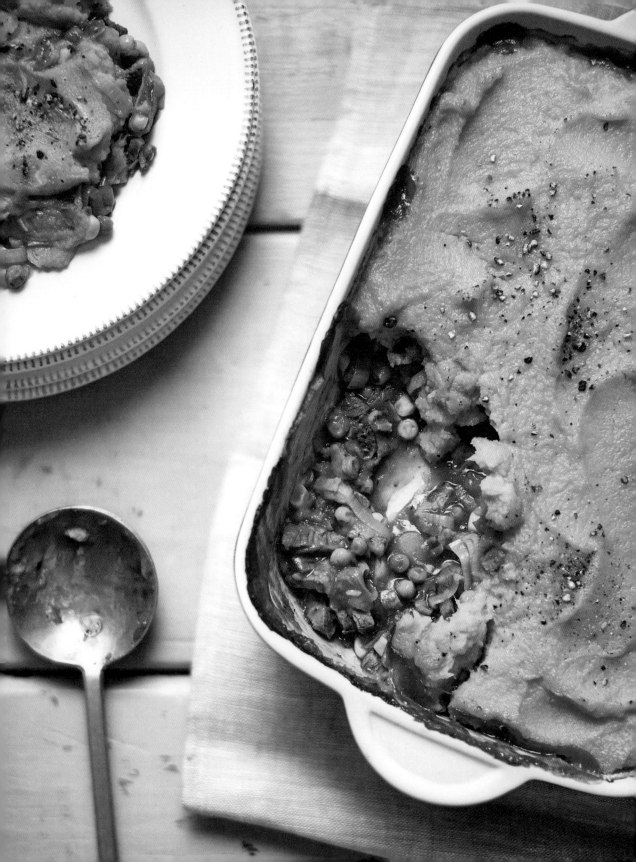

One-pan Meat and Potato Hotpot

Serves 2

This is a dish from my childhood – winter comfort food served on a Monday using the leftover roast and gravy. It was always accompanied by mushy peas – now available from supermarkets frozen and ready to cook, rather than having to be soaked overnight. They take about 30 minutes to cook, so will be ready by the time you have prepared and cooked the hotpot. Leftovers don't get better than this.

2 large handfuls of diced leftover roast beef or lamb

Leftover gravy made up to 425ml (15fl oz) with stock or water

2 large baking-sized potatoes (uncooked), peeled and diced

2 carrots, diced

2 onions, diced

Salt and freshly ground black pepper

1. Place everything in a saucepan and stir to combine.

2. Bring to the boil, then reduce the heat to medium/low and leave to bubble away, covered with a lid, for about 20 minutes or until the vegetables are cooked and the potatoes are just starting to disintegrate. Stir occasionally during cooking.

3. Season to taste with salt and pepper and serve.

Chicken Stock

Makes 1–6 portions

I make chicken stock whenever I have a leftover chicken carcass (turkey stock can be made in the same way). I also buy fresh chicken carcasses from a butcher or farmers' market. Six carcasses makes a very large pan of stock and gives enough meat picked off the bones for 1–2 meals. This stock is the simplest ever.

**Chicken carcass,
or carcasses**

Enough water to cover

1. Put the carcass or carcasses in a large pan and add enough water just to cover. Simmer for about 45 minutes. (When cooking six fresh carcasses, I fit three into a very large pan, then lift these out after 45 minutes and cook the second batch in the same liquid, topping up with more water, if necessary, to cover the carcasses.)

2. Remove the carcasses and drain the stock in a sieve to remove any debris.

3. Once it has cooled, leave the stock overnight in the fridge. This allows any fat to solidify on top of the liquid, making it easy to remove with a spoon. You can then freeze the stock in 1–6 small containers, ready for use when needed.

Creamy Chicken and Mushrooms

Serves 2

This dish can be served in so many ways. Try it with rice, buckwheat or other grains, with pasta or piled into baked potatoes.

1 small onion, finely diced

1 tbsp oil (see page 20)

8 large chestnut or white mushrooms, sliced

1 tsp mustard powder or 1 tbsp grainy mustard (see page 20)

2 level tbsps gluten-free plain flour (see page 22)

Leftover gravy made up to 425ml (15fl oz) with stock or milk

1 bay leaf

2 good handfuls of diced cooked chicken

Salt and freshly ground black pepper

1. Sweat the onion in the oil over a medium heat for about 5 minutes or until it starts to soften.

2. Add the mushrooms and continue to cook until they are beginning to brown.

3. Whisk the mustard powder and flour with the gravy and add to the pan with the bay leaf and chicken. Bring the mixture to the boil, stirring continuously, then reduce the heat and simmer for 2 minutes.

4. Remove the bay leaf and season to taste with salt and pepper.

Chicken or Turkey Chilli

Serves 2

A chilli is a really useful standby kept in the fridge for a few days or frozen for those days when you just don't feel like cooking. This is a great way of using up leftover Christmas turkey.

½ onion, finely diced

1 small carrot, finely diced

1 stick of celery, diced

½ red or yellow pepper, deseeded and finely diced

1 garlic clove, crushed

⅛–¼ tsp chilli powder

1 tsp sweet smoked paprika

½ tsp ground cumin

½ tsp ground coriander

1 x 400g (14oz) tin of chopped tomatoes

1 tbsp tomato purée

55m (2fl oz) leftover gravy or stock

2 good handfuls of chopped cooked chicken or turkey

1 handful of tinned red kidney beans, rinsed and drained

Salt and freshly ground black pepper

1. Place the vegetables in a pan with the garlic, spices, tinned tomatoes, tomato purée and gravy or stock. Bring to the boil, stirring occasionally, then reduce the heat to low, cover loosely with a lid and simmer for 20 minutes.

2. Add the meat and beans and simmer for another 5 minutes, then season to taste with salt and pepper. Serve with rice, buckwheat, millet or quinoa.

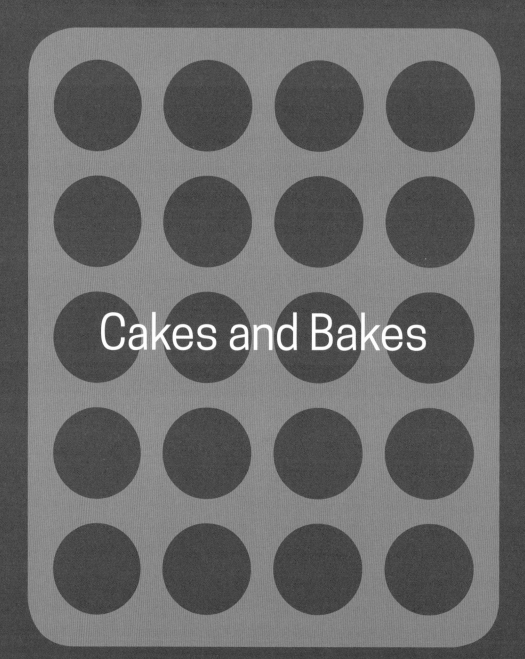

Cakes and Bakes

We all need a treat sometimes – a cake for afternoon tea or something for a special occasion. But why put something filled with sugar, dubious fat and over-processed white flour into your system when you can choose one that's full of natural goodness – dried or fresh fruit, vegetables, nuts, ground almonds, dark chocolate, spices and coconut oil? It's not about becoming obsessive – an occasional cake won't do you any harm – but continually feeding your body poor-quality ingredients will eventually tell on your system. Nowadays bought cakes are enormous, frequently eaten instead of meals and often on a daily basis. Is it any wonder we are getting bigger and sicker? Try to think of cakes as treats, and if you're eating one between meals, make sure that they are full of substantial ingredients (such as the flapjacks – pages 218–220), so that you don't cause a spike in your blood-sugar levels (see pages 8–10).

In this chapter you will find some delicious alternatives to standard cakes and bakes, showing that you can still have comfort foods without ruining your health: Rustic Fruity Scones (see page 225) when friends call unexpectedly – served hot from the oven and spread with butter; muffins (pages 211–212) for picnics and mid-afternoon treats; or a special cake to celebrate a birthday or other occasion (see pages 223–224). All are delicious – and healthy, too. I know that 'good for you' ingredients do cost more than refined sugar and flour, but you will eat less of these treats because they will support your blood sugar and you won't end up with sugar cravings.

The Chocolate Cake (see page 223) is not not what I call an everyday cake as its GI rating (see page 15) is not as low as those containing nuts, ground almonds, fruit or vegetables. However, we all occasionally need a cake for a special occasion, a birthday treat, or friends coming for a meal. The toppings included with the variations are perfect for a celebratory centrepiece if you want to wow your guests.

Careful Measuring

Measuring ingredients carefully is important when making these recipes, so make sure you have good scales, an accurate measuring jug and a set of measuring spoons. Spoon measurements are level unless otherwise stated, though 'level' is often given as a reminder where this is particularly important. An oven thermometer is also useful, as ovens do vary a lot in temperature.

Bicarbonate of Soda

I have used bicarbonate of soda in these recipes, as it helps gluten-free cakes to rise. When it interacts with an acid such as lemon juice or vitamin C powder (see page 23), carbon dioxide is released and the mixture will start to aerate with bubbles. The ingredients therefore need combining at the last minute, when the oven is hot and the baking tins are prepared, because if too much time elapses, the gases will dissipate and the baked goods will not rise. Too much bicarbonate of soda will produce an unpleasant taste, so be sure to measure correctly with a measuring spoon.

Eggs

I have also offered eggs as an option in some recipes, as eggs lower the GI rating (see page 15) of cakes and are not bad for you unless you have an intolerance.

Lining a Cake Tin

This just involves putting baking parchment in the bottom of the tin to prevent the cake from sticking. Using the base of the tin as a template, draw around it on the paper. Cut out the lining, then place it in the base of a greased tin. Alternatively, you can use ready-made cake-tin linings.

Storing and Keeping Cakes

Because these cakes do not contain sugar, they don't keep as well as standard cakes. Unless I make a cake for a special occasion, I tend to freeze it cut into slices and packed into containers interleaved with baking parchment. This serves two purposes: one, the cake is fresh when I fancy a piece; and, two, I'm not temped to keep eating a cake just because it's there.

Date Purée

Makes 6 portions

I love to use date purée instead of sugar or sugar substitutes in cakes and puddings, as the purée is not over-sweet and contains all the natural goodness and fibre from the dates. Indeed, dates have been termed a 'superfood of the ancients' and are bursting with vitamins and minerals. Ready-chopped dates are available in some wholefood shops or you could substitute moist pitted Medjool dates in recipes; they don't need soaking, just processing with a little water (see step 2 below), but they are expensive.

850g (1lb 14oz) pitted dates, finely chopped

725ml (1¼ pints) water

1. Place the dates in a pan with the water and bring to the boil, then remove from the heat, cover with a lid and leave to soak for at least 30 minutes or until the dates are soft. (I often leave dates overnight to soak, especially if they are quite dry.)

2. Drain and then blend the soaked dates until smooth in a food processor. The finished purée should have a soft, dropping consistency – in other words, lift it up on a spoon and it should easily fall off. Add a little more water if needed.

3. Divide the purée evenly between six airtight containers – weigh each portion in order to be exact – and store in the freezer, taking out a portion when you decide to bake (it defrosts quite quickly). The purée can be cut in half even when frozen where recipes call for '½ portion' or '1½ portions', as it doesn't freeze solid, or you could freeze some half portions. The purée will also keep in the fridge for a couple of weeks.

Carrot and Sultana Muffins

Makes 12 muffins

These are delicious just as they are, but for special occasions add the topping and decorate with dried cranberries and pumpkin seeds.

215g (7½oz) pitted dates, chopped, and 170ml (6fl oz) water (or 1½ portions of Date Purée – see opposite)

310g (11oz) gluten-free plain flour (see page 22)

1 tsp bicarbonate of soda

1 level tsp gluten-free baking powder

2 level tsps mixed spice

8 parings of lemon rind, finely diced

2 tbsps lemon juice

200ml (7fl oz) rice bran oil

200–250ml (7–9fl oz) dairy-free milk or water

110g (4oz) sultanas

110g (4oz) grated carrot

For the topping (optional)

50g (2oz) dried pears or 75g (3oz) dried apricots, finely diced

55ml (2fl oz) boiling water

110g (4oz) ground almonds or ground cashews

40g (1½oz) coconut oil

½ tsp ground cinnamon

2 tbsps lemon juice

12-hole muffin tin

1. Place the chopped dates in a pan with the water and bring to the boil. Remove from the heat, cover with a lid and leave to soak for about 30 minutes or until the dates are soft.

2. If making the topping, soak the pears or apricots in another container with their water and leave until needed.

3. Preheat the oven to 190°C (170°C fan), gas mark 5. Prepare the muffin tin by either greasing (using a little extra oil) and lining the bases with circles of baking parchment or by inserting muffin cases.

4. Sift together the flour, bicarbonate of soda and baking powder, then add the mixed spice and lemon rind.

5. Blend the date mixture in a food processor, then add the lemon juice, oil and 200ml (7fl oz) of milk or water and process to mix.

6. Add the flour mixture to the date mixture and process again, adding more liquid if needed, to make a very soft, dropping consistency (almost like a thick batter).

7. Using a plastic processor blade, mix in the sultanas and grated carrot (or mix together by hand in the pan used to soak the dates) and divide the mixture between the muffin moulds or paper cases (they will be quite full).

8. Bake in the oven for about 20 minutes or until the mixture is risen and springy to touch.

9. Leave the muffins to cool in the tin for 10 minutes before transferring them to a wire rack to cool down completely.

10. While the muffins are cooling, finish making the topping. Place the pears or apricots and any remaining soaking liquid in the food processor with the remaining ingredients and blend until smooth and creamy. Spread the topping on the cooled muffins. If you like you can sprinkle the surface of each with a few dried cranberries and pumpkin seeds.

Blueberry Bakewell Muffins

Makes 12 muffins

These moist, almondy muffins work well with blackcurrants or halved raspberries instead of blueberries. You can also use freeze-dried fruit instead of the fresh fruit, but you will need less as the flavour is intense; 25g (1oz) is sufficient. Don't put any on top, though, as they burn easily. The mixture makes 12 large muffins, but would easily stretch to 15 if you make them slightly smaller.

215g (7½oz) pitted dates, finely chopped, and 170ml (6fl oz) water (or 1½ portions of Date Purée – see page 210)

200g (7oz) gluten-free plain flour (see page 22)

½ level tsp bicarbonate of soda

1½ level tsps gluten-free baking powder

75g (3oz) ground almonds

75g (3oz) polenta (medium maize meal)

200ml (7fl oz) rice bran oil

1 tbsp lemon juice or ¼ tsp vitamin C powder (see page 23)

1½tsps almond extract

225–275ml (8–10fl oz) dairy-free milk or water

75g (3oz) blueberries, plus extra to decorate

12-hole muffin tin

1. Place the chopped dates in a pan with the water and bring to the boil. Remove from the heat, cover with a lid and leave to soak for about 30 minutes or until the dates are soft.

2. Preheat the oven to 190°C (170°C fan), gas mark 5. Prepare the muffin tin by either greasing (using a little extra oil) and lining the bases with circles of baking parchment or by inserting muffin cases.

3. Sift together the flour, bicarbonate of soda and baking powder, then mix with the ground almonds and polenta.

4. Blend the date mixture in a food processor, then add the oil, lemon juice or vitamin C powder, almond extract and 225ml (8fl oz) of milk or water and process to mix.

5. Add the flour mixture to the date mixture and process quickly to combine, adding more liquid if needed, to make a very soft, dropping consistency (almost like a thick batter).

6. Roughly stir in the blueberries, then divide the mixture between the muffin moulds or paper cases (they will be quite full) and press 3–4 of the extra blueberries into the surface of each muffin.

7. Bake in the oven for about 20 minutes or until the mixture is risen and springy to touch.

8. Leave the muffins to cool in the tin for 10 minutes before transferring them to a wire rack.

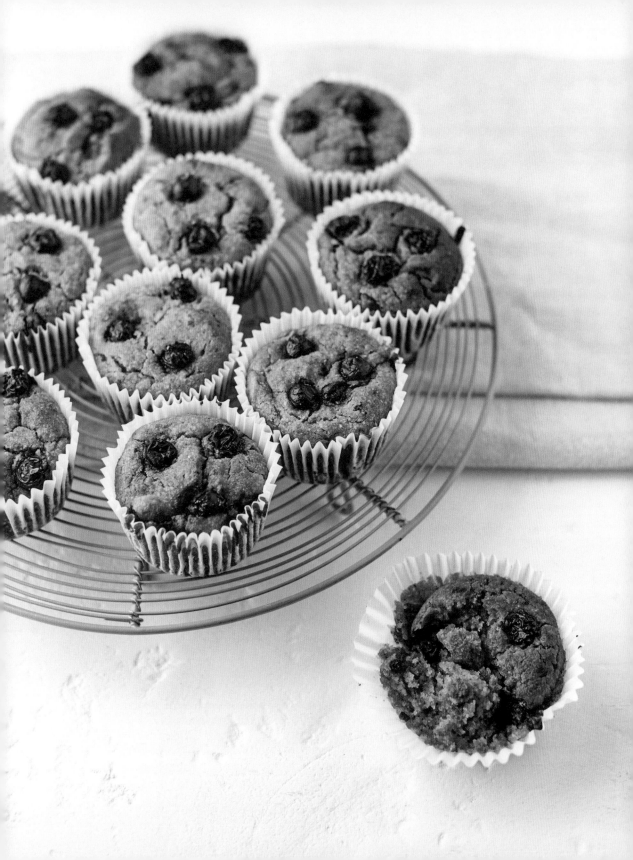

Rich Fruitcake with Marzipan Topping

Serves 8–10

This fruit cake, with its marzipan topping, is ideal to make for celebrations such as Easter and Christmas, though I love it so much I make it throughout the year. If you can't tolerate nuts use extra flour instead of the ground almonds and miss out the marzipan.

350g (12oz) mixed dried fruit

110ml (4fl oz) water

2 tbsps lemon juice

Grated rind of 1 lemon

1 tbsp blackstrap molasses

200g (7oz) gluten-free plain flour (see page 22)

½ level tsp bicarbonate of soda

1 level tsp gluten-free baking powder

1 tsp ground cinnamon

60g (2½oz) ground almonds

2 level tbsps ground flaxseed in 75ml (3fl oz) boiling water (or 2 eggs)

150ml (5fl oz) rice bran oil

1 tbsp grated fresh root ginger

75g (3oz) finely grated carrot

30–55ml (1–2fl oz) milk or water (if needed)

1 quantity of Marzipan (see opposite) (optional)

20cm (8in) deep-sided round cake tin

1. Place the dried fruit (cut into small pieces in the case of apricots or prunes) in a large saucepan with the water, lemon juice, lemon rind and molasses. Bring to the boil, then remove from the heat, cover with a lid and leave the fruit for about 20 minutes to soak up the liquid.

2. Preheat the oven to 170°C (150°C fan), gas mark 3½, and grease (using a little extra oil) and line (see page 209) the base of the cake tin.

3. Sift together the flour, bicarbonate of soda, baking powder and cinnamon, then mix with the ground almonds.

4. Whisk the flaxseed mixture until it doubles in size (or beat the eggs, if using).

5. Mix the oil, ginger, grated carrot, flaxseed mixture (or beaten eggs) with the soaked fruit in the pan. Tip in the flour mixture and stir gently but quickly to combine, adding the milk or additional water, if needed, to make a very soft dropping consistency.

6. Quickly spoon the mixture into the prepared tin, level the surface and place the cake on the middle shelf of the oven to bake for 40 minutes, then lower the temperature to 145°C (125°C fan), gas mark 1½, and cook for a further 30–45 minutes or until the centre of the cake is set and slightly springy to touch. (A skewer inserted into the middle should come out dry.)

7. Allow the cake to cool in the tin for 10 minutes, then turn it out onto a wire rack and remove the lining paper. Top with marzipan (if using), ideally while the cake is still warm, and leave to cool down fully, then store in an airtight container and eat within 3–4 days or freeze.

Marzipan

Makes enough to cover a 20cm (8in) round cake

If you're making the marzipan at the same time as the fruitcake, and not using ready-prepared date purée, then it's a good idea to put the dates on to soak at the same time as you soak the dried fruit for the cake (see step 1 opposite).

60g (2½oz) pitted dates, finely chopped, and 55ml (2fl oz) water (or ½ portion of Date Purée – see page 210)

½ tsp almond extract

110g (4oz) ground almonds, plus extra for dusting

Mild-tasting runny honey, for brushing (if needed)

1. Place the dates in a pan with the water and bring to the boil, then remove from the heat, cover with a lid and leave to soak for about 30 minutes or until the dates are soft. Cool the dates if necessary by placing the pan in a bowl or tin of cold water.

2. Once cooled, blend the date mixture in a food processor, then add the almond extract and ground almonds and process again until combined.

3. Roll out the marzipan into a circle to fit the top of your cake, dusting your work surface and rolling pin with extra ground almonds to prevent the mixture from sticking.

4. Place the marzipan circle on the cake while the cake is still warm. If the cake is cool, brush it with a little honey to help the marzipan to stick. Trim the marzipan to fit the cake and roll any leftovers into balls to make decorations for the top.

Apricot, Apple and Walnut Cake

Serves 8–10

This moist cake is packed with nutrient-rich superfoods to heal and repair and supply you with energy. Not only that, it's delicious, too.

110g (4oz) dried apricots, cut into small pieces

110g (4oz) sultanas

75ml (3fl oz) water

2 tbsps lemon juice or ½ tsp vitamin C powder (see page 23)

200g (7oz) gluten-free plain flour (see page 22)

1 level tsp gluten-free baking powder

½ level tsp bicarbonate of soda

1½ level tsps cinnamon

50g (2oz) ground almonds

50g (2oz) walnut pieces

2 level tbsps ground flaxseed soaked in 75ml (3fl oz) boiling water (or use 2 eggs)

150ml (5fl oz) rice bran oil

1 tsp almond extract

110g (4oz) finely diced apple (chopped by hand)

30–75ml (1–3fl oz) milk or water (if needed)

20cm (8in) deep-sided round cake tin

1. Place the dried fruit in a large saucepan with the water and lemon juice or vitamin C powder. Bring to the boil, then remove from the heat, cover with a lid and leave the fruit for about 20 minutes to soak up the liquid.

2. Preheat the oven to 170°C (150°C fan), gas mark 3½, and grease (using a little extra oil) and line (see page 209) the base of the cake tin.

3. Sift together the flour, baking powder, bicarbonate of soda and cinnamon, then add the ground almonds and walnuts.

4. Whisk the flaxseed mixture until it doubles in size (or beat the eggs, if using).

5. Mix the oil, almond extract, diced apple, flaxseed mixture (or beaten eggs) with the soaked fruit in the pan. Tip in the flour mixture and stir quickly to combine, adding the milk or additional water, if needed, to make a very soft, dropping consistency.

6. Quickly spoon the mixture into the prepared tin and level the surface.

7. Place the cake on the middle shelf of the oven to bake for 45 minutes, then lower the temperature to 145°C (125°C fan), gas mark 1½, and cook for a further 30–45 minutes or until the centre of the cake is set and slightly springy to touch. (A skewer inserted into the middle should come out dry.)

8. Allow the cake to cool in the tin for 10 minutes, then turn it out onto a wire rack and remove the lining paper. Once cooled, store in an airtight container and eat within 4–5 days or freeze.

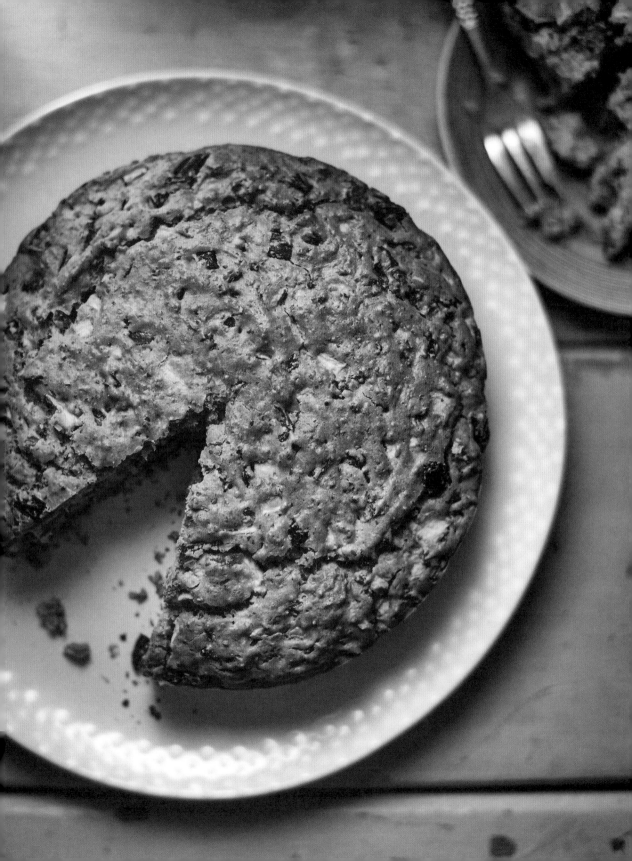

Cranberry and Coconut Flapjacks

Makes 12–16 bars

These bars, and the following two flapjack recipes, are great for healthy snacks and are so filling and nutritious that they could be used as a substitute for breakfast if you or if the kids are in a rush. I promise you won't miss the sugar, as the natural sweetness of the fruit is all that's needed. Wrap them individually and keep them in the fridge or freezer so that they are always on hand. The bars don't need to be cooked immediately, so you could prepare a batch ahead of time and then pop them in the oven when it is on.

150g (5oz) pitted dates, finely chopped, and 110ml (4fl oz) water (or 1 portion of Date Purée – see page 210)

110g (4oz) coconut oil or butter

1 tsp vanilla extract

1 eating apple, cored and grated

50g (2oz) dried cranberries

50g (2oz) raisins

50g (2oz) sunflower seeds

75g (3oz) chopped almonds

50g (2oz) desiccated coconut

200g (7oz) gluten-free oats or 225g (8oz) buckwheat flakes

20cm x 33cm (8in x 13in) brownie tin or baking tray (no need to grease)

1. Preheat the oven to 150°C (130°C fan), gas mark 2.

2. Place the chopped dates in a pan with the water and bring to the boil. Remove from the heat, add the coconut oil or butter, cover with a lid and leave to soak for about 30 minutes or until the dates are soft.

3. Once softened, blend the date mixture in a food processor or mash by hand – it doesn't need to be perfectly smooth. Add the remaining ingredients and mix well with a wooden spoon.

4. Tip the mixture out into the brownie tin or baking tray. Use the back of a spoon to spread and flatten the mixture, pressing it down firmly.

5. Bake on the middle shelf of the oven for 35–40 minutes or until golden brown.

6. Using a sharp knife, cut into 12–16 bars while warm, then leave to cool in the tin. Store in an airtight container and eat within 5 days or freeze.

Spiced Prune and Molasses Flapjacks

Makes 12–16 bars

Molasses impart a rich, treacly taste to these spiced flapjacks to make a really delicious snack.

150g (5oz) pitted prunes, finely diced

1 tbsp blackstrap molasses

110ml (4fl oz) water

110g (4oz) coconut oil or butter

75g (3oz) sunflower seeds

75g (3oz) Brazil nuts, roughly chopped

75g (3oz) sultanas

2 level tsps mixed spice

250g (9oz) gluten-free oats or 275g (10oz) buckwheat flakes

20cm x 33cm (8in x 13in) brownie tin or baking tray (no need to grease)

1. Preheat the oven to 150°C (130°C fan), gas mark 2.

2. Place the chopped prunes and molasses in a large saucepan with the water, bring to the boil and then remove from the heat. Add the coconut oil or butter, cover the pan with a lid and leave the prune mixture to soak for about 30 minutes or until the prunes are soft.

3. Once softened, blend the prune mixture in a food processor or mash by hand before adding the remaining ingredients and mixing well with a wooden spoon.

4. Tip the mixture out into the brownie tin or baking tray. Use the back of a spoon to spread and flatten the mixture, pressing it down firmly.

5. Bake on the middle shelf of the oven for 35–40 minutes or until golden brown.

6. Using a sharp knife, cut into 12–16 bars while warm, then leave to cool in the tin. Store in an airtight container and eat within 5 days or freeze.

Cherry and Chocolate Flapjacks

Makes 12–16 bars

Chop up pieces of 70–90% dark chocolate (if using) for this recipe, or use chocolate chips if you can get hold of them. Chocolate does contain some sugar, but I accept this small amount as it makes heavenly flapjacks.

150g (5oz) pitted dates, finely chopped, and 110ml (4fl oz) water (or 1 portion of Date Purée – see page 210)

1 level tbsp blackstrap molasses

110g (4oz) coconut oil or butter

2 level tbsps cocoa, cacao or carob powder

50g (2oz) ground almonds

75g (3oz) chopped almonds

50g (2oz) sunflower seeds

75g (3oz) dried cherries, halved if large

50g (2oz) 70–90% dark chocolate chips (optional)

250g (9oz) gluten-free oats or 275g (10oz) buckwheat flakes

20cm x 33cm (8in x 13in) brownie tin or baking tray (no need to grease)

1. Preheat the oven to 150°C (130°C fan), gas mark 2.

2. Place the dates in a large pan with the water, bring to the boil and then remove from the heat. Add the molasses and coconut oil or butter, cover the pan with a lid and leave the mixture to soak for about 30 minutes or until the dates are soft.

3. Once softened, blend the date mixture in a food processor or mash by hand before adding the remaining ingredients and mixing well with a wooden spoon.

4. Tip the mixture out into the brownie tin or baking tray. Use the back of a spoon to spread and flatten the mixture, pressing it down firmly.

5. Bake on the middle shelf of the oven for 35–40 minutes or until golden brown.

6. Using a sharp knife, cut into 12–16 bars while warm, then leave to cool in the tin. Store in an airtight container and eat within 5 days or freeze.

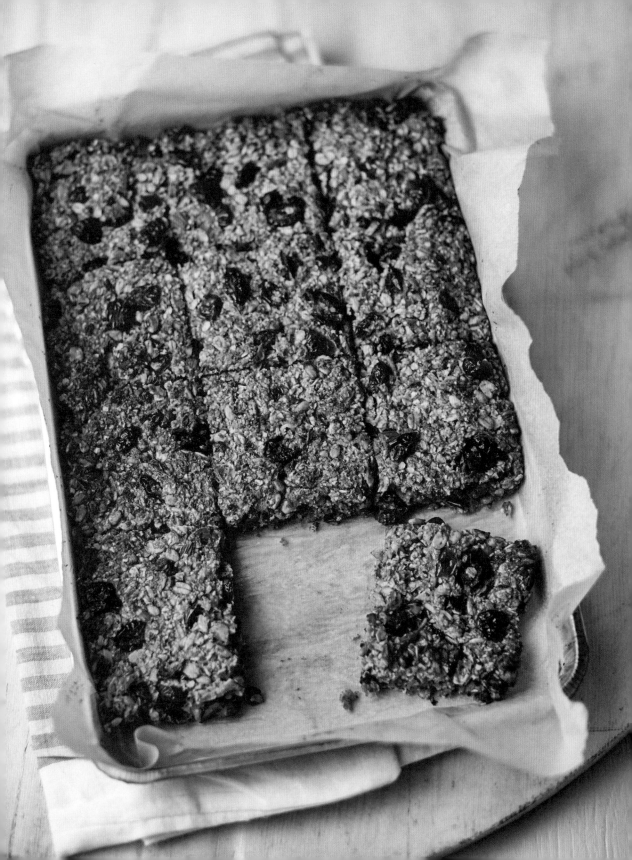

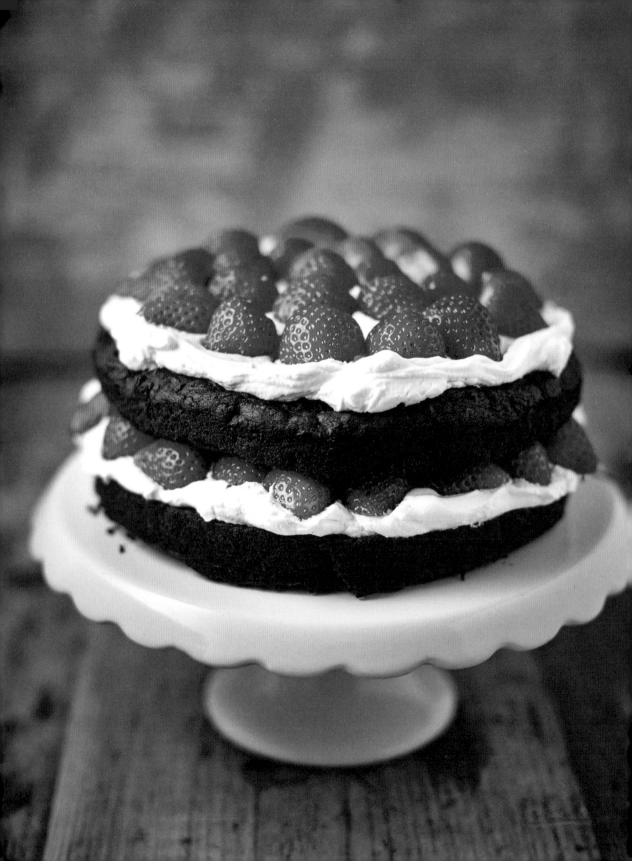

Chocolate Cake

Serves 6-8

Everyone loves a chocolate cake and this one won't disappoint. The recipe makes two sandwich cakes – ideal for assembling into a gateau (see the variations overleaf) – but can also be adapted to make one tray bake or 15 buns or muffins (see the cupcake variation overleaf). Don't try to make one thick cake, though, as the mixture won't rise so much and your cake may end up slightly soggy. The sponges freeze well, so why not save one for another day?

215g (7½oz) pitted dates, finely chopped, and 170ml (6fl oz) water (or 1½ portions of Date Purée – see page 210)

2 tsps blackstrap molasses

250g (9oz) gluten-free plain flour (see page 22)

50g (2oz) cacao, cocoa or carob powder

1 tsp bicarbonate of soda

1 tsp gluten-free baking powder

2 tsps vanilla extract

200ml (7fl oz) rice bran oil

1 tbsp lemon juice or ¼ tsp vitamin C powder (see page 23)

200-250ml (7-9fl oz) dairy-free milk or water

2 x 23cm (9in) round sandwich tins

1. Place the chopped dates in a saucepan with the water and molasses and bring to the boil. Remove from the heat, cover with a lid and leave to soak for about 30 minutes or until the dates are soft.

2. Preheat the oven to 190°C (170°C fan), gas mark 5, then grease (using a little extra oil) and line the sandwich tins with baking parchment (see page 209).

3. Sift together the flour, cacao, cocoa or carob powder, bicarbonate of soda and baking powder.

4. Blend the date mixture in a food processor, then add the vanilla extract, oil, lemon juice or vitamin C powder, and 200ml (7fl oz) of the milk or water, and mix well.

5. Add the flour mixture to the date mixture and blend quickly to combine, adding more liquid if needed, to make a very soft, dropping consistency (almost like thick batter).

6. Spoon the mixture into the prepared tins, levelling the surface, and place on the middle shelf of the oven to bake for 20-25 minutes or until the mixture is risen and springy to the touch.

7. Leave the cakes to cool in the tins for 10 minutes, then turn out onto a wire rack and remove the lining paper. Serve the cake just as it is, preferably while slightly warm, with a dollop of Whipped Coconut Cream or Cashew Cream (see page 236) and some fresh raspberries or blueberries.

Continued overleaf...

Chocolate Cake (continued)

Variations

Chocolate and Raspberry or Strawberry Gateau: Soak 1½ sheets of gelatine (see page 23) in water, squeeze dry and dissolve in 2 tablespoons of water. Add to a double quantity of Whipped Coconut Cream (see page 236) and leave to cool in the fridge until thickened and set. Spread nearly half of the cooled cream over the flat base of one of the chocolate sponges and scatter over 2 handfuls of fresh strawberries (cut if large) or raspberries. I like to top the fruit with a few more spoonfuls of cream before sandwiching together with the second sponge. The extra cream helps the second sponge to stick. Spread the remaining cream on the top of the cake, then decorate with more fruit. Keep chilled in the fridge until needed if the weather is warm.

Chocolate Ganache Gateau: Make up a double quantity of the Rich Chocolate Pot mixture on page 242 and use to sandwich the two cakes together as well as to cover the top. Decorate with some 70–90% dark chocolate, flaked, or buttons. Keep in the fridge until needed if the weather is warm.

Chocolate and Salted Caramel Cake: Make up a quadruple quantity of the salted caramel mixture on page 275 and use to sandwich the two cakes together. Top the cake with 75g (3oz) melted 70–90% dark chocolate and decorate with chopped toasted hazelnuts. Or you could use the chocolate fudge from the chocolate cupcakes recipe (see below) as an alternative topping.

Black Forest Tray Bake: Use the sponge mixture to make a tray bake in a greased and lined 20cm x 33cm (8in x 13in) brownie tin or baking tray. Cook at the same temperature for the same length of time as the sandwich cakes. When cool, drizzle with 50g (2oz) melted 70–90% dark chocolate, then sprinkle over dried cherries or cranberries, freeze-dried raspberries or strawberries, flaked chocolate, toasted almonds or chopped walnuts, or a mixture of these, while the chocolate is still soft. Allow to cool and cut into squares.

Chocolate Cupcakes: Line two 12-hole muffin tins with 15 paper cases. Divide the mixture between the cases and bake in the oven at 190°C (170°C fan), gas mark 5, for 15–20 minutes. Make chocolate fudge by melting 100g (3½oz) 70–90% dark chocolate and adding 3 tablespoons of smooth or crunchy nut butter (preferably almond or hazelnut). Spread over the cupcakes once they are cool and decorate with toasted almonds, fresh or freeze-dried berries or grated chocolate, or a mixture of these.

Rustic Fruity Scones

Makes 6 scones

These rustic, crumbly scones are meant to be eaten while still slightly warm, spread with butter. As they don't keep well, it's a good idea to assemble the dry ingredients and store in bags in the fridge or freezer so that, when you want to make some, all you have to do is add the liquid and put a batch in the oven – ideal when the children arrive home from school starving or friends pop round unexpectedly.

200g (7oz) gluten-free plain flour (see page 22)

½ level tsp bicarbonate of soda

1 level tsp gluten-free baking powder

2 level tsps mixed spice

¼ tsp salt

50g (2oz) coconut oil or butter

50g (2oz) gluten-free oats or buckwheat flakes

110g (4oz) mixed dried fruit (sultanas, currants, cranberries, candied peel)

140–200ml (5–7fl oz) dairy-free milk or water

1 tbsp lemon juice or ¼ tsp vitamin C powder (see page 23)

1 tbsp mild-tasting runny honey (optional)

1. Preheat the oven to 200°C (180°C fan), gas mark 6, and line a large tray with baking parchment.

2. Sift the flour, bicarbonate of soda, baking powder, spice and salt into a bowl or pan and rub the butter or oil into the flour using your finger tips. (You can use a food processor if you prefer.) Stir in the oats or buckwheat flakes and dried fruit.

3. Whisk 140ml (5fl oz) of the milk or water with the lemon juice or vitamin C powder and honey (if using) and pour over the dry ingredients. Stir quickly to combine, adding a little more liquid if needed, until you have very soft dough (almost a thick batter that will just hold its shape).

4. Place six heaped mounds of dough onto the prepared baking tray.

5. Bake in the middle of the oven for 12–15 minutes or until crusty and brown. Cool for 5 minutes on the baking tray before transferring to a wire rack

Brilliant Bread

I'm so pleased with my recipe for Bread with Yogurt and Chia Seeds. It makes delicious gluten-free bread that is suitable for slicing and hence sandwiches, as it doesn't fall apart and has a good springy texture. I have also offered a few alternative recipes, so hopefully you will find one to suit your needs. The mixture needs to be very soft – almost the consistency of thick batter – which means if you want to make rolls you will need to find a container to cook them in. I sometimes use a Yorkshire pudding tin, but I also have some individual tarte Tatin tins that work well, or you could make Sandwich Rounds (see page 231). It really is necessary to line the tins for this recipe or the mixture will stick; baking parchment works better than greaseproof paper here.

I have tried to be accurate with the amount of liquid you need in order that you can quickly mix the two sets of ingredients. However, you may need to adjust this amount if your scales and measures are slightly different from mine or if you are using a ready-prepared flour mix. The runnier the mixture, the more doughy your bread will be; the drier it is, the more crumbly the bread.

Bread with Yogurt and Chia Seeds

Makes 1 loaf

This recipe produces a loaf that's really tasty as well as quick and easy to make. I use a medium-thick sheep's yogurt, but you could use soya, coconut, goat's or cow's milk yogurt. It's the acid in the yogurt that helps the mixture to rise so make sure you use a live yogurt. If you can't get hold of live yogurt, add a teaspoon of lemon juice or a pinch of vitamin C powder. If your yogurt is very thick (such as coconut), water it down a little first.

For the wet ingredients

170ml (6oz) natural live yogurt

140–200ml (5–7fl oz) boiling water

1 tsp blackstrap molasses

2 tbsps olive or rice bran oil

1 tbsp chia seeds

For the dry ingredients

225g (8oz) gluten-free plain flour (see page 22)

1 level tsp mustard powder

1 level tsp gluten-free baking powder

½ level tsp bicarbonate of soda

1 scant level tsp salt

50g (2oz) gluten-free oats or buckwheat flakes

2 tbsps chia seeds, plus extra for sprinkling

450g (1lb) loaf tin

1. Preheat the oven to 200°C (180°C fan), gas mark 6, then grease the loaf tin (using a little extra oil) and line with baking parchment.

2. Whisk all the wet ingredients together, using 140ml (5fl oz) of the boiling water, and give an occasional whisk while you prepare the dry ingredients to prevent the chia seeds from clumping together.

3. Sift together the flour, mustard powder, baking powder and bicarbonate of soda. Mix in the salt, oats or buckwheat flakes, and chia seeds.

4. Combine the two sets of ingredients, adding a little more boiling water if needed, to make a very soft, dropping consistency (almost like a thick batter). You will see bubbles of gas appear as soon as you start to mix, so work quickly before they dissipate, and spoon the mixture into the prepared tin.

5. Sprinkle the bread with more seeds and bake for 35–40 minutes. The loaf should be lightly browned and crispy on the surface, but don't remove it from the oven too soon or the bread may be slightly soggy inside. Tip out onto a wire rack to cool and remove any lining paper.

Savoury Seeded Bread

Makes 1 loaf

If you make bread regularly, keep batches of ready-weighed dry ingredients in the fridge so that you can throw a loaf together at a moment's notice. You can also freeze the bread ready sliced – ideal for toast or emergency situations.

For the wet ingredients

25g (1oz) finely ground linseed

1 tsp blackstrap molasses

2 tbsps olive or rice bran oil

1 tbsp lemon juice or ¼ tsp vitamin C powder (see page 23)

140ml (5fl oz) boiling water

110–170ml (4–6fl oz) cold water

For the dry ingredients

225g (8oz) gluten-free plain flour (see page 22)

1 level tsp mustard powder

1 level tsp gluten-free baking powder

½ level tsp bicarbonate of soda

1 scant level tsp salt

50g (2oz) gluten-free oats or buckwheat flakes

3 tbsps mixed seeds (pumpkin, sunflower, sesame, hemp), plus extra for sprinkling

450g (1lb) loaf tin

1. Preheat the oven to 200°C (180°C fan), gas mark 6, then grease the loaf tin (using a little extra oil) and line with baking parchment.

2. Add the ground linseed to a bowl with the molasses, oil and lemon juice or vitamin C powder. Pour in the boiling water and whisk the ingredients together, then leave the linseeds to soak while you prepare the remaining ingredients.

3. Sift together the flour, mustard powder, baking powder and bicarbonate of soda. Mix in the salt, oats or buckwheat flakes and seeds.

4. Mix 110ml (4fl oz) of the cold water into the soaked linseed mixture and then combine the two sets of ingredients, adding more water if needed, to make a very soft, dropping consistency (almost like a thick batter). You will see bubbles of gas appear as soon as you start to mix, so work quickly before they dissipate, and spoon the mixture into the prepared tin.

5. Sprinkle the bread with more seeds and bake for 35–40 minutes. The loaf should be lightly browned and crispy on the surface, but don't remove it from the oven too soon or the bread may be slightly soggy inside. Tip out onto a wire rack to cool and remove any lining paper.

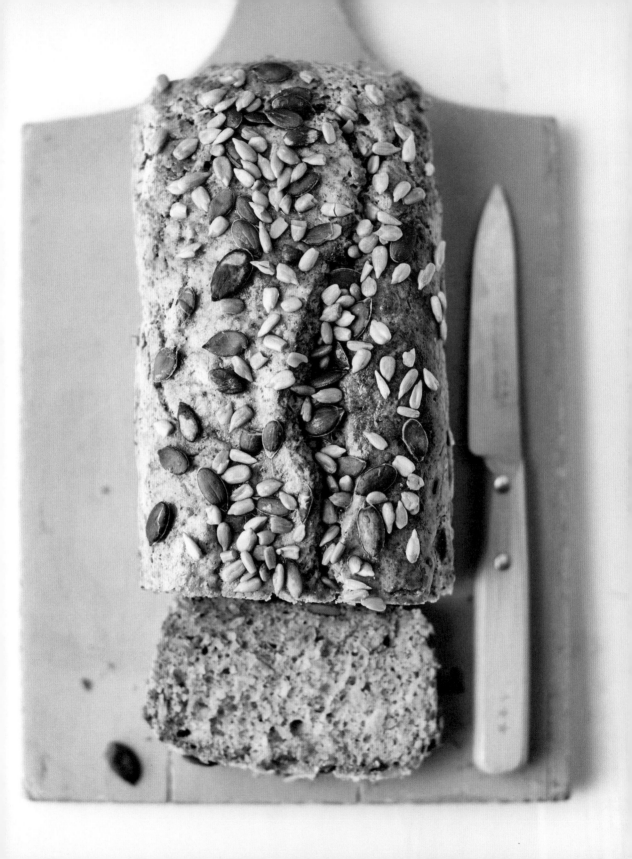

Bread with Yeast

Makes 1 loaf

For those who can tolerate yeast, this makes a really light and delicious loaf.

For the wet ingredients

7g (¼oz) packet of easy-bake yeast

1 tsp blackstrap molasses

225–250ml (8–9fl oz) warm (not hot) water

2 tbsp olive or rice bran oil

For the dry ingredients

225g (8oz) gluten-free plain flour (see page 22)

1 level tsp mustard powder

1 scant level tsp salt

50g (2oz) gluten-free oats or buckwheat flakes

1 tbsp ground linseeds

450g (1lb) loaf tin

1. Preheat the oven to 200°C (180°C fan), gas mark 6, then grease the loaf tin (using a little extra oil) and line with baking parchment.

2. Mix the yeast, blackstrap molasses and 225ml (8fl oz) of the warm water in a bowl and set aside in a warm place while you prepare the dry ingredients.

3. Sift together the flour and mustard powder and mix in the salt and oats or buckwheat flakes and linseeds.

4. When the yeast mixture starts to ferment and bubble, add the oil to the yeast mixture and then combine the two sets of ingredients, adding more warm water if needed, until you have a very soft dropping consistency (almost like a thick batter).

5. Spoon the mixture into the prepared tin, cover with cling film and leave in a warm place for about 30–45 minutes or until the loaf has increased in size by half.

6. Bake for 35–40 minutes. The loaf should be lightly browned and crispy on the surface, but don't remove it from the oven too soon or the bread may be slightly soggy inside. Tip out onto a wire rack to cool and remove any lining paper.

Brilliant Bread Variations

Use the previous bread recipes to create the following variations.

Tear and Share Flat Bread with Toppings

1. Grease and line a 20cm x 33cm (8in x 13in) brownie tin and prepare your toppings (see below) before making your chosen bread mixture.

2. Place the bread mixture in the prepared tin and press 2 good handfuls of toppings into the surface before baking the bread in the oven at 200°C (180°C fan), gas mark 6, for about 20 minutes or until risen and spongy. If you are making the yeasted bread, you will need to cover it with cling film and allow it to rise until it has increased in size by half before baking.

3. Serve while still warm, torn into pieces.

Topping ideas: Quartered olives, finely diced sun-dried tomatoes, thinly sliced red onion, blobs of dairy-free pesto (see page 90), fresh or dried rosemary and thyme.

Sandwich Rounds

These flat rounds are so simple to prepare and two of them make the perfect sandwich. Spoon the bread mix (not the yeasted) into 6–8 rounds on one or two baking sheets covered with baking parchment. Use the back of your spoon to flatten the rounds to about 1cm (½in) thick and 10cm (4in) in diameter. Sprinkle with seeds of your choice, if you like, and bake in the oven at 200°C (180°C fan), gas mark 6, for 10–14 minutes.

Artisan Crispbreads

Makes about 12 crispbreads

Finding tasty and healthy gluten-free crackers isn't easy and they are expensive. These rustic crispbreads not only look and taste good, but they are so easy to make and very moreish. They are really good to eat with dips and pâtés (see pages 76–83) or with soup.

40g (1½oz) finely ground linseed

150ml (5fl oz) boiling water

150g (5oz) gluten-free plain flour (see page 22)

½ level tsp gluten-free baking powder

1 level tsp sweet smoked paprika

2 level tsps fennel seeds

¼ tsp salt and ¼ tsp freshly ground black pepper

30ml (1fl oz) rice bran or olive oil

Sesame seeds and extra flour, for dusting

1. Preheat the oven to 200°C (180°C fan), gas mark 6.

2. Whisk the ground linseed in the boiling water and leave to soak while you prepare the remaining ingredients.

3. Sift together the flour, baking powder and paprika, then mix in the fennel seeds, salt and pepper.

4. Add the oil to the soaked linseed, then mix with the flour to form a soft dough, adding a little cold water if needed.

5. Dust a board or work surface with a mixture of flour and sesame seeds. Using your hands, roll large tablespoons of dough into balls (about 12) before rolling them out into long, thin ovals using a rolling pin. Make these as thin as the sesame seeds will allow, but don't be fussy about the shape – they are meant to look rustic.

6. Place the ovals on two large baking trays (no need to grease) and bake in the oven for 5 minutes before turning over and cooking for another 5 minutes or until crisp and golden.

7. Cool on a wire rack. Store in an airtight container once cool and eat within 5–6 days.

Variations

Vary the flavouring by replacing the smoked paprika and fennel seeds with one of the following combinations:

Cardamom and Chilli: Replace with the crushed seeds of 12 cardamom pods and ¼–½ teaspoon chilli powder.

Basil and Oregano: Replace with ½ teaspoon basil and 1 teaspoon oregano.

Cumin, Coriander and Garam Masala: Replace with 1 teaspoon of cumin seeds and ½ tsp each of ground coriander and garam masala.

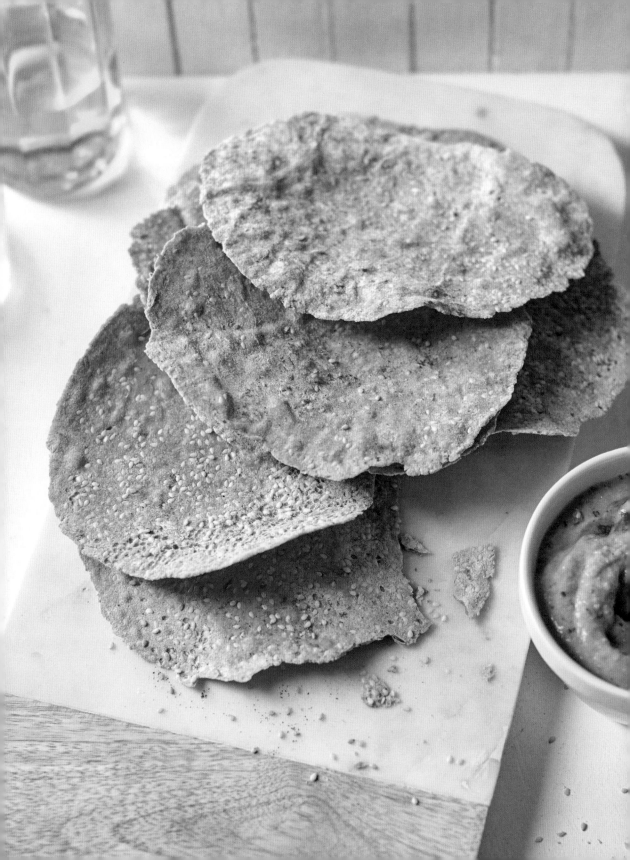

Delicious Desserts

Puddings play an important part in our social interactions, and life would be much duller and less fun if we couldn't tuck into something delicious and sweet to round off a meal when family and friends come to visit. However, delicious and sweet doesn't have to mean bad for your health or your waistline. The desserts in this section, though appealing and scrummy, all contain 'good for you' ingredients so you can indulge without feeling guilty. They are not laden with sugar or sugar substitutes and of course are dairy and gluten free. I'm really proud of my delicious cheesecakes, love my new range of ice creams and feel positively decadent eating chocolate pots and frangipane pie. There are also fruit salads made using unusual combinations of flavours, which are really good to keep in the fridge to have for breakfast, or as a snack between meals, as well as for dessert.

Toppings for Desserts

I've suggested a couple of delicious toppings to serve with cakes and desserts (see page 236), or you could use one of the ice creams in this chapter instead (see pages 254–256).

Whipped Coconut Cream

Serves 4–6

This is a delicious alternative to dairy cream and so easy to make, though you do need to refrigerate the tins of coconut milk (do not shake them) overnight. I always try to keep a couple of tins at the back of the fridge so they are ready to use. You'll need full-fat, not low-fat, coconut milk.

1 x 400ml (14fl oz) tin of full-fat coconut milk (chilled overnight in the fridge)

1 tsp mild-tasting runny honey or ¼ tsp stevia (optional)

1 tsp vanilla extract

1. Open the tins at the bottom so that you can pour off the liquid (keep this for using in smoothies or soups). Place the remaining coconut cream in a bowl and whisk for 2–3 minutes or until fluffy and creamy.

2. Add the honey or stevia (if using) and the vanilla extract and whisk again for another minute or until thick. You may need to add a little of the reserved coconut water if the cream becomes too thick. Keep in the fridge until needed and use within 3–4 days.

Almond or Cashew Cream

Serves 4–6

This sweet nut cream is full of 'good for you' essential fats and makes a healthy addition to any dessert. It is quite rich, so you won't need a lot.

110g (4oz) ground almonds or ground cashews

150ml (5fl oz) almond milk (see page 22 for how to make your own)

1 tsp mild-tasting runny honey or ¼ tsp stevia (optional)

½ tsp vanilla extract

1. Blend all the ingredients in a food processor and allow the motor to run for another minute until you have a smooth cream.

2. Refrigerate for a few hours to allow the cream to thicken. Store in the fridge and use within 3–4 days.

Prunes and Pears with Honey and Almonds

Serves 6

If you can remember to pop the prunes and water in a pan before you go to bed, then add the fruit and flavourings in the morning, you will have a delicious dessert ready and waiting for you in the evening with very little effort required.

175g (6oz) pitted prunes

400ml (14fl oz) water

3 large just-ripe pears

1 tbsp mild-tasting runny honey (optional)

1 tsp almond extract

Flaked almonds, toasted (see page 23), to decorate

1. Place the prunes and water in a pan and bring to the boil, then remove from the heat, cover with a lid and leave to soak overnight.

2. Peel and core the pears and cut into large, bite-sized chunks, then add to the soaked prunes with the honey and almond extract. Place in the fridge and leave to marinate for a few hours for the flavours to mingle.

3. Serve cold sprinkled with toasted flaked almonds.

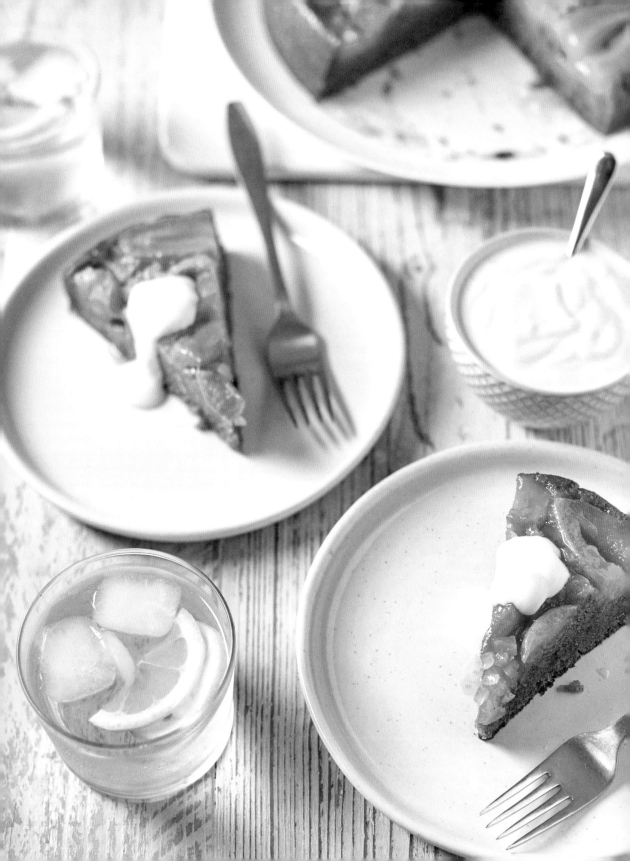

Apricot and Ginger Frangipane Pie
Serves 6

Make sure the fruits you use are not over-ripe or they will disintegrate. The crystallised ginger does contain a little sugar, so you can omit or use freeze-dried fruit instead. This pudding is best served slightly warm with a cold accompaniment, such as Whipped Coconut Cream or ice cream (see pages 236 and 254–256).

150g (5oz) pitted dates, finely diced, and 110ml (4fl oz) water (or 1 portion of Date Purée – see page 210)

8 just-ripe apricots, halved and stoned

6 pieces of crystallised ginger, diced (optional)

75g (3oz) gluten-free plain flour (see page 22)

½ tsp bicarbonate of soda

1 level tsp gluten-free baking powder

75g (3oz) ground almonds

75g (3oz) polenta or medium maize meal

1 tsp almond extract

1 tbsp lemon juice or ¼ tsp vitamin C powder (see page 23)

110ml (4fl oz) rice bran oil

150–200ml (5–7fl oz) dairy-free milk or water

25cm (10in) deep-sided round pie dish

1. Preheat the oven to 190°C (170°C fan), gas mark 5, and grease the dish (using a little extra oil).

2. Place the dates and water in a pan and bring to the boil. Remove from the heat, cover with a lid and leave to soften for about 30 minutes while you prepare the other ingredients.

3. Place the apricots in the dish, cut side down, and scatter over the ginger pieces. Sift together the flour, bicarbonate of soda and baking powder and mix with the ground almonds and polenta.

4. Place the date mixture in a food processor with the almond extract, lemon juice or vitamin C powder, oil and 150ml (5fl oz) of the milk or water, and blend until smooth. Add the flour mixture and process again, adding a little more liquid if needed, to make a very soft, dropping consistency (almost like a thick batter).

5. Spoon the mixture carefully on top of the apricots, level the surface and bake on the middle shelf of the oven for 35–45 minutes or until brown on top and springy to the touch. Serve while still slightly warm.

Variations

Plum and Orange Frangipane Pie: Substitute plums for the apricots. Sprinkle with a teaspoon of grated orange zest or 2 tablespoons of candied peel (this does contain a little sugar) before topping with the frangipane mixture.

Apple and Raspberry Frangipane Pie: Replace the apricots with 2–3 tart eating apples, unpeeled and each cut into 6–8 wedges. Sprinkle over a handful of freeze-dried raspberries before topping with the frangipane mixture.

Rhubarb and Ginger Pots

Serves 2

Rhubarb can vary in sweetness, but how you cook it makes a difference, too. By draining the rhubarb as soon as it comes to the boil you remove a lot of acidity with the water. The rhubarb can then be cooked without needing any additional liquid. Just be careful that you watch it carefully when bringing it to the boil otherwise you could end up with a pan of mush.

60g (2½oz) pitted dates, finely diced, and 55ml (2fl oz) water (or ½ portion Date Purée – see page 210)

310g (11oz) trimmed rhubarb, cut into chunks

Juice of 2 tsps finely grated fresh root ginger

75g (3oz) coconut cream (see page 22)

2 tbsps chopped crystallised ginger or toasted coconut (see page 23), to decorate

1. Place the dates and water in a pan and bring to the boil. Remove from the heat, cover the pan with a lid and leave to soak for about 30 minutes or until the dates are soft.

2. Put the rhubarb in a pan, cover with cold water and bring to the boil. As soon as it begins to boil, tip the rhubarb into a sieve to remove the liquid. Place the rhubarb back in the pan (you won't need any liquid) and simmer for 2–3 minutes or until cooked.

3. Place the date mixture in a food processor with the cooked rhubarb, ginger juice and coconut cream and blend until smooth and creamy.

4. Spoon the mixture into glasses or bowls and chill in the fridge. Decorate with crystallised ginger (though it does contain sugar) or toasted coconut before serving.

Apricot and Orange Pots

Serves 2

The velvety creaminess of this dessert makes you think that it can't be good for you, but the ingredients list tells the truth. Try to use unsulphured apricots – ones that have been allowed to go brown rather than kept orange artificially by chemical additives.

60g (2½oz) dried apricots, finely diced

55ml (4fl oz) orange juice

110g (4oz) cooked sweet potato (about 1 medium)

Grated zest of 1 orange, plus extra zest or orange slices to decorate

1 tbsp lemon juice

75g (3oz) coconut cream (the thick part from the top of the tin – see page 22)

55–75ml (2–3fl oz) water

1. Place the apricots and orange juice in a pan and bring to the boil. Remove from the heat, cover the pan with a lid and leave to soak for about 30 minutes or until the apricots are soft.

2. Place the apricot mixture in a food processor with the sweet potato, orange zest, lemon juice and coconut cream and blend until smooth and creamy, adding enough water to loosen the mixture.

3. Spoon into glasses or bowls and chill in the fridge until needed. Decorate with grated orange zest or slices before serving.

Rich Chocolate Pots

Serves 2

You will find versions of this rich chocolate treat in many recipe books. It was an inspired invention by whoever first thought of it and it is fast becoming a classic. This is my healthy take on this delicious dessert. If you make these pots with ready-made date purée (see page 210), they will be ready to eat in minutes. The block of date purée can easily be cut in half from frozen and doesn't need to be defrosted. You can make a speedier version using a large mashed banana instead of the date mixture, but it won't be quite as rich.

60g (2½ oz) pitted dates, finely diced, and 55ml (2fl oz) water (or ½ portion of Date Purée –see page 210)

Flesh of 1 large just-ripe avocado (about 175g/6oz)

25g (1oz) cacao, cocoa or carob powder

1 tsp vanilla extract

40g (1½oz) coconut oil, melted

Toasted nuts (see page 23) or 70–90% dark chocolate, flaked, to decorate

1. Place the dates and water in a pan and bring to the boil. Remove from the heat, cover the pan with a lid and leave to soak for about 30 minutes or until the dates are soft. Cool the dates if necessary by placing the pan in a bowl or tin of cold water.

2. Place the date mixture in a food processor with the avocado, cacao, cocoa or carob powder and vanilla extract and blend until smooth. With the motor running, add the melted coconut oil and process to combine. Add a little water if the mixture is too stiff.

3. Spoon the mixture into glasses or bowls and chill in the fridge until needed, then decorate just before serving.

Prune and Chocolate Tiramisu Trifle

Serves 6

I don't normally like including recipes where you have to make something else, such as a sponge cake, before you start a recipe, but as this is a special recipe for entertaining, I've made an exception. I try to keep a ready-made chocolate sponge in the freezer so that I can whip up a pudding quickly. The chocolate ganache also needs to be made first, but if you have ready-made date purée (see page 210), it will only take a few minutes to prepare. This recipe tastes best if the prunes have been soaked overnight, but you could make the recipe with ready-to-eat prunes, unsoaked, if time is short.

55g (2oz) pitted prunes, quartered

55ml (2fl oz) boiling water

½ chocolate sponge (half of a single sponge – see page 223)

40ml (1½fl oz) strong freshly brewed coffee

1 tsp Tia Maria (optional)

1 quantity of Rich Chocolate Pot mixture (see page 242)

1 quantity of Whipped Coconut Cream (see page 236)

Cacao, cocoa or carob powder, to decorate

23cm (9in) round serving or trifle dish

1. Cover the prunes with the boiling water and leave to soak for a few hours or preferably overnight.

2. Cut or break the cake into bite-sized pieces and place in the base of the serving or trifle dish. Mix the coffee and Tia Maria (if using) with the soaked prunes and spoon the mixture evenly over the chocolate cake.

3. Spread over the chocolate pot mixture, top with the coconut cream and decorate with a fine sprinkling of cacao, cocoa or carob powder.

4. Chill in the fridge for a few hours for the flavours to mingle before serving.

Variation

Chocolate and Cherry Trifle: Follow the recipe above, but use cherries instead of prunes. These could be dried cherries, soaked overnight, or you could use fresh, bottled or frozen. Add 1 tablespoon of sherry instead of the Tia Maria to the cherries, if you like, and miss out the coffee, adding a little fruit juice, if needed, to make up the liquid, then follow the recipe as before.

Raspberry and Blueberry Cheesecake

Serves 6

This deliciously creamy dessert can be made really quickly if you have ready-made date purée (see page 210), but it looks so good that everyone will think you have spent an age in the kitchen.

150g (5oz) pitted dates, finely diced, and 110ml (4fl oz) water (or 1 portion of Date Purée – see page 210)

5 sheets of gelatine (see page 23)

1 tsp vanilla extract

150g (5oz) coconut cream (the thick part from the top of the tin – see page 22)

400g (14oz) raspberries, plus 2 handfuls of raspberries and blueberries to decorate

For the base

50g (2oz) coconut oil

1 tbsp mild-tasting runny honey or ½ tsp stevia (optional)

½ tsp vanilla extract

50g (2oz) desiccated coconut

50g (2oz) finely chopped walnuts

50g (2oz) gluten-free oat or buckwheat flakes

20cm (8in) deep-sided, loose-bottomed round cake tin (no need to grease)

1. Place the dates and 110ml (4fl oz) of water in a pan and bring to the boil. Remove from the heat, cover with a lid and leave to soak for about 30 minutes or until the dates are soft. Cool the mixture, if necessary, by placing the pan in a bowl or tin of cold water.

2. In the meantime, line the base of the tin with baking parchment. Lining the sides will give a smoother finish to the cheesecake, but it isn't necessary.

3. To make the cheesecake base, melt the coconut oil with the honey or stevia (if using) in a small pan over a low heat and then add the vanilla extract. Whisk to combine, then add the desiccated coconut, walnuts and oat or buckwheat flakes. Mix until the dry ingredients are coated in the oil mixture and slightly warm.

4. Press the mixture into the base of the cake tin and chill in the fridge while you prepare the topping for the cheesecake.

5. Place the gelatine sheets in a small pan and cover with cold water to soften them.

6. Add the soaked date mixture to a food processor with the vanilla extract, coconut cream and raspberries and blend until smooth and creamy.

7. Remove the gelatine from the pan and squeeze to remove excess water. Place it back in the pan with 30ml (1fl oz) of water, bring to the boil and whisk to dissolve the gelatine.

8. With the food-processor motor running, pour the gelatine into the raspberry mixture and blend to combine, then pour the mixture onto the cheesecake base. Chill in the fridge for at least 3 hours or until set.

9. Remove the cheesecake from the tin. Place individual raspberries around the edge of the cheesecake, then pile more raspberries and the blueberries into the middle and serve.

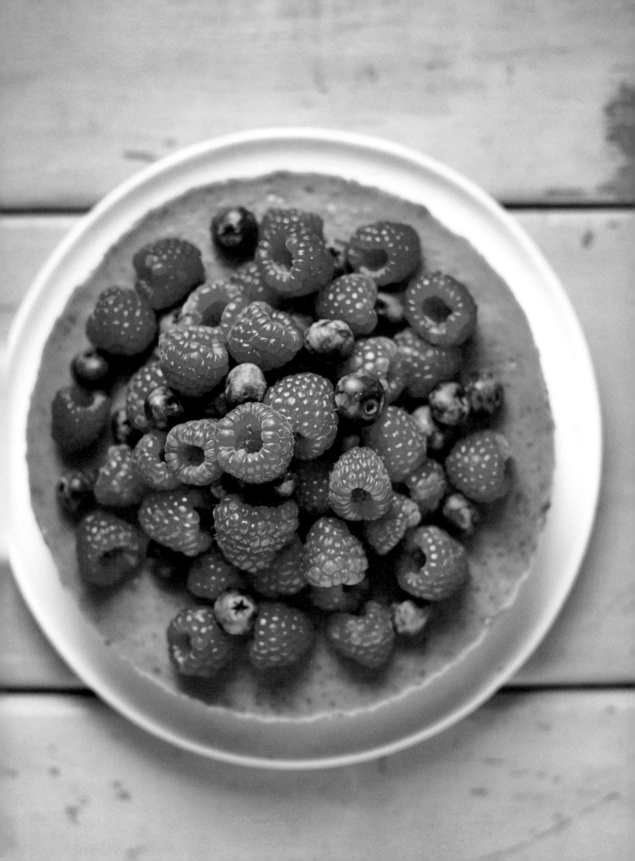

Kiwi, Lime and Coconut Cheesecake

Serves 6

Enjoy the mouth-watering combination of ingredients in this cheesecake without feeling guilty. For a brighter green coloured cheesecake substitute the dates for dried pears.

150g (5oz) pitted dates, finely diced, and 110ml (4fl oz) water (or 1 portion of Date Purée – see page 210)

3½ sheets of gelatine (see page 23)

350g (12oz) avocado flesh

150g (5oz) coconut cream (see page 22)

Grated zest of 4 limes and 8 tbsps lime juice

For the base

50g (2oz) coconut oil

1 tbsp mild runny honey or ½ tsp stevia (optional)

½ tsp vanilla extract

50g (2oz) desiccated coconut

50g (2oz) finely chopped walnuts

50g (2oz) gluten-free oats or buckwheat flakes

To decorate

2 just-ripe kiwi fruits

1 tbsp coconut flakes

20cm (8in) deep-sided, loose-bottomed round cake tin (no need to grease)

1. Place the dates in a pan with the water and bring to the boil. Remove from the heat, cover with a lid and leave to soak for about 30 minutes or until the fruit is soft. Cool the mixture, if necessary, by placing the pan in bowl or tin of cold water.

2. In the meantime, follow steps 2–4 of the Raspberry and Blueberry Cheesecake (see page 244) for making and chilling the cheesecake base.

3. Place the gelatine leaves in a small pan and cover with cold water to soften them.

4. Add the date mixture to a food processor with the avocado, coconut cream and grated lime zest and blend until smooth and creamy.

5. Remove the gelatine from the pan and squeeze to remove excess water. Place it back in the pan with the lime juice, bring to the boil and whisk to dissolve the gelatine.

6. With the food-processor motor running, pour the gelatine into the avocado mixture and blend to combine, then pour the mixture onto the cheesecake base. Chill in the fridge for at least 3 hours or until set.

7. Remove the cheesecake from the tin. Peel and thinly slice the kiwi fruit then arrange the slices around the edge of the cheesecake. Sprinkle the toasted coconut flakes in the middle before serving.

Variation

Kiwi, Lime and Coconut Mousse: You can serve the topping on its own as a mousse. Omit the cheesecake base and pour the topping into a serving bowl, or individual bowls or glasses, before chilling in the fridge as above.

Apricots and Persimmons (Sharon Fruit) with Orange and Ginger

Serves 6–8

This recipe is so easy to make, yet tastes amazing. It does take time to soak, however, so you'll need to plan ahead. Delicious for a dessert with Coconut or Cashew Cream or ice cream (see pages 236 and 254–256), it's also good spooned on top of breakfast cereal or as a mid-afternoon snack with some granola and dairy-free yogurt. For a speedier version, use shop-bought freshly squeezed orange juice and always try to keep some orange parings in the freezer ready for use.

110g (4oz) dried apricots, halved

4 parings of orange rind, finely sliced

Juice of 3–4 oranges, made up to 400ml (14fl oz) with water if necessary

1 tsp grated fresh root ginger

4 just-ripe persimmons (Sharon fruit)

1. Place the apricots in a pan with the orange rind, orange juice and the ginger. Bring to the boil, then remove from the heat, cover with a lid and leave to soak overnight.

2. Cut the persimmons into wedges and add to the apricots. Stir to combine, then leave for a few hours in the fridge for the flavours to mingle before serving.

Poached Strawberries with Pomegranate Molasses

Serves 4

I made this after a visit to France when we had been served strawberries in red wine. Pomegranate molasses is a really good substitute for red wine in both sweet and savoury dishes and it works well in this pudding. It's so simple, but very effective. This is a good recipe for using natural stevia leaves (see page 23), in place of the ½ teaspoon of stevia, as they can brought to the boil with the fruit tea bag, allowed to infuse for a couple of minutes and then removed before adding the rest of the ingredients.

575g (1¼lb) strawberries

275ml (10fl oz) water

1 fruit tea bag

1 tbsp pomegranate molasses

1 tsp grated orange zest

1 tbsp mild-tasting runny honey or ½ teaspoon stevia (optional)

1. Hull the strawberries and cut into halves or quarters depending on their size.

2. Place the water in a large pan with the fruit tea bag and bring to the boil, then remove from the heat and take out the tea bag. Add the pomegranate molasses, orange zest and honey or stevia (if using) and stir to combine.

3. Add the strawberries to the hot liquid and stir, then transfer them immediately to a serving dish, stir and leave to chill in the fridge before serving. The strawberries will soften a little and the flavours will combine.

4. Serve cold with ice cream, Cashew or Coconut Cream (see pages 254–256 and 236).

Chocolate and Salted Pecan Nut Torte

Serves 6–8

This rich and decadent dessert could grace the table at any dinner party, yet it is full of 'good for you' nutrients – antioxidants, omega-3 oils and fibre. You could add 1 tablespoon of cacao or cocoa powder to the base ingredients instead of the chocolate, if you prefer, to avoid having any sugar, but the base won't set quite as crisply.

75g (3oz) coconut oil

1 tbsp mild-tasting runny honey or ½ tsp stevia (optional)

40g (1½oz) 70–90% dark chocolate, broken into squares

½ tsp vanilla extract

75g (3oz) desiccated coconut

75g (3oz) finely chopped walnuts

75g (3oz) gluten-free oats or buckwheat flakes

2 quantities of Rich Chocolate Pot mixture (see page 242)

For the salted pecans

2 tsps mild-tasting runny honey

½ tsp salt

50g (2oz) pecan nuts

25cm (10in) round pie dish or loose-bottomed round cake tin (no need to grease)

1. Line the base of the dish or tin with baking parchment if you want to remove the torte to serve.

2. Melt the coconut oil with the honey or stevia (if using) in a pan over a low heat, then add the chocolate and vanilla extract and allow the chocolate to melt. Whisk to combine before adding the desiccated coconut, walnuts and oat or buckwheat flakes. Mix until the dry ingredients are coated in the oil mixture and warmed through.

3. Press the mixture well into the base and up the sides of the prepared pie dish or cake tin. Spread the chocolate pot mixture over the base and level the surface.

4. In a small pan, heat through the honey and salt and toss the pecan nuts in the mixture to coat. Spread the nuts on a baking tray (lined with baking parchment, if you like, to save washing up) and toast in the oven (at about 200°C/180°C fan/gas 6), or under a medium grill, until crisp and lightly browned. This will only take a few minutes, so watch them like a hawk or they will quickly burn.

5. Allow the nuts to cool a little, then use to decorate the top of the tart. Chill in the fridge for 2 hours or until ready to serve.

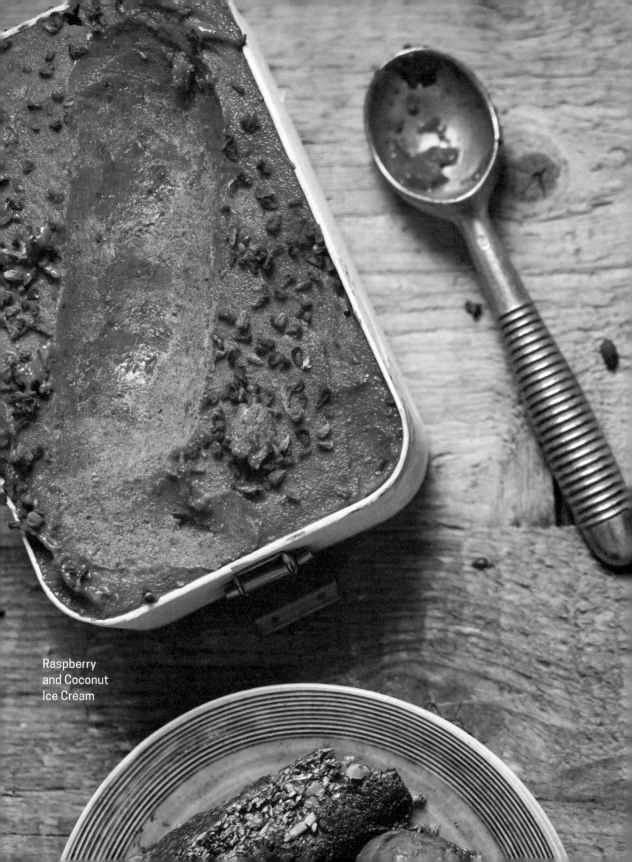

Raspberry
and Coconut
Ice Cream

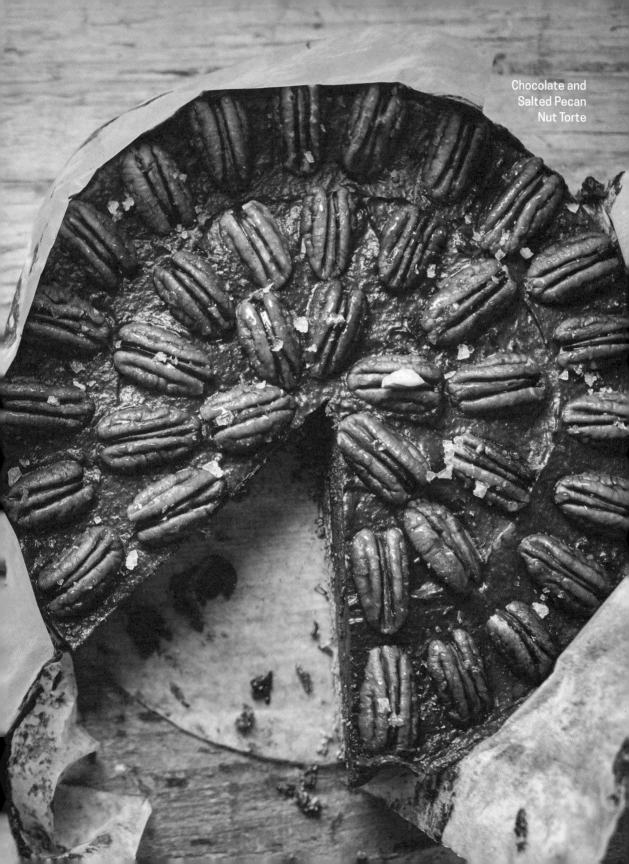

Chocolate and
Salted Pecan
Nut Torte

Banana and Chocolate Crumble

Serves 4

Fruit crumble is one of life's great pleasures; for an even more decadent dessert, push a few slivers of chocolate into the topping before baking. Don't be afraid of making substitutions, as crumble is very forgiving. Chopped Brazils or sunflower seeds work well instead of slivered almonds, or use desiccated coconut instead of ground almonds and fresh or bottled cherries instead of bananas.

275g (10oz) peeled bananas (about 4 bananas)

½ tsp ground cinnamon

½ tsp vanilla extract

For the crumble topping

110g (4oz) gluten-free plain flour (see page 22)

10g (½oz) cacao, cocoa or carob powder

½ tsp ground cinnamon

40g (1½oz) gluten-free oat or buckwheat flakes

40g (1½oz) ground almonds

40g (1½oz) slivered almonds

40g (1½oz) coconut oil

1 tbsp mild-tasting runny honey or ½ tsp stevia

½ tsp vanilla extract

1. Preheat the oven to 190°C (170°C fan), gas mark 5.

2. Slice the bananas into thick chunks and combine with the cinnamon and vanilla extract in a baking dish.

3. Sift together the flour, cocoa and cinnamon, then mix with the oat or buckwheat flakes, ground and slivered almonds.

4. Place the coconut oil in a pan with the honey or stevia and vanilla extract and melt together until runny. Add the dry ingredients and mix well to combine. Continue mixing until you have a crumbly texture.

5. Spread this mixture on top of the bananas, level the surface and bake for 25–30 minutes or until the bananas are soft and the crumble is crisp on the surface.

6. Serve with coconut cream (the thick part from the top of the tin – see page 22), ice cream or custard made with non-dairy milk.

Variation:

Apple and Cranberry Crumble: Make the recipe as above, replacing the bananas, cinnamon and vanilla extract with 3 diced, peeled apples (preferably half baking and half eating apples) and 3 tablespoons dried cranberries (or try freeze-dried raspberries). Omit the cacao/cocoa powder in the topping, increase the quantity of cinnamon to 1 teaspoon and add almond extract instead of vanilla.

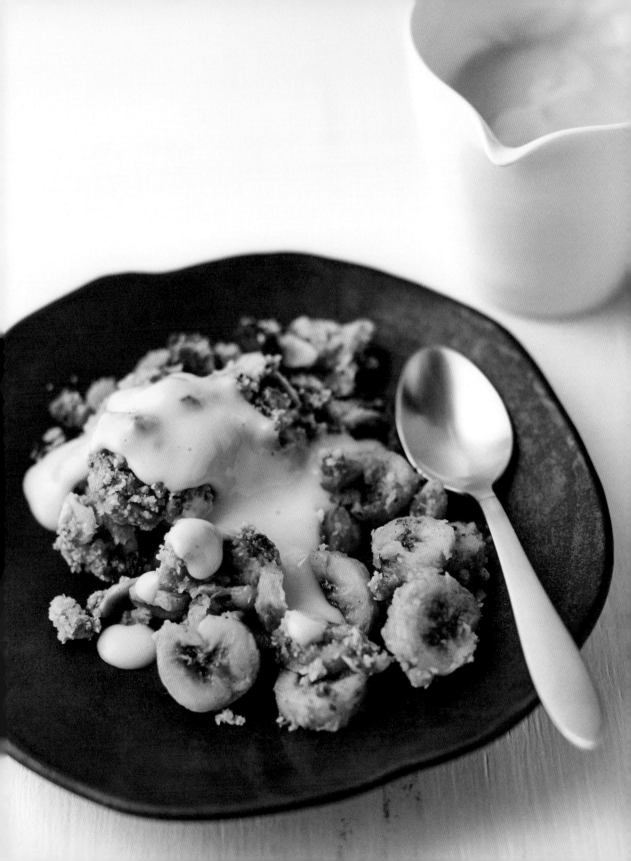

Ice Cream and Sorbets

Made from fresh fruit, these ice creams are delicious, healthy and very easy to prepare. I like to keep some fruit ready frozen to make a quick treat or dessert on a warm day. I freeze fruit when we have a glut in the garden or when it is plentiful in summer. I also freeze fruit such as bananas (slicing them up first) when I can see them ripening fast in the fruit bowl but not being eaten.

Generally, I make these ice creams and sorbets just before eating as they become quite hard if you refreeze them for more than an hour or so. But if you want them for later – if you are entertaining, for instance – you can place scoops on a tray and refreeze until needed. It is then best to allow them to soften slightly at room temperature before serving.

Banana Substitutes

I have used bananas in most of the ice cream recipes as they produce a really creamy texture, but if you cannot tolerate them, follow the recipe for Raspberry and Coconut Ice Cream (see page 256), varying the fruit according to your preferences. You could also use yogurt or dairy-free cream instead of the coconut cream in that recipe.

Banana, Vanilla and Toasted Hazelnut Ice Cream

Serves 2

You will never believe when you tuck into this ice cream that it's made with so few ingredients. For a richer version, use 75g (3oz) of coconut cream instead of the non-frozen banana.

3 large bananas (about 275g/10oz peeled weight)

1 tsp vanilla extract

1 tsp mild-tasting runny honey or ¼ tsp stevia (optional)

3 tbsps finely chopped hazelnuts, toasted (see page 23)

1. Peel and cut two of the bananas into slices, lay them on a baking tray and leave in the freezer until frozen. Place the remaining banana, unpeeled, in the fridge to keep cool.

2. Place the frozen bananas in a food processor with the banana from the fridge (peeled and sliced) and the vanilla extract and honey or stevia (if using). Blend the ice cream (pulsing at first) until the mixture is smooth and creamy. Mix in the toasted hazelnuts and serve immediately.

Chocolate Ice Cream

Serves 2

This quick and easy dessert is deliciously creamy and luxurious.

2 large bananas (about 200g/7oz peeled weight)

55ml (2fl oz) coconut cream (see page 22)

50g (2oz) 70–90% dark chocolate, broken (optional)

2 level tbsps cacao, cocoa or carob powder

3 level tbsps ground almonds (optional)

1 tsp vanilla extract

1 tsp mild-tasting runny honey (optional)

1. Peel and cut the bananas into slices, lay them on a baking tray and leave in the freezer until frozen. Keep the coconut cream in the fridge until needed.

2. Finely chop the chocolate in a food processor and set aside.

3. Place the frozen bananas in the processor with the remaining ingredients (but not the chocolate) and blend (pulsing at first) until the mixture is smooth and creamy.

4. Mix in the chopped chocolate by hand and serve immediately.

Raspberry and Coconut Ice Cream

Serves 2

I usually use frozen raspberries from the supermarket in this ice cream for a quick and easy but delicious dessert.

200g (7oz) fresh or frozen raspberries

150g (5oz) coconut cream (see page 22)

½ tsp vanilla extract

1 tsp mild-tasting runny honey or ¼ tsp stevia (optional)

3 tbsps freeze-dried raspberries, partly crushed

1. If you are using fresh raspberries, lay them on a baking tray and leave in the freezer until frozen. Place the coconut cream in the fridge (preferably overnight) to cool.

2. Place the frozen raspberries in a food processor with the vanilla extract, coconut cream and honey or stevia (if using) and blend (pulsing at first) until the mixture is smooth and creamy.

3. Add the freeze-dried fruit and mix in by hand. Serve immediately.

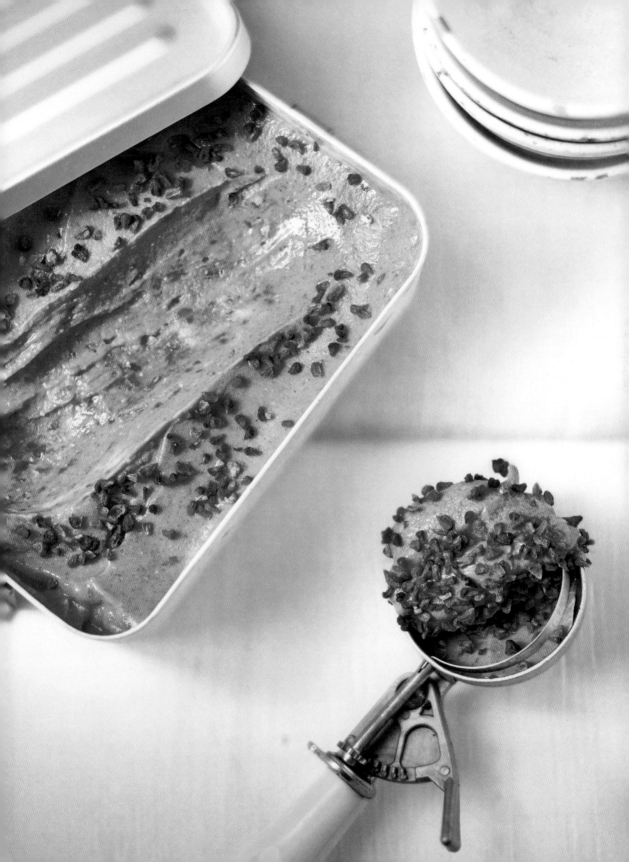

Chocolate and Cherry Sundae

Serves 2

Make this sundae, or one of the suggestions that follow, for a special treat. As well as tasting amazing, each of them is a feast for the eyes and it's hard to believe that they are full of 'good for you' ingredients. If fresh cherries are not available, you could use bottled cherries (preferably in fruit juice) or dried Morello cherries soaked overnight in water to soften.

50g (2oz) 70–90% dark chocolate, broken into squares

2 tbsps almond butter

4 scoops of Chocolate Ice Cream (see page 255)

110g (4oz) pitted fresh cherries

4 tbsps Whipped Coconut Cream (see page 236)

To decorate

1 handful of fresh cherries

70–90% dark chocolate shavings

1. Make a chocolate sauce by melting the chocolate and almond butter in a bowl set over a pan of gently simmering water. Remove from the heat and allow to cool but not set.

2. Layer the ice cream, fruit and chocolate sauce in two tall glasses.

3. Top with the coconut cream, decorate with the cherries and chocolate shavings and serve immediately.

Variations:

Peach Melba Sundae: Make a sundae using raspberry (see page 256) and/or vanilla ice cream, a sliced fresh peach and a handful of fresh raspberries layered in tall glasses. Pour over a little fresh fruit smoothie, homemade or bought (such as strawberry and banana), and top with Whipped Coconut Cream (see page 236). Decorate with raspberries and toasted flaked almonds and serve immediately.

Banana and Toasted Hazelnut Sundae: Fry 2 sliced bananas in 1 teaspoon coconut oil and ¼ teaspoon of cinnamon until browning and softening but not mushy. Allow to cool, then layer with vanilla and/or Chocolate Ice Cream (see page 255) and 2 tablespoons toasted chopped hazelnuts. Decorate with Whipped Coconut Cream (see page 236) and more toasted hazelnuts.

Strawberry and Mango Sorbet

Serves 2

If you have a supply of ready-frozen strawberries in your freezer, you can whip up a delightful dessert at a minute's notice. You could use a peeled, diced fresh peach if you don't have a mango.

250g (9oz) fresh strawberries

Flesh of ½ large ripe mango, diced

2 tsps lemon juice

1. Hull the fresh strawberries and cut into small pieces before laying them on a tray and leaving in the freezer until frozen. Place the diced mango in the fridge to keep cool.

2. Blend the strawberries, mango flesh and lemon juice in a food processor (pulsing at first) until you have a smooth sorbet. Serve immediately.

Pineapple, Orange and Mint Sorbet

Serves 2

This zingy combination works really well to produce a healthy and delicious sorbet – ideal when the weather turns hot and you want an instant cooler.

Flesh of ½ small pineapple (350g/12oz)

55ml (2fl oz) orange juice

4 parings of orange rind, finely sliced

4 mint leaves, thick stems removed

1. Dice the pineapple flesh, lay the pieces on a tray and leave in the freezer until frozen. Leave the orange juice in the fridge to keep cool.

2. Blend the pineapple, orange juice, orange rind and mint in a food processor (pulsing at first) until you have a smooth sorbet. Serve immediately.

Sweets and Treats

So many of the foods we regard as sweets and treats are not good for our health or our waistlines. In this chapter I have tried to bring together a selection of recipes made using 'good for you' ingredients that still have that indulgent feel. It's far better to hand round some homemade, sugar-free Salted Caramel Cups (see page 275) for a dinner-party nibble than to tuck into shop-bought chocolate mints, or to leave Spiced Pecan Clusters and Chocolate and Walnut Truffles (see pages 268 and 272) around at Christmas rather than commercial boxes of chocolates. Eventually you will not want to eat conventional treats, as they will taste far too sweet or sickly and leave you with the sugar blues or craving more; you'll be far happier with these homemade versions.

I often have a couple of Almond and Marzipan Cups (see page 276) or chocolate truffles when I sit down with a cuppa after my evening meal. But I have just a couple and I'm fine with that. If you have difficulty knowing when to stop, then you need to address the reasons why. Have you not eaten well enough during the day so that your blood sugar is dipping and you are craving sweet food to lift it? Is it because you have not cured your sugar addiction (see 'Why One Chocolate is Never Enough' on page 14)? If this is the case, you may need to avoid sweet foods for a few weeks to break the vicious cycle. Or are you using food as an emotional crutch? (I talk about emotions and addictions in my first book, *Cooking Without*.) If so, you may have to address any emotional issues so that your body no longer needs its sugar fixes.

Chocolate

Dairy- and soya-free chocolate is now available (see the list of suppliers on page 286), with the percentage of cocoa solids in them ranging from 70 to 90, but they do contain some sugar. I accept this small amount of sugar as I do love good-quality chocolate. They also say that nuts, soya and dairy products are used elsewhere in the factory so they may not be suitable for those with severe allergies. I have created a sugar-free version (see below) made with 100% cacao butter, which on its own is very solid and quite bitter, but you may want to search out your own or swap for a carob version.

Sugar-free Chocolate

Melt 100g (3½oz) of 100% cacao butter (available from health-food shops or online) with 50g (2oz) of coconut oil in a bowl set over a pan of hot water. Add ½ teaspoon of stevia if you want a sweeter version. (The stevia does remain a little grainy but it tastes fine.) Mix well and use to replace chocolate in recipes.

Energy Balls

Makes 25–30 balls

These tasty nuggets are full of goodness and make an ideal snack to keep you feeling satisfied. I store them in the freezer, once made, and grab a couple if I need a quick and easy treat, as they defrost quickly. You can make a more decadent version by pushing a small piece of 70–90% dark chocolate into the centre of each ball as you roll it, or you could substitute half the seeds for dried fruit (such as roughly chopped raisins or cranberries) for a sweeter version. Add these along with the dates.

10 whole pitted dates (Medjool are ideal)

125g (4½oz) mixed nuts (such as almonds, cashews, hazelnuts or walnuts)

125g (4½oz) mixed seeds (such as pumpkin, sunflower, sesame or chia)

25g (1oz) desiccated coconut

3 level tbsps nut butter (such as almond, cashew or hazelnut)

1 tbsp mild-tasting runny honey (optional)

1 tsp vanilla or almond extract (see page 23)

1 level tsp cinnamon

1. Soak the whole dates in hot water until they are soft (about 30 minutes), then squeeze out any excess water. (Medjool dates don't need soaking.)

2. Place the nuts and seeds in a food processor and blend until finely ground. Add the remaining ingredients and process again until the mixture sticks together when pressed between your fingers, adding a tablespoon of water if this is not happening.

3. Roll the mixture into balls and place on a baking tray. Allow them to dry out overnight (uncovered) in the fridge, then store in an airtight container in the fridge or freezer.

Activated Nuts or Seeds

Makes 1 bowl

Activated nuts or seeds have been soaked in water and salt for a period of time, which starts off germination and the sprouting process. They are then dehydrated at a low temperature. The nuts/seeds have an increased nutrient content and are easier to digest. They are crunchy, crisp and delicious, very quick and easy to make and work out at a fraction of the cost of bought versions. I make them up in bulk and store in the freezer. Use either nuts or seeds, rather than a mixture of both, as each will take a different amount of time to dry.

225g (8oz) nuts (such as almonds, cashews, hazelnuts or walnuts) or seeds (such as sunflower or pumpkin)

½ tsp salt

1. Soak the nuts or seeds overnight in double their volume of water and the salt.

2. Rinse and drain the soaked nuts/seeds and spread them on a baking tray, then place the tray in a warm but not hot place. You could try the lowest setting on your cooker or a gas cooker with the pilot light on (machines called dehydrators are also available); I use the top of my boiler, which is enclosed and always warm. It should be no hotter than 50°C. The nuts/seeds take 12–48 hours to dry depending on the level of heat. They are ready when they are crisp and crunchy. Store in an airtight container in the fridge or freezer.

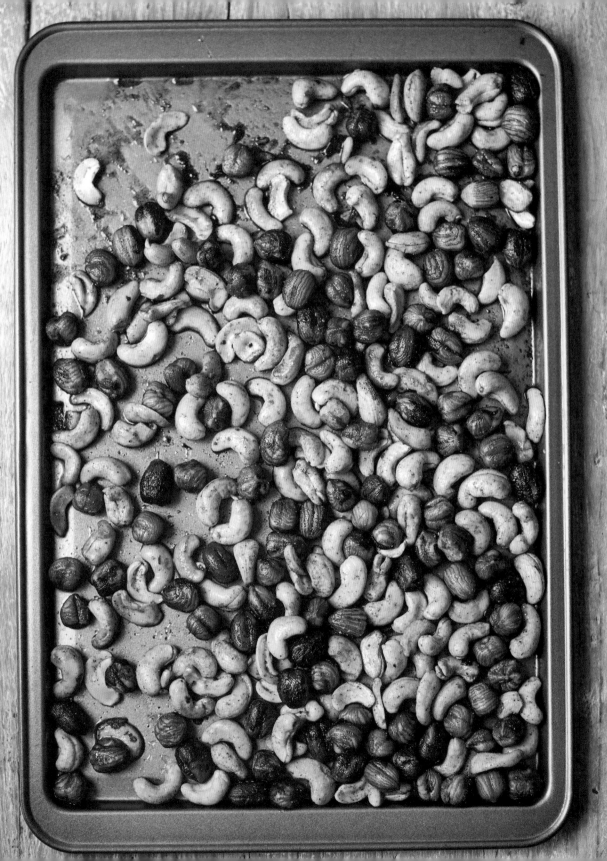

Activated Nuts or Seeds with Salt and Paprika

Makes 1 bowl

In this recipe, activated nuts or seeds are coated in a spicy dressing before drying, for a savoury twist on the basic recipe (see page 264).

200g (7oz) nuts (such as almonds, cashews, hazelnuts or walnuts) or seeds (such as sunflower or pumpkin)

1 tbsp tomato purée

1 tsp sweet smoked paprika

½ tsp salt

1 tbsp olive oil

1 tsp sesame oil

1. Soak the seeds or nuts overnight in double their volume of water, then rinse and drain.

2. Whisk together the tomato purée, smoked paprika, salt and oils and toss with the soaked nuts or seeds.

3. Spread on a baking tray and place in a warm but not hot place. You could try the lowest setting on your cooker or a gas cooker with the pilot light on (machines called dehydrators are also available); I use the top of my boiler, which is enclosed and always warm. It should be no hotter than 50°C. The nuts/seeds take 12–48 hours to dry depending on the level of heat. They are ready when they are crisp and crunchy. Store in an airtight container in the fridge or freezer.

Activated Nuts or Seeds with Chinese Five-spice

Makes 1 bowl

I adore these sweet and salty spiced nuts. They are very moreish, yet full of 'good for you' ingredients.

200g (7oz) nuts (such as almonds, cashews, hazelnuts or walnuts) or seeds (such as sunflower or pumpkin)

1 tsp mild-tasting runny honey

1 tsp coconut oil

1 tsp ginger juice (squeezed from grated fresh root ginger)

1½ tsps Chinese five-spice powder

½ tsp vanilla extract

½ tsp salt

1. Soak the seeds or nuts overnight in double their volume of water, then rinse and drain.

2. Melt the honey and oil together, then whisk in the ginger juice, Chinese five spice, vanilla extract and salt, and toss together with the soaked nuts or seeds.

3. Spread on a baking tray and place in a warm but not hot place. You could try the lowest setting on your cooker or a gas cooker with the pilot light on (machines called dehydrators are also available); I use the top of my boiler, which is enclosed and always warm. It should be no hotter than 50°C. The nuts/seeds take 12–48 hours to dry depending on the level of heat. They are ready when they are crisp and crunchy. Store in an airtight container in the fridge or freezer.

Spiced Pecan Clusters

Makes 1 bowl

Serve these clusters in bowls for people to dip in and help themselves. I like to make them to leave around over Christmas. You can also ring the changes very easily: try replacing the pecans with walnuts, cranberries with sultanas, candied peel with crystallised ginger and mixed spice with cinnamon. Candied peel does contain some sugar: the overall quantity will be small, but try the sugar-free variation below if you prefer.

60g (2½oz) pitted dates, finely chopped, and 55ml (2fl oz) water (or ½ portion of Date Purée – see page 210)

150g (5oz) pecan nuts, broken into quarters

1 tsp mixed spice

50g (2oz) candied peel

40g (1½oz) dried cranberries

Salt and freshly ground black pepper

1. Preheat the oven to 145°C (125°C fan), gas mark 1½.

2. Place the dates and water in a pan and bring to the boil. Remove from the heat, cover with a lid and leave for about 30 minutes or until the dates are soft.

3. Mix the pecan nuts with the mixed spice, dried fruit and a good sprinkling of salt and pepper.

4. Blend the dates in a food processor until smooth, then add to the fruit and nut mixture. Stir to coat the fruit and nuts in the date mixture – it will not bind but form clusters.

5. Spread the mixture evenly on a baking tray and bake on the middle shelf of the oven for 30 minutes, then reduce the temperature to 120°C (100°C fan), gas mark ½, and cook for another 15–20 minutes or until the mixture is almost dried out and crisp but not browning too much (it will continue to dry out a little more on cooling). You may need to turn the mixture during cooking if the sides start to cook before the middle.

6. Allow the clusters to cool on the tray, then store in an airtight container in the fridge (they will keep like this for a few weeks) or freezer.

Variation

Sugar-free Spiced Pecan Clusters: For a completely sugar-free but still Christmassy version, soak the dates in fresh orange juice and add the grated zest of an orange to the mixture and some sultanas instead of the candied peel.

Spiced Chilli Nut Clusters

Makes 1 bowl

A more savoury version of the Spiced Pecan Clusters (see page 268), these are full of antioxidants, vitamins and minerals, making them highly nutritious as well as very tasty. Vary the chilli powder if you prefer more or less heat and try sunflower seeds instead of pumpkin or raw peanuts instead of pistachios for a variation on this recipe.

60g (2½oz) pitted dates, finely chopped, and 55ml (2fl oz) water (or ½ portion of Date Purée – see page 210)

40g (1½oz) dried apricots, finely diced

50g (2oz) sultanas

75g (3oz) pumpkin seeds

75g (3oz) pistachio nuts

75g (3oz) whole almonds, roughly chopped

⅛–¼ tsp chilli powder

1 tsp ground coriander

½ tsp garam masala

½ tsp salt and ½ tsp freshly ground black pepper

Juice from 1 tbsp grated fresh root ginger

1 tbsp tomato purée

1. Preheat the oven to 145°C (125°C fan), gas mark 1½.

2. Place the dates and water in a pan and bring to the boil. Remove from the heat, cover with a lid and leave for about 30 minutes or until the dates are soft.

3. Mix the dried fruit with the seeds, nuts, spices, salt and pepper.

4. Blend the dates, ginger juice and tomato purée in a food processor until smooth, then add this to the fruit and nut mixture. Stir to coat the fruit and nuts with the date mixture – it will not bind but form clusters .

5. Spread the mixture evenly on a baking tray and bake on the middle shelf of the oven for 30 minutes, then reduce the temperature to 120°C (100°C fan), gas mark ½, and cook for another 15–20 minutes or until the mixture is almost dried out and crisp but not browning too much (it will continue to dry out a little more on cooling). You may need to turn the mixture during cooking if the sides start to cook before the middle.

6. Allow the clusters to cool on the tray, then store in an airtight container in the fridge (they will keep like this for a few weeks) or freezer.

Kale Crisps

Serves 4

So simple to make, this snack is a powerhouse of super-nutrients – and it's delicious, too. Children will love this way of eating their greens.

1 bunch of kale (about 200g/7oz)

1 tbsp oil (see page 20), melted if necessary

Salt

1. Preheat the oven to 150°C (130°C fan), gas mark 2

2. Remove the stalks from the kale and roughly tear the flesh into crisp-sized pieces. Wash and dry the kale pieces, if necessary, and place in a bowl or pan with the oil. Toss in the oil, using your fingers to massage the oil evenly into the kale pieces until they are coated. Spread the kale out on one or two baking trays, spacing the pieces so that they don't overlap, and sprinkle with salt.

3. Bake for 15–20 minutes or until they are crisp and dry. Keep your eye on them during cooking and remove any pieces from around the edge of the tray that are ready first. Kale crisps are best eaten soon after making, as they will soften if you try to store them.

Chocolate and Morello Cherry Fridge Cake

Makes about 16 squares

This treat takes only minutes to make, yet it's really yummy. Make substitutions according to your needs and preferences. Other nut butters can be used, other dried or freeze-dried fruit substituted, and toasted seeds or coconut flakes used instead of nuts, or try making it with unsweetened popcorn instead of puffed rice.

110g (4oz) 70–90% dark chocolate, broken into squares

2 rounded tbsps smooth almond or peanut butter

75g (3oz) dried cherries, chopped if large

75g (3oz) chopped or slivered almonds, toasted (see page 23)

110g (4oz) puffed rice cereal

20cm x 33cm (8in x 13in) brownie tin or baking tray (no need to grease)

1. Melt the chocolate and nut butter together in a large bowl set over a pan of hot water (removed from the heat) and stir to combine.

2. Add the cherries, almonds and puffed rice and mix well until all the ingredients are coated in the chocolate mixture.

3. Spread the mixture in the brownie tin or baking tray and level the surface with the back of a spoon. Chill in the fridge for 3 hours or in the freezer for 1 hour if you are short of time.

4. Using a sharp knife, cut into squares, or just break into chunks once set, and store in an airtight container in the fridge. Eat within 5 days or store in the freezer.

Chocolate and Walnut Truffles
Makes 25–30 truffles

I love these truffles and the fact that I can have a treat knowing that I'm eating ingredients that are good for me. I usually freeze them once made so they will keep, but you can eat them almost as soon as they come out of the freezer – so no need to wait long!

150g (5oz) pitted dates, finely chopped, and 110ml (4fl oz) water (or 1 portion of Date Purée – see page 210)

2 tsps blackstrap molasses

½ tsp vanilla extract

75g (3oz) ground almonds

25g (1oz) cacao, cocoa or carob powder

75g (3oz) chopped walnuts

Extra ground almonds, chopped walnuts, cocoa powder or desiccated coconut, for dusting

1. Place the dates, water and molasses in a pan and bring to the boil. Remove from the heat, cover with a lid and leave to soak for about 30 minutes or until the dates have softened.

2. Bend the dates in a food processor, then add the vanilla extract, ground almonds and cacao, cocoa or carob powder. Process the ingredients to combine, then mix in the walnuts by hand or using a plastic processor blade.

3. Roll by hand into 25–30 balls and roll each in extra ground almonds, chopped walnuts, cocoa powder or desiccated coconut to coat.

4. Place the truffles on a tray and leave overnight in the fridge to dry out a little. Store in an airtight container in the fridge and eat within one week or freeze.

Variations

Chocolate Chip Truffles: Roughly chop 50g (2oz) 70–90% dark chocolate with a sharp knife and add to the mixture once it is cool. (If the date mixture is still hot, the chocolate will melt.)

Coconut and Vanilla Truffles: Replace the chopped walnuts with 25g (1oz) desiccated coconut.

Fruit and Nut Truffles: Add 50g (2oz) of sultanas, raisins, dried cranberries or dried cherries (chopped if large) to the mixture and vary the chopped nuts according to your preference. Try almonds or hazelnuts, for instance.

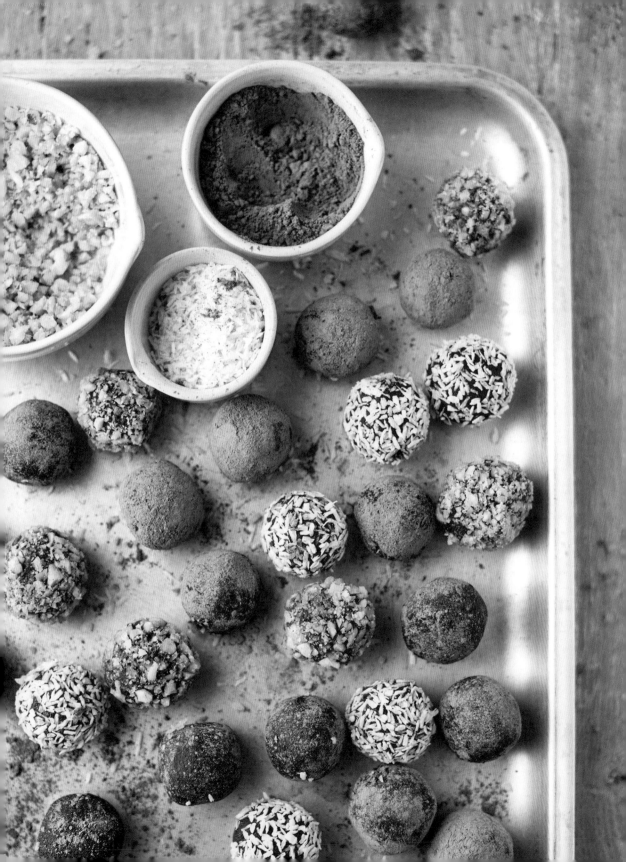

Chocolate-coated Seed and Nut Bars

Makes 16–20 bars

Just look at the list of ingredients in this recipe – impressively healthy, yet these seed and nut bars are delicious and decadent. Having treats such as these to tuck into has enabled me to stay on a healthy regime, because I never feel deprived.

60g (2½oz) coconut oil

1 tbsp mild-tasting runny honey (optional)

1 tsp vanilla extract

40g (1½oz) sunflower or hemp seeds

40g (1½oz) pumpkin seeds

40g (1½oz) almonds

40g (1½oz) Brazil nuts

75g (3oz) cashews

75g (3oz) desiccated coconut

150g (5oz) 70–90% dark chocolate, broken into squares

20cm x 33cm (8in x 13in) brownie tin or baking tray (no need to grease)

1. Melt the oil and honey with the vanilla extract in a pan over a medium heat.

2. Pulse the seeds and nuts (but not the desiccated coconut) in a food processor until finely chopped but not ground.

3. Add the chopped seeds and nuts to the oil mixture with the desiccated coconut and stir well to combine. Leave on the heat for 1 more minute, stirring, until the mixture has warmed through.

4. Press the mixture well into the brownie tin or baking tray and place in the fridge or freezer to cool.

5. Melt the chocolate in a bowl over a pan of hot water (removed from the heat) and spread it over the base. Leave in the fridge or freezer until set.

6. Heat a knife in boiling water and cut the nut mixture into squares. Store in an airtight container in the fridge for up to a week or freeze.

Salted Caramel Cups

Makes about 30 sweets

These chocolate cups are crispy on the outside and soft and gooey in the middle. If you don't have Medjool dates, just soak standard whole dates in hot water until they soften, then squeeze out any excess water.

175g (6oz) 70-90% dark chocolate, broken into squares

3 tbsps roughly chopped or 30 whole hazelnuts, toasted (see page 23)

For the salted caramel

60g (2½oz) whole soft pitted dates (Medjool are ideal)

25g (1oz) coconut oil, melted

25g (1oz) coconut cream (the thick part from the top of the tin – see page 22)

½ tsp vanilla extract

½ tsp fine salt

30 sweet paper cases

1. To make the salted caramel, blend all the ingredients in a food processor until smooth and creamy and then freeze the mixture until it thickens and sets. Once it has set, you can use a teaspoon to scoop out enough of the mixture to fit each paper case (this is easy to do, as it doesn't set solid) and roll it quickly into small balls.

2. Melt the chocolate in a small bowl set over a pan of hot water (removed from the heat).

3. Place a good ½ teaspoon of melted chocolate in each paper case and add a piece of frozen salted caramel on top, pressing it down a little so that the top of the caramel flattens and the chocolate squidges up the sides of the paper case.

4. Drizzle more chocolate over the top of the salted caramel so that it covers the surface and runs down the sides of the caramel to meet the layer beneath.

5. Place toasted hazelnuts on top and press into the chocolate. Put the sweets in the fridge to set and either store in the fridge for up to a week or freeze for later.

Almond and Marzipan Cups

Makes about 30 sweets

These individual sweets look so professional, but they are unbelievably simple to make and so delicious. If you don't have Medjool or very soft dates, just soak whole dates in hot water until they soften, then squeeze out any excess moisture.

40g (1½oz) whole soft pitted dates (Medjool are ideal)

60g (2½oz) ground almonds, plus extra for dusting

¼ tsp almond extract

175g (6oz) 70–90% dark chocolate, broken into squares

3 tbsps slivered almonds or 30 whole almonds, toasted (see page 23)

30 sweet paper cases

1. Blend the dates in the small bowl of a food processor or using a hand-held stick blender. Add the ground almonds and almond extract and mix to combine.

2. Sprinkle a board with some ground almonds and, using your hands, squeeze and roll the marzipan into a sausage shape with its diameter roughly the same size as the base of the paper cases. Cut the marzipan into 1cm (½in) lengths.

3. Melt the chocolate in a small bowl set over a pan of hot water (removed from the heat).

4. Place a good ½ teaspoon of melted chocolate in each paper case and add a piece of marzipan on top, pressing it down a little so that the top of the marzipan flattens and the chocolate squidges up the sides of the paper case.

5. Drizzle more chocolate over the top of the marzipan so that it covers the surface and runs down the sides of the marzipan to meet the layer beneath.

6. Place toasted almonds on top and press into the chocolate. Put the sweets in the fridge to set and either store in the fridge or freeze for later.

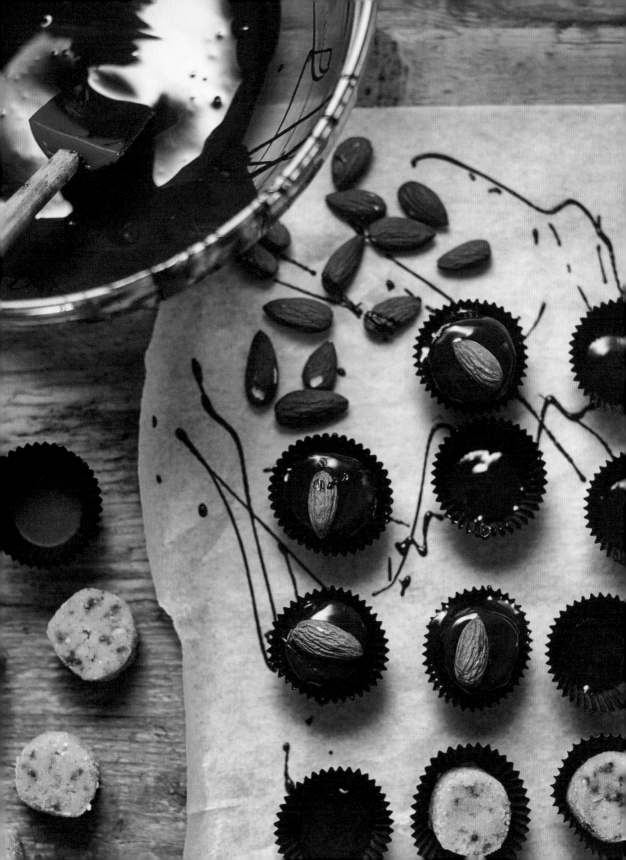

Index and Suppliers

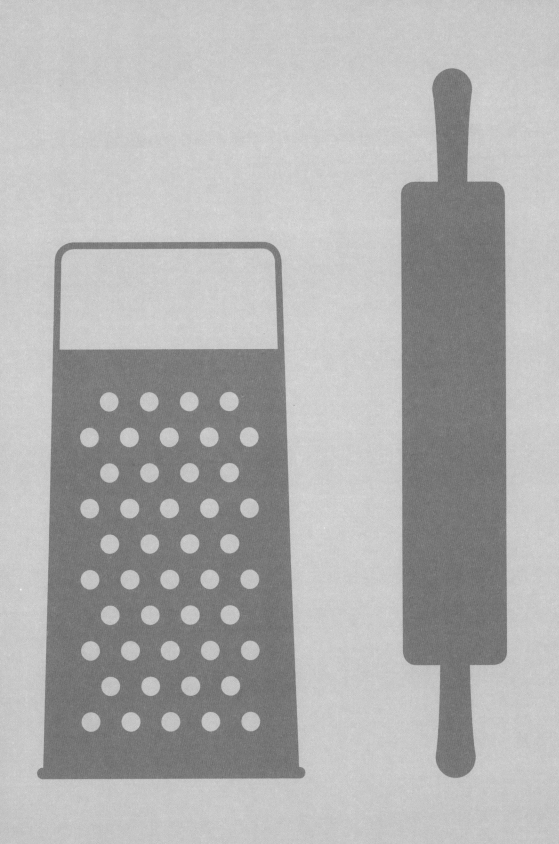

INDEX

SUPPLIERS

www.abelandcole.co.uk
preservative-free bacon
(does contain sugar)

www.brindisa.com
additive-free chorizo made
with pork, spices and salt

www.buywholefoodsonline.co.uk
a wide range of wholefoods,
including stevia in ground-leaf form

www.clonakiltyblackpudding.ie
additive- and gluten-free black pudding
(available from Waitrose)

www.coyo.co.uk
coconut yogurt

www.dovesfarm.co.uk
organic and gluten-free flours,
cereals and pasta

www.frontiercoop.com
alcohol-free almond extract
(also available from Amazon)

www.graigfarm.co.uk
organic meats and fish, plus
additive-free sausages

www.healthysupplies.co.uk
wholefoods online

www.laverstokepark.co.uk
preservative-free bacon and sausages,
plus organic meat (some available
from Ocado)

www.lindt.co.uk
dairy- and soya-free chocolate

www.marigoldhealthfoods.com
pomegranate molasses

www.montezumas.co.uk
dairy- and soya-free chocolate

www.yourorganicsources.com
alcohol-free vanilla powder

www.sumawholesale.com
a wide range of wholefoods for bulk buying

www.sunitafoods.co.uk
dairy-free pesto and organic
lemon juice with no additives

www.tiana-coconut.com
dairy-free butter spread and
other coconut products

www.tyrrellscrisps.co.uk
popcorn with just salt added

www.yorktest.com
testing for food intolerances
using a pin-prick blood sample

ACKNOWLEDGEMENTS

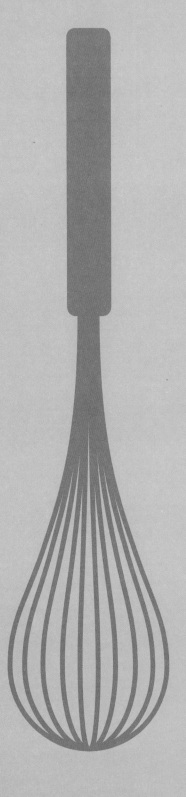

Thanks go to my family and friends who have supported me over the years, even though some of my ideas must have seemed quite radical at times – like cutting out added sugar more than 25 years ago. They have frequently been the guinea pigs, testing those recipes that didn't work as well as the ones that made it into my books. I'd also like to thank those people who have bought my previous books and who have helped to keep the 'Cooking Without' series in print since 1990. I have received a lot of positive feedback, which has helped me to continue creating recipes.

Thanks also go to the staff, past and present, at Thorsons, who have always believed in me. A special thanks to those who have worked so patiently with me on this last book. Between us, I feel we have produced an exciting piece of work. I hope that you do too.

Best wishes,

Barbara

Thorsons

An imprint of HarperCollins*Publishers*
1 London Bridge Street
London SE1 9GF

www.harpercollins.co.uk

First published by Thorsons 2016

13 5 7 9 10 8 6 4 2

Text © Barbara Cousins 2016
Photography © Tom Regester 2016
Food Styling © Katie Giovanni 2016
Illustrations © Simeon Greenaway 2016

© Barbara Cousins 2016
Barbara Cousins asserts the moral right to be identified as the author of this work

A catalogue record of this book is available from the British Library

ISBN 9780008156831

Printed and bound in China by RR Donnelley APS

MIX
Paper from
responsible sources
FSC C007454
www.fsc.org

FSC™ is a non-profit international organisation established to promote the
responsible management of the world's forests. Products carrying the FSC
label are independently certified to assure consumers that they come from
forests that are managed to meet the social, economic and ecological needs
of present and future generations, and other controlled sources.

Find out more about HarperCollins and the environment at
www.harpercollins.co.uk/green

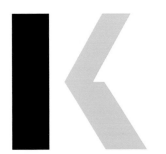

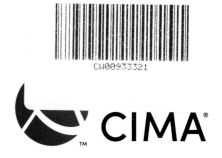

CW00933321

How to access your on-line resources

Kaplan Financial students will have a MyKaplan account and these extra resources will be available to you online. You do not need to register again, as this process was completed when you enrolled. If you are having problems accessing online materials, please ask your course administrator.

If you are not studying with Kaplan and did not purchase your book via a Kaplan website, to unlock your extra online resources please go to www.en-gage.co.uk (even if you have set up an account and registered books previously). You will then need to enter the ISBN number (on the title page and back cover) and the unique pass key number contained in the scratch panel below to gain access.

You will also be required to enter additional information during this process to set up or confirm your account details.

If you purchased through the Kaplan Publishing website you will automatically receive an e-mail invitation to register your details and gain access to your content. If you do not receive the e-mail or book content, please contact Kaplan Publishing.

Your code and information

This code can only be used once for the registration of one book online. This registration and your online content will expire when the final sittings for the examinations covered by this book have taken place. Please allow one hour from the time you submit your book details for us to process your request.

Please scratch the film to access your unique code.

Please be aware that this code is case-sensitive and you will need to include the dashes within the passcode, but not when entering the ISBN.

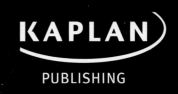

CIMA

Subject E1

Managing Finance in a Digital World

Study Text

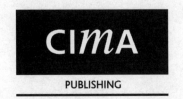

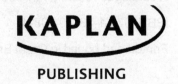

Published by: Kaplan Publishing UK

Unit 2 The Business Centre, Molly Millars Lane, Wokingham, Berkshire RG41 2QZ

Acknowledgements

We are grateful to the CIMA for permission to reproduce past examination questions. The answers to CIMA Exams have been prepared by Kaplan Publishing, except in the case of the CIMA November 2010 and subsequent CIMA Exam answers where the official CIMA answers have been reproduced. Questions from past live assessments have been included by kind permission of CIMA,

Notice

The text in this material and any others made available by any Kaplan Group company does not amount to advice on a particular matter and should not be taken as such. No reliance should be placed on the content as the basis for any investment or other decision or in connection with any advice given to third parties. Please consult your appropriate professional adviser as necessary.

Kaplan Publishing Limited and all other Kaplan group companies expressly disclaim all liability to any person in respect of any losses or other claims, whether direct, indirect, incidental, consequential or otherwise arising in relation to the use of such materials.

Kaplan is not responsible for the content of external websites. The inclusion of a link to a third party website in this text should not be taken as an endorsement.

Kaplan Publishing's learning materials are designed to help students succeed in their examinations. In certain circumstances, CIMA can make post-exam adjustment to a student's mark or grade to reflect adverse circumstances which may have disadvantaged a student's ability to take an exam or demonstrate their normal level of attainment (see CIMA's Special Consideration policy). However, it should be noted that students will not be eligible for special consideration by CIMA if preparation for or performance in a CIMA exam is affected by any failure by their tuition provider to prepare them properly for the exam for any reason including, but not limited to, staff shortages, building work or a lack of facilities etc.

Similarly, CIMA will not accept applications for special consideration on any of the following grounds:

- failure by a tuition provider to cover the whole syllabus
- failure by the student to cover the whole syllabus, for instance as a result of joining a course part way through
- failure by the student to prepare adequately for the exam, or to use the correct pre-seen material
- errors in the Kaplan Official Study Text, including sample (practice) questions or any other Kaplan content or
- errors in any other study materials (from any other tuition provider or publisher).

British Library Cataloguing in Publication Data

A catalogue record for this book is available from the British Library.

ISBN: 978-1-78740-708-4

Printed and bound in Great Britain

Contents

Introduction

How to use the Materials

These official CIMA learning materials have been carefully designed to make your learning experience as easy as possible and to give you the best chances of success in your objective tests.

The product range contains a number of features to help you in the study process. They include:

- a detailed explanation of all syllabus areas

- extensive 'practical' materials

- generous question practice, together with full solutions.

This Study Text has been designed with the needs of home study and distance learning candidates in mind. Such students require very full coverage of the syllabus topics, and also the facility to undertake extensive question practice. However, the Study Text is also ideal for fully taught courses.

The main body of the text is divided into a number of chapters, each of which is organised on the following pattern:

- **Detailed learning outcomes.** These describe the knowledge expected after your studies of the chapter are complete. You should assimilate these before beginning detailed work on the chapter, so that you can appreciate where your studies are leading.

- **Step-by-step topic coverage.** This is the heart of each chapter, containing detailed explanatory text supported where appropriate by worked examples and exercises. You should work carefully through this section, ensuring that you understand the material being explained and can tackle the examples and exercises successfully. Remember that in many cases knowledge is cumulative: if you fail to digest earlier material thoroughly, you may struggle to understand later chapters.

- **Activities.** Some chapters are illustrated by more practical elements, such as comments and questions designed to stimulate discussion.

- **Question practice.** The text contains three styles of question:

  - Exam-style objective test questions (OTQs).

  - 'Integration' questions – these test your ability to understand topics within a wider context. This is particularly important with calculations where OTQs may focus on just one element but an integration question tackles the full calculation, just as you would be expected to do in the workplace.

- – 'Case' style questions – these test your ability to analyse and discuss issues in greater depth, particularly focusing on scenarios that are less clear cut than in the objective tests, and thus provide excellent practice for developing the skills needed for success in the Operational Level Case Study Examination.

- **Solutions.** Avoid the temptation merely to 'audit' the solutions provided. It is an illusion to think that this provides the same benefits as you would gain from a serious attempt of your own. However, if you are struggling to get started on a question you should read the introductory guidance provided at the beginning of the solution, where provided, and then make your own attempt before referring back to the full solution.

If you work conscientiously through this Official CIMA Study Text according to the guidelines above you will be giving yourself an excellent chance of success in your objective tests. Good luck with your studies!

Quality and accuracy are of the utmost importance to us so if you spot an error in any of our products, please send an email to mykaplanreporting@kaplan.com with full details, or follow the link to the feedback form in MyKaplan.

Our Quality Co-ordinator will work with our technical team to verify the error and take action to ensure it is corrected in future editions.

Icon explanations

Definition – These sections explain important areas of knowledge which must be understood and reproduced in an assessment environment.

Supplementary reading – These sections will help to provide a deeper understanding of core areas. The supplementary reading is **NOT** optional reading. It is vital to provide you with the breadth of knowledge you will need to address the wide range of topics within your syllabus that could feature in an assessment question. **Reference to this text is vital when self-studying.**

Test your understanding – Following key points and definitions are exercises which give the opportunity to assess the understanding of these core areas.

Illustration – To help develop an understanding of particular topics. The illustrative examples are useful in preparing for the Test your understanding exercises.

Study technique

Passing exams is partly a matter of intellectual ability, but however accomplished you are in that respect you can improve your chances significantly by the use of appropriate study and revision techniques. In this section we briefly outline some tips for effective study during the earlier stages of your approach to the objective tests. We also mention some techniques that you will find useful at the revision stage.

Planning

To begin with, formal planning is essential to get the best return from the time you spend studying. Estimate how much time in total you are going to need for each subject you are studying. Remember that you need to allow time for revision as well as for initial study of the material.

With your study material before you, decide which chapters you are going to study in each week, and which weeks you will devote to revision and final question practice.

Prepare a written schedule summarising the above and stick to it!

It is essential to know your syllabus. As your studies progress you will become more familiar with how long it takes to cover topics in sufficient depth. Your timetable may need to be adapted to allocate enough time for the whole syllabus.

Students are advised to refer to the examination blueprints (see page P.13 for further information) and the CIMA website, www.cimaglobal.com, to ensure they are up-to-date.

The amount of space allocated to a topic in the Study Text is not a very good guide as to how long it will take you. The syllabus weighting is the better guide as to how long you should spend on a syllabus topic.

Tips for effective studying

(1)   Aim to find a quiet and undisturbed location for your study, and plan as far as possible to use the same period of time each day. Getting into a routine helps to avoid wasting time. Make sure that you have all the materials you need before you begin so as to minimise interruptions.

(2)   Store all your materials in one place, so that you do not waste time searching for items every time you want to begin studying. If you have to pack everything away after each study period, keep your study materials in a box, or even a suitcase, which will not be disturbed until the next time.

(3)   Limit distractions. To make the most effective use of your study periods you should be able to apply total concentration, so turn off all entertainment equipment, set your phones to message mode, and put up your 'do not disturb' sign.

(4)   Your timetable will tell you which topic to study. However, before diving in and becoming engrossed in the finer points, make sure you have an overall picture of all the areas that need to be covered by the end of that session. After an hour, allow yourself a short break and move away from your Study Text. With experience, you will learn to assess the pace you need to work at. Each study session should focus on component learning outcomes – the basis for all questions.

(5)   Work carefully through a chapter, making notes as you go. When you have covered a suitable amount of material, vary the pattern by attempting a practice question. When you have finished your attempt, make notes of any mistakes you made, or any areas that you failed to cover or covered more briefly. Be aware that all component learning outcomes will be tested in each examination.

(6)   Make notes as you study, and discover the techniques that work best for you. Your notes may be in the form of lists, bullet points, diagrams, summaries, 'mind maps', or the written word, but remember that you will need to refer back to them at a later date, so they must be intelligible. If you are on a taught course, make sure you highlight any issues you would like to follow up with your lecturer.

(7)   Organise your notes. Make sure that all your notes, calculations etc. can be effectively filed and easily retrieved later.

Progression

There are two elements of progression that we can measure: how quickly students move through individual topics within a subject (for example within the individual topics of the E1 subject); and how quickly they move from one subject to the next (for example, from E1 to E2). We know that there is an optimum for both, but it can vary from subject to subject and from student to student. However, using data and our experience of student performance over many years, we can make some generalisations.

A fixed period of study set out at the start of a course with key milestones is important. This can be within a subject, for example 'I will finish this topic by 30 June', or for overall achievement, such as 'I want to be qualified by the end of next year'.

Your qualification is cumulative, as earlier papers provide a foundation for your subsequent studies, so do not allow there to be too big a gap between one subject and another. For example, E1 *Managing finance in a digital world* builds on your knowledge of the finance function from certificate level and lays the foundations for E2 *Managing performance* and all strategic papers particularly E3 *Strategic management* and P3 *Risk management*.

Also, it is important to realise that the Operational Case Study (OCS) tests knowledge of all subjects within the Operational level. Please note that candidates will need to return to this material when studying OCS as it forms a significant part of the OCS syllabus content.

We know that exams encourage techniques that lead to some degree of short term retention, the result being that you will simply forget much of what you have already learned unless it is refreshed (look up Ebbinghaus Forgetting Curve for more details on this). This makes it more difficult as you move from one subject to another: not only will you have to learn the new subject, you will also have to relearn all the underpinning knowledge as well. This is very inefficient and slows down your overall progression which makes it more likely you may not succeed at all.

In addition, delaying your studies slows your path to qualification which can have negative impacts on your career, postponing the opportunity to apply for higher level positions and therefore higher pay.

You can use the following diagram showing the whole structure of your qualification to help you keep track of your progress. Make sure you seek appropriate advice if you are unsure about your progression through the qualification.

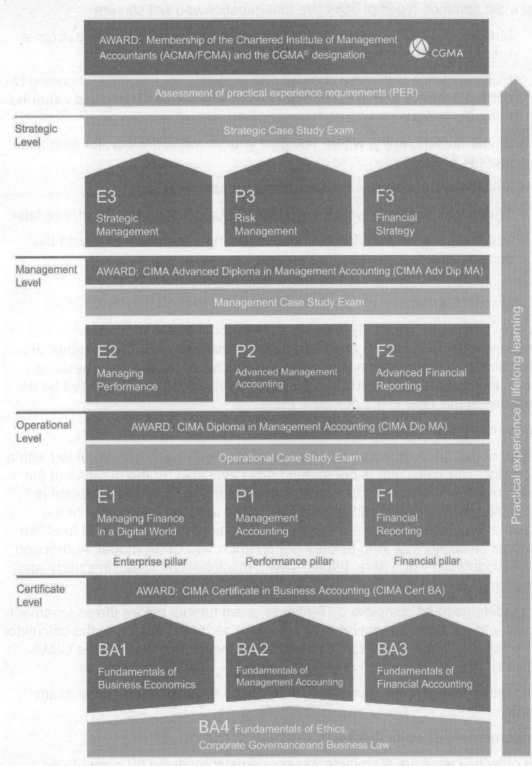

Reproduced with permission from CIMA

Objective test

Objective test questions require you to choose or provide a response to a question whose correct answer is predetermined.

The most common types of objective test question you will see are:

- Multiple choice, where you have to choose the correct answer(s) from a list of possible answers. This could either be numbers or text.

- Multiple choice with more choices and answers, for example, choosing two correct answers from a list of eight possible answers. This could either be numbers or text.

- Single numeric entry, where you give your numeric answer, for example, profit is $10,000.

- Multiple entry, where you give several numeric answers.

- True/false questions, where you state whether a statement is true or false.

- Matching pairs of text, for example, matching a technical term with the correct definition.

- Other types could be matching text with graphs and labelling graphs/diagrams.

In every chapter of this Study Text we have introduced these types of questions, but obviously we have had to label answers A, B, C etc. rather than using click boxes. For convenience, we have retained quite a few questions where an initial scenario leads to a number of sub-questions. There will be no questions of this type in the objective tests.

Guidance re CIMA on-screen calculator

As part of the CIMA objective test software, candidates are now provided with a calculator. This calculator is on-screen and is available for the duration of the assessment. The calculator is available in each of the objective tests and is accessed by clicking the calculator button in the top left hand corner of the screen at any time during the assessment. Candidates are permitted to utilise personal calculators as long as they are an approved CIMA model. Authorised CIMA models are listed here: https://www.cimaglobal.com/Studying/study-and-resources/.

All candidates must complete a 15-minute exam tutorial before the assessment begins and will have the opportunity to familiarise themselves with the calculator and practise using it. The exam tutorial is also available online via the CIMA website.

Candidates may practise using the calculator by accessing the online exam tutorial.

Fundamentals of objective tests

The objective tests are 90-minute assessments comprising 60 compulsory questions, with one or more parts. There will be no choice and all questions should be attempted. All elements of a question must be answered correctly for the question to be marked correctly. All questions are equally weighted.

CIMA syllabus 2019 – Structure of subjects and learning outcomes

Details regarding the content of the new CIMA syllabus can be located within the CIMA 2019 professional syllabus document.

Each subject within the syllabus is divided into a number of broad syllabus topics. The topics contain one or more lead learning outcomes, related component learning outcomes and indicative knowledge content.

A learning outcome has two main purposes:

(a)   To define the skill or ability that a well prepared candidate should be able to exhibit in the examination.

(b)   To demonstrate the approach likely to be taken in examination questions.

The learning outcomes are part of a hierarchy of learning objectives. The verbs used at the beginning of each learning outcome relate to a specific learning objective, e.g.

Calculate the break-even point, profit target, margin of safety and profit/volume ratio for a single product or service.

The verb '**calculate**' indicates a level three learning objective. The following tables list the verbs that appear in the syllabus learning outcomes and examination questions.

The examination blueprints and representative task statements

CIMA have also published examination blueprints giving learners clear expectations regarding what is expected of them.

The blueprint is structured as follows:

*   Exam content sections (reflecting the syllabus document)

*   Lead and component outcomes (reflecting the syllabus document)

*   Representative task statements.

A representative task statement is a plain English description of what a CIMA finance professional should know and be able to do.

The content and skill level determine the language and verbs used in the representative task.

CIMA will test up to the level of the task statement in the objective tests (an objective test question on a particular topic could be set at a lower level than the task statement in the blueprint).

The task statements in the blueprint are representative and are not intended to be (nor should they be viewed as) an all-inclusive list of tasks that may be tested on the Examination. It also should be noted that the number of tasks associated with a particular content group or topic is not indicative of the extent such content group, topic or related skill level will be assessed on the test.

The format of the objective test blueprints follows that of the published syllabus for the 2019 CIMA Professional Qualification.

Weightings for content sections are also included in the individual subject blueprints.

CIMA VERB HIERARCHY

CIMA place great importance on the definition of verbs in structuring objective tests. It is therefore crucial that you understand the verbs in order to appreciate the depth and breadth of a topic and the level of skill required. The objective tests will focus on levels one, two and three of the CIMA hierarchy of verbs. However, they will also test levels four and five, especially at the management and strategic levels.

Skill level	Verbs used	Definition
Level 5 **Evaluation** How you are expected to use your learning to evaluate, make decisions or recommendations	Advise	Counsel, inform or notify
	Assess	Evaluate or estimate the nature, ability or quality of
	Evaluate	Appraise or assess the value of
	Recommend	Propose a course of action
	Review	Assess and evaluate in order, to change if necessary
Level 4 **Analysis** How you are expected to analyse the detail of what you have learned	Align	Arrange in an orderly way
	Analyse	Examine in detail the structure of
	Communicate	Share or exchange information
	Compare and contrast	Show the similarities and/or differences between
	Develop	Grow and expand a concept
	Discuss	Examine in detail by argument
	Examine	Inspect thoroughly
	Interpret	Translate into intelligible or familiar terms
	Monitor	Observe and check the progress of
	Prioritise	Place in order of priority or sequence for action
	Produce	Create or bring into existence
Level 3 **Application** How you are expected to apply your knowledge	Apply	Put to practical use
	Calculate	Ascertain or reckon mathematically
	Conduct	Organise and carry out
	Demonstrate	Prove with certainty or exhibit by practical means
	Prepare	Make or get ready for use
	Reconcile	Make or prove consistent/compatible

Skill level	Verbs used	Definition
Level 2 Comprehension What you are expected to understand	Describe	Communicate the key features of
	Distinguish	Highlight the differences between
	Explain	Make clear or intelligible/state the meaning or purpose of
	Identify	Recognise, establish or select after consideration
	Illustrate	Use an example to describe or explain something
Level 1 Knowledge What you are expected to know	List	Make a list of
	State	Express, fully or clearly, the details/facts of
	Define	Give the exact meaning of
	Outline	Give a summary of

Information concerning formulae and tables will be provided via the CIMA website, www.cimaglobal.com.

SYLLABUS GRIDS

E1: Managing Finance in a Digital World

How the finance function is organised

Content weighting

Content area	Weighting
A Role of the finance function	20%
B Technology in a digital world	20%
C Data and Information in a digital world	20%
D Shape and structure of the finance function	20%
E Finance Interacting with the organisation	20%
	100%

E1A: Role of the finance function

This section examines the roles that finance plays in organisations and why. It describes in detail the activities that finance professionals perform to fulfil these roles. Consequently, it is the foundation of the whole qualification and answers the question: what do finance professionals do and why? It provides links with other topics within the subject and what is covered in other areas of the Operational Level.

Lead outcome	Component outcome	Topics to be covered	Explanatory notes	Study Text Chapter
1. Explain the roles of the finance function in organisations.	Explain how the finance function: a. Enables organisations to create and preserve value b. Shapes how organisations create and preserve value c. Narrates how organisations create and preserve value	• The fast-changing and unpredictable contexts in which organisations operate • Enabling value creation through planning, forecasting and resource allocation • Shaping value creation through performance management and control • Narrating the value creation story through corporate reporting • The role of ethics in the role of the finance function	Describe the increasingly disruptive contexts in which organisations and their finance teams operate and how these contexts shape the role of finance. Take each role and show how finance performs it in a typical organisational setting. The coverage should be introductory and brief. It is meant to set the scene for subsequent sections and draw a link between the roles and the topics that will be covered in other areas of the Operational Level.	1
2. Describe the activities that finance professionals perform to fulfil the roles.	Describe how the finance function: a. Collates data to prepare information about organisations b. Provides insight to users by analysing information c. Communicates insight to influence users d. Supports the implementation of decisions to achieve the desired impact e. Connects the different activities to each other	• How data is collected, cleaned and connected by finance • Types of analysis to produce insights • How finance communicates to influence key stakeholders (audiences, frequency, format, etc.) • How finance uses resource allocation and performance management to enable organisations to achieve their objectives • Potential impact of technology	Use 'information to impact' framework to describe the primary activities finance professionals perform. Relate it to how data is generated, transformed and used. Link it to how technology could be used to improve the productivity of finance professionals in these areas and the threat of automation.	2

E1B: Technology in a digital world

This section focuses on the technologies that define and drive the digital world in which finance operates. It provides awareness of the technologies used in organisations and deepens understanding of the impact of the technologies on what finance does. It draws on the issues raised in the previous section about the role of finance and the activities finance performs to fulfil these roles. Given that the digital world is underpinned by technology and the use of data, this section provides a foundation to the next section on data.

Lead outcome	Component outcome	Topics to be covered	Explanatory notes	Study Text Chapter
1. Outline and explain the technologies that affect business and finance.	a. Outline the key features of the fourth industrial revolution. b. Outline and explain the key technologies that define and drive the digital world.	• Characteristics and dynamics of the fourth industrial revolution • Cloud computing • Big data analytics • Process automation • Artificial intelligence • Data visualisation • Blockchain • Internet of things • Mobile • 3-D printing	The aim is to create awareness of the technologies that drive the digital world and how they interact with each other. The technologies outlined by the major advisory firms and the World Economic Forum digital transformation initiative provide the material on which learning and related activities can be based.	5
2. Examine how the finance function uses digital technologies to fulfil its roles.	Examine how finance uses the following to guide how it performs its roles: a. Digital technology b. Digital mindsets c. Automation and the future of work d. Ethics of technology usage	• How finance uses technologies listed above • Areas of finance susceptible to automation and why • New areas for finance to focus on • Digital mindsets for finance • Ethics of the use of technology	Examine how finance professionals use the relevant technologies to fulfil their roles. Explain how the technologies affect various activities finance professionals perform in the 'information to impact' framework. The intention is to move from creating awareness to generating understanding of how finance can use these technologies to increase its value and relevance to organisations.	6

E1C: Data and information in a digital world

This section draws out one of the major implications of using technology in organisations and the finance function – namely the collection and processing of information can be done more effectively by machines rather than by people. It asserts that the role of finance professionals should be to use data to create and preserve value for organisations. Five ways of using data are examined. The key competencies required to use data in these ways are also highlighted. The primary objective is to help finance professionals understand what they can do with data and how to build the skills needed to use data.

Lead outcome	Component outcome	Topics to be covered	Explanatory notes	Study Text Chapter
1. Describe the ways in which data is used by the finance function.	Identify the ways in which the finance function uses data: a. In a general sense b. Specifically in each of the primary activities of finance	Using data for: • Decision-making • Understanding the customer • Developing customer value proposition • Enhancing operational efficiency • Monetising data • Ethics of data usage	Build on the previous section on technology to explain why, in the digital world, finance professionals must place more focus on using information than on collecting and/or processing information. Outline and describe the various uses of information. Link them to the primary activities that the finance function performs and to the topics to be covered in other modules of the Operational Level.	7
2. Explain the competencies required to use data to create and preserve value for organisations.	Explain the competencies that finance professionals need in: a. Data strategy and planning b. Data engineering, extraction and mining c. Data modelling, manipulation and analysis d. Data and insight communication	• Assessment of data needs • Extraction, transformation and loading (ETL) systems • Business Intelligence (BI) systems • Big data analytics • Data visualisation	Highlight and explain the data competencies required in the digital world. Locate where finance has a competitive advantage and where finance will need to work with data scientists.	8

E1D: Shape and structure of the finance function

This section brings together the implications of the previous sections. It reveals how the finance function is structured and shaped. This structure and shape enables finance to perform its role in the organisation and with other internal and external stakeholders. In this sense, it prepares candidates for the next section, which looks at how finance interacts with key internal stakeholders in operations, marketing and human resources.

Lead outcome	Component outcome	Topics to be covered	Explanatory notes	Study Text Chapter
1. Describe the structure and shape of the finance function.	Describe the: a. Evolution of the shape of the finance function b. Shape of the finance function in the digital era	• Structure of the finance function from the roles that generate information to the roles that turn information into insight and communicate insight to decision-makers • Hierarchical shape of finance function • Shared services and outsourcing of finance operations • Retained finance • Automation and diamond shape of finance function	Introduce candidates to the structure of the finance function and outline the broad areas of finance such as finance operations, external reporting, financial planning and analysis (FP&A), decision support etc. Describe the evolving shape of the finance function from the triangle to the diamond shape. Link the description to the impact of digital technology and automation on the finance function.	3
2. Explain what each level of the finance function does.	Explain the activities of: a. Finance operations b. Specialist areas including financial reporting and financial planning and analysis (FP&A) c. Strategic partnering for value d. Strategic leadership of the finance team	• Finance operations to generate information and preliminary insight • FP&A, taxation, corporate reporting, decision support to produce insight • Business partnering to influence organisation to make appropriate decisions • Leading the finance team to create the required impact for the organisation	The focus is the diamond shape and the four levels within this shape. Explain what each level does, the relationship between the levels, and the link between the levels and the basic finance activities covered under the role of finance.	4

E1E: Finance interacting with the organisation

The finance function is not the only area of activity in organisations. Finance joins with others to create and preserve value for their organisations. This section brings together what has been learned in the previous section to describe how finance can interact with other parts of the organisation to achieve the objectives of finance, those other areas and crucially the objectives of the whole organisation. The aim is to show how finance can work collaboratively in a connected (and joined-up) organisation and not in isolation.

Lead outcome	Component outcome	Topics to be covered	Explanatory notes	Study Text Chapter
1. Describe how the finance function interacts with operations.	Describe: a. Main role of operations b. Areas of interface with finance c. Key performance indicators	• Process management • Product and service management • Supply chain management	Describe how finance plays its role by interacting with the rest of the organisation. Bring together the issues raised in the previous sections and link them to what the other areas of the organisations do. For example, address how finance and marketing interact using data and collaborative technology to achieve organisational goals and the individual functional goals of both finance and marketing. Describe how the use of KPIs influence these interactions and how the KPIs of finance and these areas can be aligned to ensure they work together effectively.	9
2. Describe how the finance function interacts with sales and marketing.	Describe: a. Main role of sales and marketing b. Areas of interface with finance c. Key performance indicators	• Market segmentation • Big data analytics in marketing • Channel management • Sales forecasting and management		10
3. Describe how the finance function interacts with human resources.	Describe: a. Main role of human resources b. Areas of interface with finance c. Key performance indicators	• Staff acquisition • Staff development • Performance management • Motivation and reward systems		11
4. Describe how the finance function interacts with IT.	Describe: a. Main role of IT b. Areas of interface with finance c. Key performance indicators	• IT infrastructure • IT systems support • Costs and benefits of IT systems		12

P.22

The roles of the finance function in organisations

Chapter learning objectives

Lead	Component
A1: Explain the roles of the finance function in organisations.	Explain how the finance function: (a) Enables organisations to create and preserve value (b) Shapes how organisations create and preserve value (c) Narrates how organisations create and preserve value

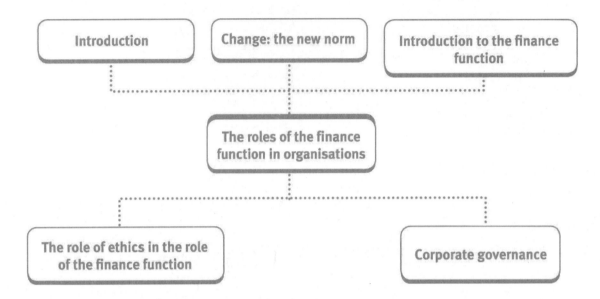

1   Introduction

Before we look at the roles of the finance function in organisations, it is useful to understand the overall purpose of E1 and how it fits within CIMA's Professional Qualification.

1.1   The CIMA Professional Qualification

The CIMA Professional Qualification will give you the skills that you need to work as a confident and competent management accountant in an age where change is the new norm so that you can guide and lead your organisation's success.

We live in an age of technological advancements and innovation and these factors are transforming the way in which we work and live. The World Economic Forum calls it the **4ᵗʰ Industrial Revolution** and this revolution is having a huge impact on the finance function and, as a result, the skillset of a management accountant.

1.2   The Operational Level

'Finance' runs through the Operational level:

- **P1** – focuses on '**what**' the finance function does
- **F1** – focuses on '**what**' the finance function does and its **implications**
- **E1** – focuses on '**how**' the finance function is organised

At the Operational level the emphasis will be on **remembering** and **understanding** but **some insight** regarding specific problems or situations may also be required. On completion of this level you will be able to work with others in the organisation to use appropriate data and technology to translate medium-term decisions into short-term actionable plans.

1.3 Paper E1: Managing Finance in a Digital World

There are five connected areas to the syllabus:

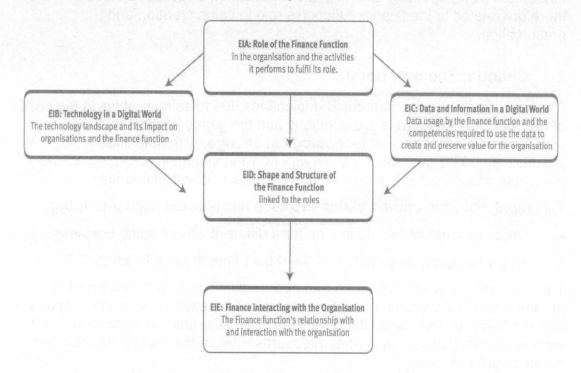

EIA: Role of the Finance Function
in the organisation and the activities
it performs to fulfil its role.

EIB: Technology in a Digital World
The technology landscape and its impact on
organisations and the finance function

EIC: Data and Information in a Digital World
Data usage by the finance function and the
competencies required to use the data to
create and preserve value for the organisation

EID: Shape and Structure of
the Finance Function
linked to the roles

EIE: Finance Interacting with the Organisation
The Finance function's relationship with
and interaction with the organisation

1.4 The roles of the finance function in organisations

This chapter covers **syllabus area A1**, '**explain the roles of the finance function in organisations**'. It describes in detail the activities that finance professionals perform to fulfil these roles. Consequently it is the foundation of the whole qualification and answers the question 'what do finance professionals do and why?'. It provides links with other syllabus areas and what is covered in other modules of the Operational level.

By the end of this chapter you should understand how the finance function enables, shapes and narrates value creation through its **roles** of:

- planning
- forecasting
- resource allocation
- performance management and control and
- financial (corporate) reporting.

These roles are changing due to the **continuous change** that is impacting all organisations and so before introducing the roles of the finance function we will begin our discussion of this syllabus area by briefly looking at change.

The chapter concludes with a discussion of **ethics**, **corporate social responsibility** and **corporate governance** since these areas will be fundamental underpinning factors in an organisation's sustained value and are therefore related to the finance function's role in value creation and preservation.

2   Change: The new norm

Change is the new norm in many organisations due to seismic shifts in the level of **competition**, customers' expectations and the global political outlook combined with a fast pace of **technological change** (with machines increasingly taking over routine tasks and new technologies emerging across the global economy this is considered to be the key driver of change).

This **rapid** and often **unpredictable** evolution has resulted huge **disruption**:

- Organisations are having to plan for a different way of doing business.

- There has been an evolution of the roles of the finance function.

These changes present both risks and opportunities and will be explored in greater depth in subsequent chapters but before we explore what the changes are and how they will impact the organisation and the finance function within it, we need to firstly understand what the overall roles of the finance function are within an organisation.

Illustration 1 – Change and impact on organisations

Extraordinary economic changes are happening at such a fast pace driven by technology innovations and advances. The digital world created has been cited as the main reason just over half of companies on the Fortune 500 have disappeared since the year 2000. Those companies that have disappeared, such as Blockbusters in 2010 and Kodak in 2012, may well have been using outdated 20th century business thinking and concepts trying to build sustainable organisations in the 21st century digital world.

3   Introduction to the finance function

Before focusing on the finance function it is useful to remind ourselves of the different types of organisations that exist and also of the different functions that exist within an organisation.

3.1 Different types of organisation

As we know from our earlier studies, there are many different types of organisation:

- **Profit seeking organisations, i.e. businesses** include companies (Ltd or plc), partnerships and sole traders. Their primary objective is the maximisation of the wealth of their owners.

- **Not-for-profit organisations (NFPOs)** include public sector organisations (such as schools and hospitals) and private sector organisations (such as charities and non-governmental organisations (NGOs)). These organisations do not see profit as their primary objective but exist to maximise the benefit to beneficiaries.

Throughout the text the concepts that are introduced are done so mainly in relation to businesses. However, it is worth noting that much of the discussion is just as relevant to NFPOs.

Types of NFPO

Two main types of NFPO exist:

- **Public sector organisations** are operated by the government and exist to provide a service for the population and the community.

- **Private sector organisations** are operated by the private sector (i.e. not the government). There are two sub-types:

  - **Third sector organisations** aim to make a different to society and include charities, community groups/clubs and social enterprises.

  - **Non-governmental organisations (NGOs)** are local, national or international voluntary groups that aim to address issues (such as health, human rights or the environment) to support the public good. Examples include Amnesty International and Save the Children.

Test your understanding 1

Which THREE of the following are not-for-profit organisations?

A   private school

B   medical research charity

C   local publically funded hospital

D   sole trader who is making a loss

E   private limited company

F   local government agency

3.2 The functions of an organisation

The main functions of a business are:

- operations
- sales and marketing
- human resources (HR)
- IT and
- **finance**.

This reflects the model of the business as taking three basic types of resource – material, labour and money – to produce goods and services which generate profit.

It is a major part of the finance function's work to look after the business's money. The finance function's role in managing the financial resources of the organisation and providing information to help economic decision making will be integral to the effectiveness of the finance function.

3.3 The roles of the finance function in organisations

The finance function plays **three key roles**. A finance function:

- **ENABLES** an organisation to create and preserve value though planning, forecasting and resource allocation:

  - **Planning:** the finance function will have an important role in preparing plans to assist the organisation in achieving its objectives and formulating relevant strategies. One of the main types of planning carried out at the operational level will be budgeting.

  - **Forecasting:** the preparation of forecasts, for example of future sales or material prices, will be an important role of the finance function at the operational level.

  - **Resource allocation:** an important role of the finance function will be in working out which resources (for example, labour, material, machinery, finance) the organisation will require to achieve its objectives.

  In the CIMA Professional Qualification, the 'enables' element is encompassed in the Enterprise pillar.

- **SHAPES HOW** an organisation creates and preserves value through performance management and control:

  - **Performance management:** the finance function has an important role in the management of performance and the achievement of the organisation's plans and budgets.

For example, it will help to prepare information for internal management such as performance measures. These measures will assist in monitoring the performance of the organisation. The performance measures may be quantitative, i.e. numerical (such as sales, profit or units produced) or may be qualitative, i.e. non-numerical (such as customer satisfaction or levels of innovation).

– **Control:** this will be an important part of effective performance management; actual performance will be compared to planned performance to identify any differences. Variance analysis may be carried out as part of this role. The identification of these differences may result in a reassessment or amendment of the original plans, strategies or budgets.

In the CIMA Professional Qualification, the 'shapes how' element is encompassed in the Performance pillar.

- **NARRATES HOW** an organisation creates and preserves value through financial (corporate) reporting:

  – Financial reporting (also called corporate reporting): an important role of the finance function is in preparing comprehensive reports intended to give information to shareholders and/or other interested people about the organisation's activities and performance throughout the year.

  In the CIMA Professional Qualification, the 'narrates how' element is encompassed in the 'Financial' pillar.

If it plays these roles effectively, then finance professionals are valuable to organisations.

Important note: This is a brief introduction to the roles of the finance function. However, this area is highly examinable and will be returned to and built upon in subsequent chapters. It will underpin much of the discussion in these later chapters.

4 The role of ethics in the role of the finance function

4.1 The ethical responsibilities of the organisation and individuals

As mentioned previously (in section 1.4), ethics will be a fundamental underpinning factor in the organisation's sustained value creation.

The roles that the finance function performs should be carried out in an ethical way, with integrity and professionalism.

The professional accountant has a special role in promoting ethical behaviour throughout the business.

Ethics, business ethics and ethical dilemmas

Ethics is the system of moral principles that examines the concept of right and wrong.

Business ethics is the application of ethical values to business behaviour.

An **ethical dilemma** involves a situation where a decision-maker has to decide what is the 'right' or 'wrong' thing to do. Examples of ethical dilemmas can be found throughout all aspects of business operations:

Accounting issues

- Creative accounting to boost or suppress reported profits.

- Directors' pay arrangements – should directors continue to receive large pay packets even if the company is performing poorly?

- Should bribes be paid to facilitate contracts, especially in countries where such payments are commonplace?

- Insider trading, where for example directors may be tempted to buy shares in their company knowing that a favourable announcement about to be made should boost the share price.

Production issues

- Should the company produce certain products at all, for example guns, pornography, tobacco, alcoholic drinks aimed at teenagers?

- Should the company be concerned about the effects on the environment of its production processes?

- Should the company test its products on animals?

Sales and marketing issues

- Price fixing and anti-competitive behaviour may be overt and illegal or may be more subtle.

- Is it ethical to target advertising at children, for example for fast food or for expensive toys at Christmas?

- Should products be advertised by junk mail or spam email?

Personnel (HRM) issues

- Employees should not be favoured or discriminated against on the basis of gender, race, religion, age, disability, etc.

- The contract of employment must offer a fair balance of power between employee and employer.

- The workplace must be a safe and healthy place to operate in.

4.2 CIMA's ethical guidelines

Management accountants have a duty to observe the highest standards of conduct and integrity, and to uphold the good standing and reputation of their profession.

The Code of Ethics for Professional Accountants, published by The International Federation of Accountants (IFAC), forms the basis for the ethical codes of many accountancy bodies, including CIMA.

CIMA's Code of Ethics, based on IFAC's five ethical principles, seeks to help management accountants in their day to day role. It helps management accountants to identify areas where ethical pressures may exist and provides a recommended course of action for their resolution.

In order to achieve the objectives of the accounting profession, professional accountants have to observe five fundamental principles:

Fundamental Principle	Interpretation
Integrity	Integrity means being straightforward, honest and truthful in all professional and business relationships.
Objectivity	Objectivity means not allowing bias, conflict of interest, or the influence of other people to override your professional judgement.
Professional competence and due care	This is an ongoing commitment to maintain your level of professional knowledge and skill so that your client or employer receives a competent professional service. Work should be completed carefully, thoroughly and diligently, in accordance with relevant technical and professional standards.
Confidentiality	This means respecting the confidential nature of information you acquire through professional relationships such as past or current employment. You should not disclose such information unless you have specific permission or a legal or professional duty to do so. You should also never use confidential information for your or another person's advantage.
Professional behaviour	This requires you to comply with relevant laws and regulations. You must also avoid any action that could negatively affect the reputation of the profession.

> ### Test your understanding 2
>
> John is a CIMA Member in Practice, and advises a range of individual clients and organisations. John has been asked, by his brother, to prepare the accounts for his brother's company. John's brother says that he wants the reported profit to be as high as possible, as he will soon be applying to the bank for loan finance.
>
> **To do this would be in breach of which fundamental ethical principle (according to CIMA's Code of Ethics)?**
>
> A   integrity
>
> B   objectivity
>
> C   professional competence and due care
>
> D   confidentiality
>
> E   professional behaviour

4.3 Why business ethics are important

In addition to the professional accountant having a role in promoting ethical behaviour within an organisation, the organisation as a whole, and all of the individuals within it, are expected to act in an ethical way.

Businesses are part of society. Society expects its individuals to behave properly, and similarly expects companies to operate to certain standards. Acceptable business ethics may comprise as a minimum:

- paying staff **decent wages** and pensions
- providing **good working conditions** for staff
- **paying suppliers** in line with agreed terms
- **sourcing supplies** carefully
- using sustainable or **renewable sources**
- being **open and honest** with customers.

However, apart from any moral duty to be ethical, the prime purpose of a company is to maximise shareholder wealth and the chance of this happening is increased by the adoption of ethical behaviour since:

- Ethical behaviour is likely to be favoured by:
  - customers: resulting in higher sales volumes and/or prices.
  - employees: resulting in the attraction/retention of the best employees and increased employee productivity.
  - business collaborators: resulting in increased opportunities for profitable projects.

- Ethical behaviour reduces risk and gives access to cheaper funds which, in turn, increase project profitability.

- Unethical behaviour will, at some point be discovered resulting in a damage to reputation and potential legal charges.

Illustration 2 – Why business ethics are important

The Fairtrade mark is a label on consumer products that guarantees that disadvantaged producers in the developing world are getting a fair deal. For example, the majority of coffee around the world is grown by small farmers who sell their produce through a local co-operative. Fairtrade coffee guarantees to pay a price to producers that covers the cost of sustainable production and also an extra premium that is invested in local development projects.

Consumers in the developed world may be willing to pay a premium price for Fairtrade products, knowing that the products are grown in an ethical and sustainable fashion.

Test your understanding 3

Which of the following would potentially be ethical concerns for a cosmetics manufacturer? Choose all that apply.

A   The amount of chemicals included in their products.

B   The quality of the cosmetics.

C   How much it pays its staff.

D   How much its supplier pays its staff.

E   The way the cosmetics are advertised.

4.4   Corporate codes of ethics

Most companies (especially if they are large) have approached the concept of business ethics by creating a written code of ethics (a set of internal policies) and instructing employees to follow them. These policies can either be **broad** generalisations (**a corporate ethics statement**) or can contain **specific** rules (**a corporate ethics code**).

There is no standard list of contents – it will vary between different organisations. Typically, however, it may contain guidelines on issues such as honesty, integrity and customer focus.

It is becoming more commonplace for organisations (particularly those that are larger and/or those that operate in sectors such as finance or healthcare) to appoint **Ethics Officers** (also known as Compliance Officers). The Ethics Officer monitors the application of the policies and is available to discuss ethical dilemmas with employees where needed.

4.5 Corporate social responsibility

This follows on from our discussion of ethics but before we review 'corporate social responsibility', we need to define the term 'stakeholder'.

 A **stakeholder** is a group or individual, who has an interest in what the organisation does, or an expectation of the organisation.

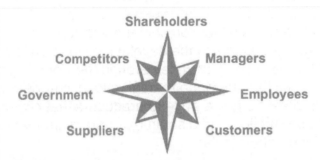

Stakeholders can be broadly categorised into three categories; internal, connected and external.

Internal

Internal stakeholders are intimately connected to the organisation, and their objectives are likely to have a strong influence on how it is run. Internal stakeholders include:

Stakeholder	Need/expectation
employees	pay, working conditions and job security
managers/directors	status, pay, bonus, job security

Connected

Connected stakeholders either invest in or have dealings with the firm. They include:

Stakeholder	Need/expectation
shareholders	dividends and capital growth and the continuation of the business
customers	value-for-money products and services
suppliers	paid promptly
finance providers	repayment of finance

External

These stakeholders do not tend to have a direct link to the organisation but can influence or be influenced by its activities. They include:

Stakeholder	Need/expectation
community at large	will not want their lives to be negatively impacted by business decisions
environmental pressure groups	the organisation does not harm the external environment
government	provision of taxes and jobs and compliance with legislation
trade unions	to take an active part in the decision-making process

The needs/expectations of different stakeholder groups may conflict. In the event of conflict, an organisation will need to decide which stakeholders' needs are more important. This will commonly be the most dominant stakeholder. If the organisation is having difficulty deciding who the dominant stakeholder is, they can use **Mendelow's power-interest matrix**.

Level of interest

		Low	High
Level of power	Low	Minimal effort	Keep informed
	High	Keep satisfied	Key players

By plotting each stakeholder according to the power that they have over an organisation and the interest they have in a particular decision, the dominant stakeholder(s), i.e. the key player(s) can be identified. The needs of the key players must be considered during the formulation and evaluation of new strategies.

Illustration 3 – Stakeholders' influence

The airline, Ryanair, has regular labour relations problems with pilots, cabin attendants and check-in staff. For example, in recent years pilots at Ryanair threatened a mass strike (and possible desertion to a competitor airline) if there were not significant improvements in pay and conditions. Ryanair cannot operate without these staff so these employees have great power and have shown that they are willing to exercise that power.

Example of stakeholder management

R is a high-class hotel situated in a thriving city. It is part of a worldwide hotel group owned by a large number of shareholders. Individuals hold the majority of shares, each holding a small number, and financial institutions hold the rest. The hotel provides full amenities, including a heated swimming pool, as well as the normal facilities of bars, restaurants and good quality accommodation. There are many other hotels in the city, all of which compete with R. The city in which R is situated is old and attracts many foreign visitors, especially in the summer season

The main stakeholders with whom relationships need to be established and maintained by management and the importance of maintaining these relationships is as follows.

Internal stakeholders

The employees and the managers of the hotel are the main link with the guests and the service they provide is vital to the quality of the hotel as guests' experience at the hotel will be determined by their attitude and approach.

Managers should ensure that employees deliver the highest level of service and are well trained and committed.

Connected stakeholders

The shareholders of the hotel will be concerned with a steady flow of income, possible capital growth and continuation of the business. Relationships should be developed and maintained with the shareholders, especially those operating on behalf of institutions. Management must try to achieve improvements in their returns by ensuring that customers are satisfied and are willing to return.

Each guest will seek good service and satisfaction. Different types of guests, for example business versus tourist, will have different needs and managers should regularly analyse the customer database to ensure that these needs are met.

Suppliers should be selected very carefully to ensure that services and goods provided (for example, food and laundry) continue to add to the quality of the hotel and to customer satisfaction. Suppliers will be concerned with being paid promptly for goods. Maintaining a good relationship with suppliers will ensure their continued support of the hotel.

External stakeholders

The management of the hotel must maintain close relationships with the authorities to ensure they comply with legislation. Examples of external stakeholders include fire and safety authorities and food hygiene authorities. Failure to do so could result in the hotel being closed down.

Stakeholder conflict

The needs/expectations of the different stakeholder groups may conflict. Some of the typical conflicts are shown below:

Stakeholders	Conflict
Employees versus managers	Jobs/wages versus bonus
Customers versus shareholders	Product quality/service levels versus profits/dividends
General public versus shareholders	Effect on the environment versus profit/dividends
Managers versus shareholders	Independence versus growth by merger/takeover

It is important that an organisation meets the needs of the most dominant stakeholders, but the needs of the other stakeholders should also be considered – nearly every decision becomes a compromise. For example, the firm will have to earn a satisfactory return for its shareholders whilst paying reasonable wages.

Now that we understand what we mean by 'stakeholders' we can introduce the concept of 'corporate social responsibility'.

 Corporate social responsibility (CSR) refers to the idea that a company should be sensitive to the needs and wants of all the stakeholders in its business operations, not just the shareholders.

As such, business ethics are just one dimension of CSR.

A socially responsible company may consider:

- the environmental impact of production or consumption, for example due to the use of non-renewable resources or non-recyclable inputs

- the health impact for consumers of certain products, for example tobacco and alcohol

- the fair treatment of employees

- whether it is right to experiment on animals

- the safety of products and production processes.

Traditionalists argue that companies should operate solely to make money for shareholders and that it is not a company's role to worry about social responsibilities.

The **modern view** is that by aligning the company's core values with the values of society, the company can improve its reputation and ensure it has a long-term future due to the following:

- **Differentiation** (making the product/service different from its competitors) – the firm's CSR strategy (for example with regards to the environment, experimentation on animals or to product safety) can act as a method differentiation.

- **High calibre staff** will be attracted and retained due to the firm's CSR policies.

- **Brand strengthening** – due to the firm's honest approach.

- **Lower costs** – can be achieved in a number of ways, for example due to the use of less packaging or energy.

- The identification of **new market opportunities** and of **changing social expectations**.

An overall **increase in profitability** should be achieved as a result of the above – good CSR should hopefully contribute to an increase in revenue and a reduction in costs in the long-term.

Illustration 4 – Responsibilities of businesses to stakeholders

888.com is an internet gambling site that is listed on the London Stock Exchange. Its headquarters are in Gibraltar and it operates under a licence granted by the Government of Gibraltar.

It has responsibilities to the following stakeholders:

- **Shareholders** – since it is listed on the London Stock Exchange it must comply with the rules of that exchange, including adopting the Corporate Governance Code (the code is discussed later in this chapter).

- **Employees** – to be a good employer to all its members of staff.

- **Customers** – to offer a fair, regulated and secure environment in which to gamble.

- **Government** – to comply with the terms of its licence granted in Gibraltar.

- **The public** – the company chooses to sponsor several sports teams as part of strengthening its brand. The company also tries to address public concerns about the negative aspects of gambling, for example by identifying compulsive gamblers on their site and taking appropriate action.

Test your understanding 4

Voluntarily turning away business

Why should a gambling company like 888.com voluntarily choose to turn away certain business, for example known compulsive gamblers, gamblers who may be under-age, gamblers in certain countries etc?

Test your understanding 5

Humes plc adopts a socially responsible approach.

This means that the company seeks to:

A   Meet the minimum obligations it owes to its shareholders

B   Exceed the minimum obligations it owes to its shareholders

C   Meet the minimum obligations it owes to its stakeholders

D   Exceed the minimum obligations it owes to its stakeholders

5   Corporate governance

The discussion of corporate governance touches upon and builds upon aspects of business ethics and CSR.

5.1   Why corporate governance?

Corporate governance has become a major business issue driven by a succession of public 'scandals'.

In the early nineties, the collapse of London Stock Exchange listed company Polly Peck International, the Mirror Group collapse (and the associated Maxwell pension scandal) and the liquidation of BCCI (The Bank of Credit and Commerce International) led to the formation of the **UK Corporate Governance Code**.

Illustration 5 – Why corporate governance?

Polly Peck International

Asil Nadir, the owner of Polly Peck International (PPI) built the company from very little but by the end of the 1980s it was worth over £2bn. However, the company collapsed in 1991 following the discovery of huge theft by Nadir from his own company, totalling £29m.

The Mirror Group

In 1991 the Mirror Group collapsed amid allegations that £440m had been defrauded from the company's pension scheme by its owner, the late Robert Maxwell. An enquiry concluded that Robert Maxwell and his son Kevin had a heavy responsibility for the collapse of the company but that City Institutions were also to blame.

> **BCCI**
>
> In 1991 BCCI was forced to shut its doors by the Bank of England amid identification of huge fraud. Hard hit were 35 local UK councils who lost approximately £90m in investments.

More recently, the 2008 financial crisis, which claimed Lehman Brothers, Northern Rock, Bradford & Bingley and many others, saw the code revised and radical changes to how risks are assessed within financial institutions.

The **need for corporate governance** arises because, in all but the smallest of organisations, there is a separation of ownership and control.

 The **separation of ownership and control** refers to the situation in a company where the people who own the company (the shareholders) may not be the same people as those who run the company (the board of directors).

This separation can bring benefits (for example, specialist managers can often run the company more efficiently than those who own the company). However, there is a risk that the directors may run the company in their own interests, rather than those of the shareholders and the other stakeholders. This is referred to as the '**agency problem**'.

Illustration 6 – The agency problem in a company

The directors of a large quoted company may hold a board meeting and vote themselves huge bonuses and salaries even if only modest profit targets are achieved and may also put contractual terms in place granting them huge compensation payments if they are sacked. Those votes are in the selfish best interests of the directors, and not in the best interests of the shareholders who own the company and whose interests the directors are meant to be looking after.

5.2 The meaning of corporate governance

 Corporate governance is the set of processes and policies by which a company is directed, administered and controlled. It includes the appropriate role of the board of directors and the auditors of the company.

Corporate governance is concerned with the overall control and direction of a business so that the business's objectives are achieved in an acceptable manner by **ALL** stakeholders.

The following **symptoms** can indicate that there is poor corporate governance:

- **Domination of the board** by a single individual or group

- **No involvement by the board, for example** meeting irregularly, failing to consider systematically the organisation's activities and risks, or basing decisions on inadequate information

- **An inadequate control function**, for instance no internal audit, or a lack of adequate technical knowledge in key roles, or a rapid turnover of staff involved in accounting and control

- Lack of **supervision** of employees

- Lack of independent scrutiny by **external or internal auditors**

- Lack of **contact with shareholders**

- Emphasis on **short-term profitability**, leading to concealment of problems or errors, or manipulation of financial statements to achieve desired results

- **Misleading financial statements and information**

5.3 The principles of corporate governance

One of the main debates surrounding corporate governance regulation is whether it should be:

- A set of **best practice** guidelines – as in the UK with its principles based approach requiring companies to adhere to the spirit rather than the letter of the law.

- A **legal** requirement – as in the US with appropriate penalties for transgression.

The US Sarbanes-Oxley Act 2002 (SOX)

In 2002, following a number of corporate governance scandals such as Enron and WorldCom, tough new corporate governance regulations were introduced in the US by SOX.

SOX is only applicable in the US and for subsidiaries of US-based companies.

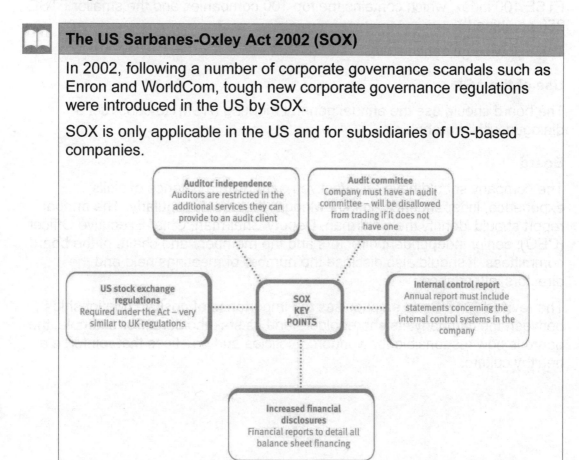

5.4 Features of the UK corporate governance code

In the UK, company law sets out a great many of the rules on corporate governance, especially with regards to the following:

- The **board of directors**

- **Directors' powers and duties**

- The **relationship of the company with directors**, such as loans to directors and the interests of directors in company contracts

- Accountability for stewardship and financial reporting via the **financial statements**

- Rules on meetings and resolutions

The Financial Reporting Council (FRC) is the body responsible for promoting high standards of corporate governance in the UK. All companies listed on the London Stock Exchange are required to apply the principles of the **UK Corporate Governance Code** (last revised in 2018) and must produce a disclosure statement confirming compliance with the code and explaining any departures from it.

Smaller listed companies, i.e. those not in the FTSE 350 can take a more flexible approach to applying the code. (**Note:** The FTSE 350 is an index of the top 350 companies by capitalisation and includes the more commonly used FTSE 100 index, which contains the top 100 companies and the smaller FTSE 250 combined.)

The following guidance exists:

Use of the AGM

The board should use the annual general meeting (AGM) to construct a dialogue with shareholders.

Board

The company should have an effective board (with a balance of skills, experience, independence and knowledge) that meets regularly. The annual report should identify the Chairman, Deputy Chairman, Chief Executive Officer (CEO), senior independent directors and the members and chairs of the board committees. It should also disclose the number of meetings held and the directors' attendance.

The revised 2018 Code emphasises the importance of positive relationships between the company, its shareholders and its stakeholders. For example, the board is now responsible for workforce policies and practices that reinforce a healthy culture.

Chairman and Chief Executive Officer (CEO)

The positions of the Chairman (person responsible for leadership and board effectiveness) and the CEO (the person in charge of running the company) should be separated. This is to ensure that no one individual has too much power within the company. The Chairman should be independent on appointment.

Non-executive directors (NEDs)

Directors who are involved in the execution of day-to-day management decisions are called **executive directors (EDs)**. Those who primarily only attend board meetings (and the meetings of board committees) are known as **NEDs.**

Current guidance is that NEDs should as far as possible be 'independent' so that their oversight role can be effectively and responsibly carried out. NEDs must not:

- have been an employee of the company in the last five years

- have had a material business interest in the company for the last three years either directly or indirectly (for example, as an employee of an organisation that has a relationship with the business)

- participate in the company's share options, performance-related pay scheme or pension schemes

- have close family ties with company directors or senior employees

- serve as a NED for more than nine years with the same company

- hold cross directorship (i.e. two or more directors sit on the board of the same third party company) or have significant links with other directors through involvement in other organisations.

If any of these apply to a NED, their independence will be seriously compromised.

Typical recommendations include:

- At least half of the board (excluding the chairman) should comprise independent NEDs. A smaller company should have at least two independent NEDs.

- One of the NEDs should be appointed the 'senior independent director'. Shareholders can contact them if they wish to raise matters outside the normal executive channels of communication.

Test your understanding 6

Independent NED

Mr X retires from the post of finance director at AB plc. The company is keen to retain his experience, so invite him to become a NED of the company.

Can he qualify as an independent non-executive?

Nomination committees

Appointments to the board should be made via a nominations committee. Over 50% of this committee should be made up of NEDs. This is to provide some independence from the current board members and to ensure that all appointments are based on merit and suitability and that the composition of the board is balanced.

The revised 2018 Code states that the committee is responsible for effective succession planning when developing a more diverse board and that the gender balance of senior management and their direct reports should be reported.

Remuneration committees

It is an important principle of corporate governance that no director should be involved in setting the level of their own remuneration.

 A remuneration committee is a committee made up of NEDs (at least three for FTSE 350 companies and at least two for smaller listed companies) which is responsible for deciding on the pay and incentives offered to executive directors (including pension rights and compensation payments). The Chairman can be a member but cannot chair the committee. The chair must have been a committee member for at least 12 months.

Remuneration should be sufficient to attract, retain and motivate quality directors but shouldn't be more than necessary. A significant proportion of director's pay should be performance related.

The revised 2018 Code states that there should be clear reporting on remuneration and how its helps the organisation to achieve its strategy and long-term success and its alignment to workforce remuneration.

 Remuneration committee

Advantages of having a remuneration committee:

- It avoids the agency problem of directors determining their own levels of remuneration.

- It leaves the board free to make strategic decision about the future.

Disadvantages of having a remuneration committee:

- There is a danger that NEDs may recommend high remuneration for the executive directors in the hope that the executives will recommend high remuneration for the NEDs.

- There will be a cost involved in preparing for and holding the meetings

---

Test your understanding 7

Remuneration of NEDs

On what basis should NEDs be remunerated for their service to the company?

Test your understanding 8

Which one of the following can non-executive directors accept as remuneration from the company?

A   A fixed daily rate for their time

B   Shares

C   Pension payments

D   Equity options

Audit committees

An audit committee consists solely of independent NEDs (at least three for FTSE 350 companies and at least two for smaller listed companies) who are responsible for monitoring and reviewing the company's financial controls and the integrity of the financial statements.

The board should review the effectiveness of risk management and internal controls at least annually and report to shareholders covering all material controls.

The audit committee acts as an interface between the board of directors on one side and the internal and external auditors on the other side. They:

- review the work and effectiveness of the internal audit function

- monitor the external auditor's independence and objectivity

- short-list external audit firms when a change is needed.

An audit committee should be the first point of contact for auditors, improving the independence and the overall quality of the audit functions.

The role of the audit committee

Responsibilities include the following:

- Reviewing accounting policies and financial statements as a whole to ensure that they are appropriate and balanced.

- Review systems of internal controls and risk management within the organisation. (Note that risk management may be dealt with by a separate committee – the risk committee.)

- Agreement of the work agenda for the internal audit department, as well as reviewing the results of internal audit work.

- Liaising with the external auditors, including dealing with problems in the audit as they arise as well as the appointment and removal of external auditors.

Test your understanding 9

Composition of audit committee

Why are the members of an audit committee required to be NEDs rather than executive directors?

6   Chapter summary

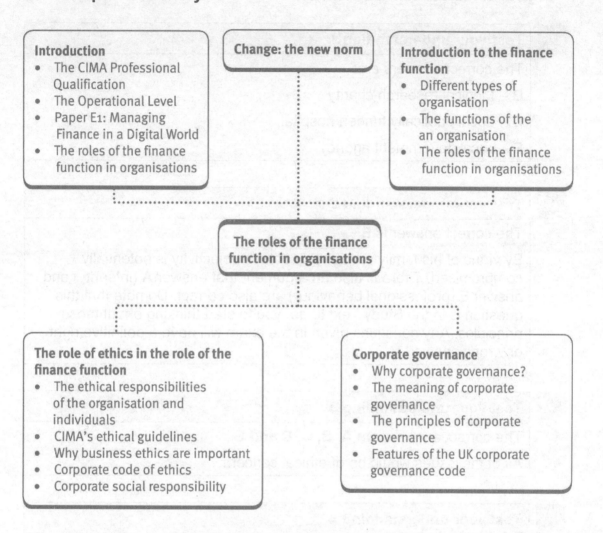

Introduction
- The CIMA Professional Qualification
- The Operational Level
- Paper E1: Managing Finance in a Digital World
- The roles of the finance function in organisations

Change: the new norm

Introduction to the finance function
- Different types of organisation
- The functions of the an organisation
- The roles of the finance function in organisations

The roles of the finance function in organisations

The role of ethics in the role of the finance function
- The ethical responsibilities of the organisation and individuals
- CIMA's ethical guidelines
- Why business ethics are important
- Corporate code of ethics
- Corporate social responsibility

Corporate governance
- Why corporate governance?
- The meaning of corporate governance
- The principles of corporate governance
- Features of the UK corporate governance code

Test your understanding answers

Test your understanding 1

The correct answers are:

B – Medical research charity

C – Local publically funded hospital

F – Local government agency

Test your understanding 2

The correct answer is **B**

By virtue of his family relationship John's objectivity is potentially compromised. There is also an argument that answer A (integrity) and answer E (professional behaviour) are also correct. Do note that this question is in the Study Text to get you to start thinking about these principles. Any questions given in the exam will have a definitive right or wrong answer.

Test your understanding 3

The correct answers are **A, B, C, D and E**

All of the issues would be of ethical concern.

Test your understanding 4

Either you could argue that such action was ethically correct (with the company wanting to 'do the right thing'), or you could argue that a concentration on short-term profits is likely to store up problems in the longer term. If under-age gamblers are seen to be gambling on a particular website, then the public reputation of that site will be damaged and its long term profitability could be in jeopardy if governments or customers turn against it.

Test your understanding 5

The correct answer is **D**

A socially responsible organisation seeks to exceed their obligations they owe to all stakeholders not just the shareholders.

Test your understanding 6

It is very unlikely that Mr X can be independent since he has been an employee of the company within the last five years. If the board believes that Mr X is independent despite his recent employment then they must state the reasons for this determination.

Test your understanding 7

NEDs should be paid fees that reflect the time commitment and the responsibilities of the role, for example a fixed daily rate for when they work for the company. Share options should not be granted to the NEDs since this could detract from their independent judgement.

Test your understanding 8 – OTQ

The correct answer is **A**

NEDs should be paid fees that reflect the time commitment and the responsibilities of the role, for example a fixed daily rate for when they work for the company. Share options should not be granted to NEDs since this would detract from the detached judgement that they should bring, and it would also prevent them from being identified as 'independent' NEDs.

Test your understanding 9

NEDs have no day-to-day operating responsibilities, so they are able to view the company's affairs in a detached and independent way and liaise effectively between the main board and both sets of auditors.

2

The activities performed by finance professionals to fulfil the roles

Chapter learning objectives

Lead	Component
A2: Describe the activities that finance professionals perform to fulfil the roles.	Describe how the finance function: (a) Collates data to prepare information for organisations (b) Provides insight to users by analysing information (c) Communicates insight to influence users (d) Supports the implementation of decisions to achieve the desired impact (e) Connects the different activities to each other

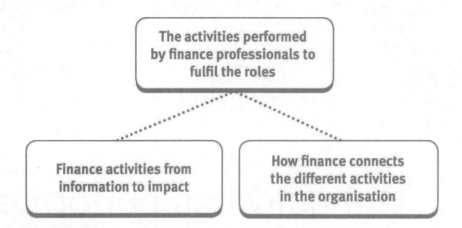

1 Introduction

In the previous chapter we discussed the roles of the finance function in organisations – understanding how the finance function **enables**, **shapes** and **narrates** value creation and preservation through planning, forecasting, resource allocation, performance management and control, and financial (corporate) reporting.

In Chapter 2 we will focus on the **activities** that finance professionals perform to fulfil these roles.

2 Finance activities from information to impact

2.1 The information to impact framework

The structure of the finance function and the activities that finance professionals perform can be best understood in the context of the basic finance activities that form the backbone of all the work of finance professionals.

These basic activities can be summarised using the **'information to impact framework'**.

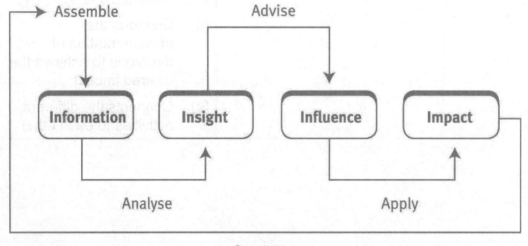

The finance professionals' basic activities are the **5 A's – assemble, analyse, advise, apply, acumen**:

Finance activity	Explanation
Assembling information	**Collates data to prepare information about the organisation** Finance professionals collect and assemble data from a range of internal and external sources (see section 2.2). Data is defined as facts or figures in a raw, unprocessed form. To become useful in the organisation this data needs to be turned into information. Information is data that has been processed in such a way that is has a meaning and use to the person who receives it. This processing may involve: • cleaning the data, i.e. identifying incomplete, inaccurate or irrelevant data and then replacing, modifying or deleting it • connecting different sources of data. Examples of assembled information would be: • management information in an accessible format for managers • accounts and returns prepared in a prescribed format for external reporting. (See section 2.3 for more detail on 'information'). This activity can also be viewed as the broad role of **REPORTING**.
Analysing for insights	**Provides insight to users by analysing information** Finance professionals analyse both financial (for example, sales information) and non-financial (for example, customer satisfaction information) information to draw out patterns and relevant insights for those who use the information. This could take the form of a comparison of the information with budgeted or historical figures. (See section 2.4 for more detail on the 'types of information'). This activity can also be viewed as the broad role of **QUESTIONING**.

Finance activity	Explanation
Advising to influence	**Communicates insight to influence users** Finance professionals then: • communicate these insights and • contribute an objective and responsible perspective to influence the organisation's decision making. This activity can also be viewed as the broad role of **DEVELOPING SOLUTIONS**.
Applying for impact (also called **'execute'**)	**Supports the implementation of decisions to achieve the desired impact** Finance professionals apply the information to harness value for the organisation through their impact on, for example: • strategic plans • budgeting and resource allocation • performance measures • performance reviews. This activity can also be viewed as the broad role of **DEPLOYING SOLUTIONS**.
Acumen	**Connects the different activities to each other** Finance professionals prepare valuable information (such as reports and analysis) on the outcomes achieved from different initiatives to help inform future proposals. (**Note:** The information to impact framework may not always show 'acumen' but it will always be an important activity of the finance function.)

Note: These activities will be explored in more detail in Chapter 4.

Test your understanding 1

Using the 'Information to Impact' framework, match the following descriptions to the activities they are describing and put them into the correct order.

Activity	Description
Advising to influence	Providing insights that will be useful for future decisions.
Assembling information	Using information to create value for the organisation.
Applying for impact	Interpreting information to find patterns and trends that may not have been previously known.
Acumen	Processing data into meaningful, useful information.
Analysing for insights	Developing solutions to influence the decisions made by the organisation.

The **information to impact framework can be expanded** as follows:

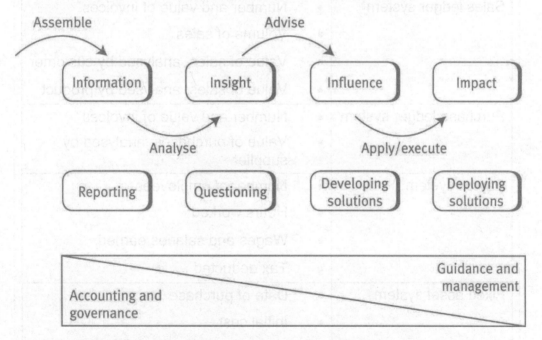

Moving from left to right there is a shift in emphasis between:

- **accounting and governance** (for example, financial (corporate) reporting, management accounting, regulatory compliance, risk management and corporate governance) and

- **guidance and management** (for example, helping the organisation to forecast and analyse trends to reach profitable growth goals).

2.2 Sources of data

As discussed, finance professionals assemble data from a range of internal and external sources.

Internal sources

Internal sources of data may be taken from a variety of areas such as:

- accounting records including sales ledger data (such as the volume of sales), purchase ledger data (such as the value of purchases for each supplier) and fixed asset data (such as the depreciation method and rate)

- payroll data such as the number of employees and the hours worked and paid

- production data such as the number of rejected units

- sales and marketing data such as market research results.

Examples of internal sources of data	
Examples of internal data:	

Source	Data
Sales ledger system	• Number and value of invoices • Volume of sales • Value of sales, analysed by customer • Value of sales, analysed by product
Purchase ledger system	• Number and value of invoices • Value of purchases, analysed by supplier
Payroll system	• Number of employees • Hours worked • Wages and salaries earned • Tax deducted
Fixed asset system	• Date of purchase • Initial cost • Location • Depreciation method and rate • Service history • Production capacity

External sources

In addition to internal data sources, there is much data to be obtained from external sources such as:

- suppliers (for example, product prices)

- customers (for example, product requirement and price sensitivity)

- the internet, newspapers and journals (for example, data on competitors, technological developments, discussion groups)

- the government (for example, inflation rate).

External data may be limited in its usefulness to finance professionals. The **limitations of using externally generated data** are as follows:

- External data may not be accurate.

- External data may be out of date.

- The company publishing the data may not be reputable.

- External data may not meet the exact needs of the business.

- It may be difficult to gather external data, for example, from customers or competitors.

Examples of external sources of information		
External source	**Information**	
Suppliers	• Product prices	
	• Product specifications	
Newspapers, journals	• Share price	
	• Information on competitors	
	• Technological developments	
	• National and market surveys	
Government	• Industry statistics	
	• Taxation policy	
	• Inflation rates	
	• Demographic statistics	
	• Forecasts for economic growth	

Customers	• Product requirements
	• Price sensitivity
Banks	• Information on potential customers
	• Information on national markets
Business enquiry agents	• Information on competitors
	• Information on customers
Internet	• Almost everything via databases (public and private), discussion groups and mailing lists

2.3 Information

As discussed in section 2.1, to become useful in the organisation, the data needs to be turned into information.

The organisation needs **'good'** information for planning and decision making and in order to manage and control the organisation effectively.

One way of looking at the qualities of good information is to use the acronym **'accurate'**. This is explained using the illustration below.

Illustration 1 – Qualities of management reports ACCURATE

The 'accurate' acronym is explained in the context of the management reports produced by an information system. The reports from an information system should allow the organisation to run the business effectively both today and in the future. Management reports should have the following characteristics:

Characteristic	Explanation
Accurate	For example, figures should add up and there should be no typographical errors.
Complete	The reports should include all the information that is needed by the readers of the report and should be aligned to the overall objectives of the report or of the organisation.
Cost < benefit (i.e. **C**ost effective)	The benefit of having the information must be greater than the cost of providing it.
Understandable	The readers of the report must be able to understand the contents and use the contents to fulfil their needs. Presentation should be clear and in line with best practice.

Relevant	Information that is not needed by the reader(s) of the report should be omitted. Information overload can be a huge problem and can detract from the usefulness of the report. The problem of information overload may be overcome using, for example, drill-down reports (provide users with the capability to look at increasingly detailed information about a particular item) and exception reports (which are only triggered when a situation is unusual or requires management action).
Adaptable	The output reports should have the capability of being adapted to meet the needs of the user or the organisation. (Note: this 'A' can also be for 'Accessible' meaning that the information is accessible via the appropriate channel of communication (verbally, via reports, via emails etc) and is reported to the relevant person).
Timely	The information should be provided when needed and should not be provided too frequently (this can result in information overload and the cost of providing the information exceeding the benefit).
Easy to use	Information should be presented in a form recommended by the industry or organisation's best practice. It should not be too long (to prevent information overload) and it should be sent using the most appropriate communication channel to ensure user needs are met.

Technology will play a key role in capturing this information. Automation involving complex machines can now do the collection of data much more effectively and much more efficiently than humans.

Information can now be produced at a press of a button, in real time and in a format the suits the needs of the organisation.

Illustration 2 – Visualisation

Visualisation is becoming a mainstream feature of many organisations' finance functions. Visualisation is about using technology to turn increasing amounts of raw data into useful information for the organisation. Traditional spreadsheet content is turned into pictures and infographics, making important organisational stories much easier to understand for the lay person who sit outside of the finance function.

Technology should not be viewed by the finance function as a threat but rather as an opportunity. For the finance professional, the automation of repetitive tasks will free up their time to concentrate on creating and preserving organisational value.

Important note: This is only a brief introduction as to how technology is impacting business and finance. This area will be explored and built upon in subsequent chapters.

2.4 Types of information

As discussed in section 2.1, finance professionals will **analyse** a range of information to draw out patterns and relevant insights for those who use the information. Information may include the following:

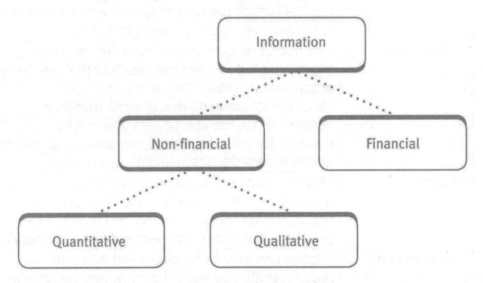

Quantitative and qualitative information will be discussed in a little more detail below.

Quantitative information

 Quantitative information is information that can normally be expressed in numerical terms

Financial information will be quantitative (for example total sales information). Non-financial information will be partly quantitative (for example, number of complaints).

There are a number of common mistakes that finance professionals could make when analysing quantitative information for insights. For example:

- **Presentation of information** – the choice of, say, graph or chart may be inappropriate. For example, a graph may indicate dramatic changes but only because of the scale chosen.

- **Failure to evaluate the figures using a suitable comparator or benchmark** – finance professionals may report an increase in sales of 20% on the last year but this may indicate poor performance if the market grew by 30% over the same period.

- **Collection of data** – an organisation often uses sampling to collect data and establish statistics. However, it is difficult to collect a random sample and a sample that is big enough to be representative of the whole population. This will result in poor information being produced and then analysed by finance professionals.

Qualitative information

 Qualitative information is information that cannot normally be expressed in numerical terms

Qualitative information is often in the form of opinions, for example:

- **employees** – who will be affected by certain decisions which may threaten their continued employment, or cause them to need re-training

- **customers** – who will be interested to know about new products, but will want to be assured that service arrangements, etc. will continue for existing products

- **suppliers** – who will want to be aware of the entity's plans, for example, a move to a just-in-time (JIT) environment (i.e. holding no or minimal inventory).

The fact that qualitative information is often in the form of opinions presents a problem since the information is **subjective** in nature. For example, in assessing quality of service, customers have different expectations and priorities and so are unlikely to be consistent in their judgements. One way to reduce the effect of subjectivity is for finance professionals to look at **trends** in performance since the biases will be present in each individual time period but the trend will show relative changes in quality.

It is difficult to record and process data of a qualitative nature but qualitative factors still need to be considered when making a decision. These include:

- **The effects on the environment:** certain decisions may affect emissions and pollution of the environment. The green issue and the entity's responsibility towards the environment may seriously affect its public image.

- **Legal effects:** there may be legal implications of a course of action, or a change in law may have been the cause of the decision requirement.

- **Political effects:** government policies, in both taxation and other matters, may impinge on the decision.

- **Timing of decision:** the timing of a new product launch may be crucial to its success.

These factors must be considered before making a final decision. Each of these factors is likely to be measured by opinion. Such opinions must be collected and coordinated into meaningful information. Qualitative data will often be transformed into quantitative information (for example, by applying a 1 to 5 scale when assessing customer satisfaction). However, it will never escape from the problem of being judgemental and subjective.

3 How finance connects the different activities in the organisation

The finance function does not work in isolation. Rather the contemporary finance function works with and alongside the other functions of the business and helps to connect the different activities that they perform.

- It provides information and insight to other functions **enabling** them to create and preserve value.

Illustration 3 – Resource allocation

The finance function can use **resource allocation** to enable the organisation to achieve its objectives.

For example, it may assist the sales and marketing function in understanding the potential impact of its promotional spend. The sales and marketing function will be need to decide which products/services it should focus promotion on, the potential benefit of the different promotional tools available and the cost of these tools. The finance function can assist in providing this information and in recommending how the resources available for promotional activity should be allocated.

- It works with other functions to **shape how** the function creates and preserves value.

Illustration 4 – Performance management

The finance function can use **performance management** to assist the organisation in achieving its objectives. 'What gets measured gets done', i.e. the things that are measured get done much more often than the things that are not measured.

For example, finance may work with the operations function to set appropriate performance measures to capture what the operations function needs to do in order to achieve its objectives. Examples of measures could include the time taken to deliver a customer's order or the percentage wastage rate. The finance function can help to assemble the relevant performance measurement information, report it to those people who need it and question and understand any deviations between the actual and the planned performance. In this way, the operations function (and the organisation) can be assisted in achieving its objectives.

- It works with other functions to achieve the desired organisational impact for this function, **narrating how** the finance function creates and preserves value.

The finance function will communicate insight to influence stakeholders, getting value from financial and non-financial data in order to help the organisation to, for example:

- make better future decisions

- enhance future operational efficiency

- better understand its customers.

The focus will be very much on what the organisation will need to do in the future to preserve and to create value.

Important note: This is a brief introduction only. Chapters 9 to 12 will discuss in greater detail how finance interacts with the organisation.

4 Chapter summary

```
                    ┌──────────────────────────┐
                    │   The activities performed │
                    │  by finance professionals to │
                    │        fulfil the roles     │
                    └──────────────────────────┘
```

Finance activities from information to impact
- The information to impact framework
- Sources of data
- Information
- Types of information

How finance connects the different activities in the organisation

Test your understanding answers

Test your understanding 1

Using the 'Information to Impact' framework, match the following descriptions to the activities they are describing and put them into the correct order.

Activity	Description
1 Assembling information	Processing data into meaningful, useful information.
2 Analysing for insights	Interpreting information to find patterns and trends that may not have been previously known.
3 Advising to influence	Developing solutions to influence the decisions made by the organisation.
4 Applying for impact	Using information to create value for the organisation.
5 Acumen	Providing insights that will be useful for future decisions.

The structure and shape of the finance function

Chapter learning objectives

Lead	Component
D1: Describe the structure and shape of the finance function.	Describe the: (a) Evolution of the shape of the finance function (b) Shape of the finance function in the digital era

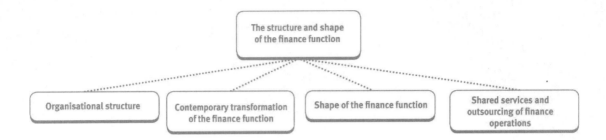

1   Introduction

In the previous chapters we looked at the different roles of the finance function and the activities that finance professionals perform to fulfil these roles. We also discussed the importance of ethics, CSR and corporate governance for an organisation and its people and, more specifically, for the finance function.

In this chapter we are going to continue to learn about the finance function, with a focus on the structure and shape of the finance function and how this enables finance to perform its role in the organisation. We will learn about the traditional shape and structure of the finance function and we will then look at the contemporary transformation of this shape and structure and the reasons for this transformation.

Before we learn about these areas it is useful to begin by understanding the different structures that the organisation as a whole may adopt.

2   Organisational structure

 Organisational structure is formed by the grouping of people into departments or sections and the allocation of responsibility and authority.

2.1   Mintzberg's effective organisation

Mintzberg suggested that an organisation can be analysed into **six building blocks** and that effective **co-ordination** will be needed to integrate the building blocks into one cohesive unit.

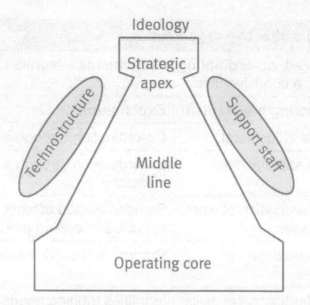

Operating core – this is the basic work of the organisation, i.e. the individuals who perform the task of producing the product or providing the service. In a small organisation this will represent nearly all the organisation, but larger organisations will require more complex arrangements.

Strategic apex – higher levels of management responsible for formulating the strategy and long-term plans.

Middle line – this links the strategic apex to the operating core and includes middle and lower level management.

Technostructure – this is responsible for designing procedures and standards. The technostructure includes accountants, computer specialists and engineers.

Support staff – provide services to the organisation which support operations/production.

Ideology – this is the organisation's values and beliefs (culture).

Test your understanding 1
The technostructure:
A   is dedicated to the technical side of product and process development
B   is the board of directors who decide on the financial structure and technicalities of a business
C   are departments such as accounting and personnel which provide support for technical structures by co-ordinating and standardising work
D   are functions to purchase materials and process them for distribution

Mintzberg's effective organisation

As mentioned, **co-ordinating mechanisms** integrate the building blocks into a cohesive unit:

Co-ordinating mechanism	Explanation
1 Mutual adjustment	Co-ordination through informal contact
2 Direct supervision	Co-ordination through a formal hierarchy
3 Standardisation of work processes	Standardisation of work processes and specified operating procedures
4 Standardisation of outputs	Product and service specifications
5 Standardisation of skills and knowledge	Identifies training needs and the necessary skills base to do the work
6 Standardisation of norms	Cultural norms and expectations

The building blocks and the co-ordinating mechanisms vary significantly from business to business. Mintzberg **combined the building blocks and co-ordinating mechanisms in different ways** and identified **five main structural configurations**.

Structural configuration (and example)	Key building block	Key co-ordinating mechanism
Simple structure (newsagent)	Strategic apex	Direct supervision
Machine bureaucracy (heavily unionised organisation)	Techno structure	Standardisation of work
Professional bureaucracy (hospital, Kaplan)	Operating core	Standardisation of skills
Divisionalised (organisation split into business units for each product sold)	Middle line	Standardisation of outputs
Adhocracy/Innovative (advertising agency)	Operating core/ Support staff	Mutual adjustment

2.2   Types of structure

Different categories of structure exist and will be appropriate to businesses at the various phases of their lives. A typical pattern of structural change would be as follows:

- entrepreneurial structure
- functional structure
- divisional structure
- matrix structure.

Entrepreneurial structure

- The structure is built around the owner-manager – typical of small companies (early stages of development).

- The structure is totally centralised with all key decisions being made by the strategic leader (often the owner/entrepreneur in an owner-managed business).

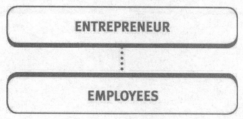

Advantages	Disadvantages
• **Fast decision making** – Only one person is making decisions • **Good control** – The small size and few layers of management means that the entrepreneur has good control over the workforce and all decisions within the organisation, leading to better goal congruence • **More responsive to market** – As soon as an element in the market changes the entrepreneur should recognise it and be quick to react • **Close bond to workforce** – The entrepreneur and employees work closely together.	• **Success is dependent on the capabilities of the owner-manager** • **Lack of career structure** for employees due to the small size of the organisation • **Cannot cope with diversification/growth** – The owner-manager will not be able to cope with, for example, the increased volume of decisions.

Functional structure

- Common in organisations that have outgrown the entrepreneurial structure, therefore need to group together employees that undertake similar tasks into departments.

- Most appropriate to smaller companies with few products and locations and which exist in a relatively stable environment.

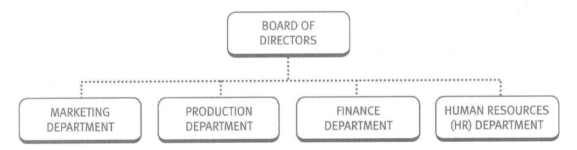

Advantages	Disadvantages
• **Economies of scale** – Roles and activities are grouped together and not duplicated leading to lower costs	• **Empire building and conflicts between function** – Functional managers may make decisions to increase their own power or that are in the best interests of their function, rather than working in the best interests of the company overall
• **Standardisation of outputs and systems** – Similar activities are grouped together resulting in standardisation and a focus on optimum quality	
• **Specialists more comfortable** – People with similar skills are grouped together and do not feel isolated	• **Slow to adapt to market changes** – Decision making is slow due to the long chain of command
• **Career opportunities** – Employees can work their way up through the function.	• **Cannot cope with rapid growth or diversification** – For example, specialists in the production function may not be able to cope with making a new product.

Divisional structure

- This structure occurs where an organisation is split into several **divisions** (strategic business units) – each one autonomously overseeing a **product** line/brand or **geographical** location.

- Headed by general managers who take responsibility for their own resources.

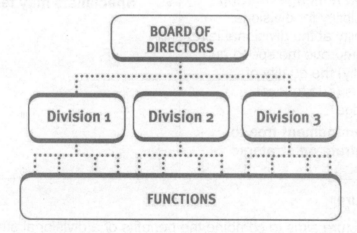

Illustration 1 – Divisional structure

AB is a company that manufactures two different products – toasters and televisions. The products require different components and require different advertising and sales and staffing.

AB therefore operates a divisional structure, with a toasters division and a television division. Each division has its own sales, purchasing, HR and advertising divisions.

The finance department, however, is still operated centrally.

Advantages	Disadvantages
• **Enables product or geographical growth** – The structure can be easily adapted for further growth and diversification	• **Duplication of business functions** – Each division will have its own functions. This will result in more managers
• **Clear responsibility** – Divisional managers should be able to see clearly where their area of responsibility lies	• **Lack of goal congruence** – Divisions may make decisions to benefits themselves to the detriment of the overall company
• **Training of general managers** – Less focus on specialisation should result in managers having a wider view of the organisation's operations	• **Potential loss of control** due to the autonomy given to the divisions and its managers
• **Decision making** – Placing responsibility for divisional profitability at the divisional level should improve the speed and (hopefully) the quality of decisions (due to local knowledge)	• **Allocation of central costs can be a problem**
• **Top management free to concentrate on strategic matters.**	• **Specialists may feel isolated.**

Matrix structure

- This structure aims to combine the benefits of a divisional structure and a functional structure.

- Usually found in multi-product and multi-functional organisations with significant interrelationships and interdependencies.

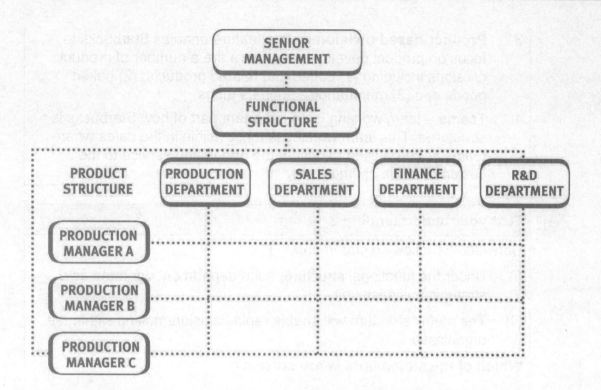

Advantages	Disadvantages
• **Advantages of both functional and divisional structures** • **Flexibility** – The matrix structure offers the flexibility to co-ordinate the tasks and people required in more complex situations • **Encourages teamwork and the exchange of opinions and expertise.**	• **Dual command** – Team members may be answerable to a product manager and a functional manager resulting in potential confusion, stress, conflict • **Dilution of functional authority** • **Time-consuming meetings**

 Illustration 2 – Starbucks' matrix structure

Starbucks Coffee Company has a matrix structure with the following four features:

1 **Functional groups** – the company is split into a number of functions including human resources (HR), finance and marketing. The functions are hierarchical so, for example, the company's HR function implements policies applicable to all of the company's cafes and these are then monitored and controlled by senior management.

2 **Geographical divisions** – these are based on the physical location of operations, with each division head being given the flexibility to adjust strategies and policies to reflect the local market. Starbucks has three geographical divisions: (1) Americas, (2) China and Asia-Pacific and (3) Europe, Middle East and Africa.

3   **Product-based divisions** – this feature enables Starbucks to focus on product development. There are a number of product divisions including (1) coffee and related products, (2) baked goods and (3) merchandise such as mugs.

4   **Teams** – team working is an important part of how Starbucks is structured. This team working is most visible in the cafes where teams are organised to deliver the goods and service to the customer in the optimum way.

Test your understanding 3

Consider the following statements:

(i)   Under the functional structure, each department operates as a strategic business unit.

(ii) The matrix structure will enable rapid decision-making within the organisation.

Which of the statements is/are correct?

A   (i) only

B   (ii) only

C   Both

D   Neither

Test your understanding 4

M is a large company that operates in country G. It manufactures several different products, each of which is highly complex and extremely specialised. Its sales have grown significantly over the last several years, with each of its products producing a roughly equal amount of M's overall revenue.

Which organisational structure is most likely to be appropriate for M?

A   Geographic

B   Divisional

C   Functional

D   Entrepreneurial

2.3 Centralisation and decentralisation

Another method of analysing structures is by reference to the degree of autonomy or the level at which decisions are made.

 In a **centralised structure,** the upper levels of an organisation's hierarchy retain the authority to make decisions.

 In a **decentralised structure,** the authority to make decisions is passed down to units and people at lower levels.

 Factors affecting the amount of (de)centralisation

The following factors will affect the amount of (de)centralisation:

- **Management style** – for example, managers who want to retain control may operate a centralised structure.

- **The ability of management/employees** – for example, the more able the employees, the more decisions they can be entrusted with and the greater the level of decentralisation.

- **Geographical spread** – this may make central control more difficult resulting in a decentralised structure.

- **The size of the organisation** – small organisations can retain a level of central control relatively easily.

In reality most organisations will operate a degree of both centralised and decentralised decision making; the extent of each will be influenced by the factors above.

 Illustration 3 – A centralised organisation

A good example of a centralised business would be a multinational fast food chain such as McDonalds or Burger King. The majority of the locations of these international fast-food chains are privately owned franchises (a franchise is the purchase of the right to exploit a business brand in return for a capital sum and a share of the profit or turnover).

A centralised structure enables control and consistency to be maintained across thousands of outlets thus protecting its brand and reputation, while saving on overheads such as local payroll and accounting functions, through economies of scale.

The advantages and disadvantages of decentralisation are:

Advantages of decentralisation	Disadvantages of decentralisation
• Senior management free to concentrate on strategy • Better local decisions due to local expertise • Better motivation due to increased empowerment of employees and a more defined career path • Quicker responses/flexibility due to reduced bureaucracy and increased autonomy	• Loss of control by senior management and lack of standardisation • Dysfunctional decisions due to a lack of goal congruence • Poor decisions made by inexperienced managers • Training costs • Duplication of roles within organisation • Extra costs in obtaining information since it is stored in several locations

(**Note:** The advantages and disadvantages of centralisation have not been discussed but are largely the opposite of the points above).

Test your understanding 5

Which of the following is not a likely additional cost to an organisation caused by decentralisation?

A   Additional training costs are often required in a decentralised organisation

B   Duplication of roles, leading to higher costs

C   Extra costs of gathering information from various sources and locations

D   Lost sales due to a lack of local knowledge and expertise

2.4   Tall and flat organisations

Organisations can also be classed as tall or flat depending on the length of the scalar chain and the breadth of the span of control.

   The **scalar chain** is the line of authority which can be traced up or down the chain of command, from the most senior member of staff to the most junior. It therefore relates to the number of levels of management within an organisation.

Illustration 4 – British Army chain of command

The British Army is a good example of an organisation with a long chain of command. There are two main groups of staff with a ranking system existing within each group:

1 **Commissioned officers** are ranked from top to bottom as follows – Field Marshal, General, Lieutenant General, Major General, Brigadier General, Colonel, Lieutenant Colonel, Major, Captain, Lieutenant, Second Lieutenant.

2 **Other ranks and non-commissioned officers** are ranked from top to bottom as follows – Regimental Sergeant Major, Company Quarter Master Sergeant, Company Sergeant Major, Staff Sergeant, Sergeant, Corporal, Lance Corporal, Private.

The **span of control** considers how many people report to one superior.

Factors that influence the span of control

The factors that influence the span of control include the:

- **Nature of the work** – the more repetitive or simple the work, the wider the span of control can be.

- **Type of personnel** – the more skilled and motivated the managers and other staff members are, the wider the span of control can be.

- **Location of personnel** – if personnel are all located locally, it takes relatively little time and effort to supervise them. This allows the span of control to become wider.

Test your understanding 6

Consider the following statements:

(i) The scalar chain relates to the number of people over whom a manager has authority.

(ii) A business with highly skilled, motivated members of staff will tend to have a wider span of control than a business with demotivated employees.

Which of these statements is/are correct?

A (i) only

B (ii) only

C Both

D Neither

A '**tall**' organisation has many levels of management (a long scalar chain) and a narrow span of control.

 A '**flat**' organisation has few levels of management (a short scalar chain) and a wide span of control.

 Illustration 5 – A move by organisations to a flatter structure

Many organisations are adopting (and seeing the benefits of) a flatter structure. For example, Google's core values from the beginning were to have a flat organisation, a lack of hierarchy and a collaborative environment. This flatter organisation encourages employees to take initiative without needing approval from multiple managers. They empower employees to take charge, help make decisions and feel responsible for the company's success.

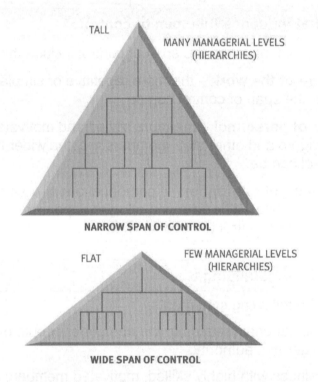

It is worth noting that **tall** organisations tend to be **more bureaucratic** and take **longer to make decisions**, due to the large number of levels of management that need to be involved.

However, **flat** organisations are not without their problems. These organisations tend to have **weaker control** and **fewer chances for employees to progress** or be promoted within the organisation.

> ## Test your understanding 7
>
> If a managerial structure has many levels of management, is it likely to have a narrow or wide span of control at each level of management?

2.5 Contemporary transformation of organisations

- It is worth noting that the **discussion above has focused on the historical organisational configurations and structural dimensions** that an organisation may adopt.

- Although much of this is still relevant, the changing expectations of customers, competitive pressures, a changing political and economic landscape and huge technological innovations have changed many of the traditional organisational forms and boundaries.

- Organisations have adopted new forms, for example outsourcing many aspects of the organisation's work to specialist providers, and have focused on factors such as flexibility rather than having a more rigid set of organisational boundaries in place.

> ## Illustration 6 – Nike
>
> The sports good manufacturer, Nike, outsources production activities but retains total control over design and quality specifications.

This contemporary transformation will be reviewed in the remainder of this chapter, with a specific focus on the contemporary transformation of the finance function.

> ## Illustration 7 – General Electric
>
> The term 'boundaryless' organisation originated from Jack Welch in the early 1990s when he was Chairman of General Electric. He recognised that the modern environment was subject to continuous innovation and change, thus requiring management to develop more flexible organisations. He aimed to achieve competitive advantage by replacing vertical hierarchies with horizontal networks; linking together traditional functions into inter-functional teams and forming strategic alliances with suppliers, customers and even competitors.

3 Contemporary transformation of the finance function

3.1 Introduction

In Chapter 2 we discussed the finance activities from information to impact. The basic activities of the finance function are still relevant in today's organisations but there has been a shift in emphasis regarding the importance of each of the activities.

Historically, the overall mandate of the finance function was to focus on organisational efficiencies and to reduce operational costs. This focus has resulted in organisations achieving optimum operational efficiency.

Technology has, to a large extent, replaced the historical mandate of the finance function, with machines being capable of monitoring operational costs and patterns of organisational efficiency.

If we relate this back to the information to impact framework this has resulted in **automation** of much of the '**assembly**' and '**analysis**'.

Illustration 8 – Automation of the finance function's activities

> Advances in technology are providing opportunities to automate many of the activities of the finance function. For example, robotic process automation (RPA) is providing opportunities to automate many routine, clerical 'assembly' activities.
>
> RPA is a software-based approach that replicates user actions to reduce or eliminate human intervention in mundane, repetitive and manually intensive processes.
>
> RPA started off in manufacturing (for example, with robotic vehicle assembly lines) but is now used across other functions such as finance. Rapid strides in the development of this technology mean machines are now encroaching on activities previously assumed to require human judgement and expense, such as data entry, automated formatting, reconciliations and foreign exchange transactions.
>
> This allows finance staff to re-focus on higher value, customer-focused activities.

Finance professionals should not view this automation as a threat but as an opportunity. The core accounting role will still be an essential foundation of the finance function but enabled by new technologies, the function can now be a more influential player in the organisation.

Technology allows the contemporary finance function to refocus its energy on revenue and value creation.

The finance function will no longer work largely in isolation but will work with others from across the organisation to drive business transformation that creates shareholder value.

To do this the **finance function** will need to reallocate its resources to the '**advising**' and '**applying/executing**' activities in the information to impact framework.

Note: The use of technology by the finance function is explored in more detail in Chapter 6.

Test your understanding 8

Read the following statements and decide if each one is true or false.

A   Because of advancements in technology the basic activities of the finance function are no longer relevant

B   Technology allows the contemporary finance function to refocus its energy on value creation

C   Technology has meant that a large amount of the assembly and analysis activities can be automated

D   Technology has meant that a large amount of the advising and applying activities can be automated

3.2 Can the finance function cope with this shift?

Traditionally, organisational finance functions have proved their worth because of particular areas of expertise. These have centred on the generation of information. With digital and technological capabilities increasing, these functions are recognising a need to develop new areas of expertise (for example, communicating insights) and build upon these to develop particular competencies.

However, the finance function is well positioned to meet this changing mandate since:

- it has a unique end-to-end view of the organisation, understanding that every activity has a financial consequence

- its accounting information is trusted and credible

- it already provides a framework for performance management, for example through management accounting

- it brings professional, evidence based objectivity to decision making.

3.3 The information to impact framework revisited

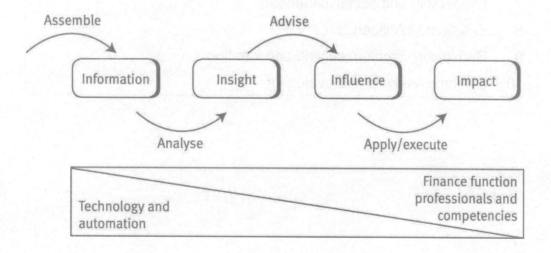

The information to impact framework clearly shows that:

- **Technology and automation** will play an important role in all of the activities of the finance function but will have the largest impact on the '**assembly**' and '**analysis**' activities.

- This will 'free up' the resource of the **finance function professionals** who can now place greater focus on the '**advising**' and '**applying/executing**' activities.

- The finance function will need to develop its **competencies**:
  - firstly, so that they are able to **use the up to date technology** and
  - secondly, so that they have the **necessary skills to provide the influence and impact required**.

Illustration 9 – New competencies required by finance function

The World Economic Forum published a 'Future of Jobs' report in 2018. This report concluded that by 2022 each individual within the finance function will require an extra 101 days of learning.

Competencies will not only be around technology but will also focus on business skills, leadership skills, people skills and more traditional technical skills (all of which will be underpinned by ethics, integrity and professionalism).

The survey identified ten key competencies:

1   Analytical thinking and innovation

2   Active learning and learning strategies

3   Creativity, originality and initiative

4   Technology design and programming

5   Critical thinking and analysis

6   Complex problem-solving

7   Leadership and social influence

8   Emotional intelligence

9   Reasoning, problem solving and ideation

10   Systems analysis and evaluation

Test your understanding 9

Which of the following THREE activities are likely to be the most impacted by technology and automation?

A	Processing data into information
B	Producing monthly variance reports
C	Developing solutions to influence the decisions of an organisation
D	Analysing non-financial information for insights
E	Using information to create value for the organisation

4 Shape of the finance function

4.1 Introduction

In this section we are going to look at the shape of the finance function and how this shape is evolving as a result of advances in technology, the changing mandate of the finance function and the changing capabilities of the finance function.

The evolution of the shape of the finance function is as follows:

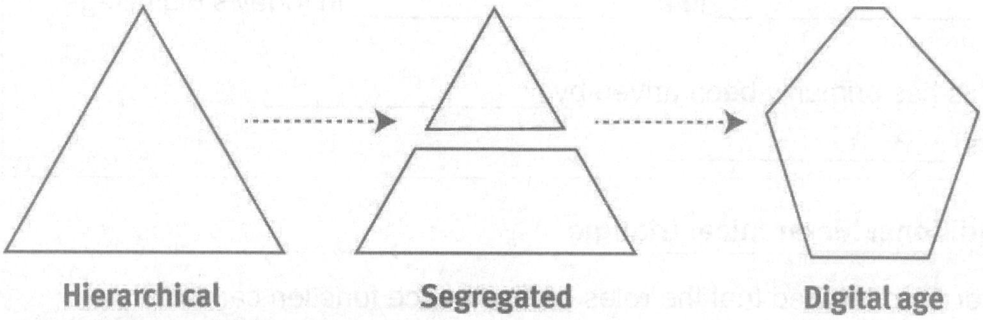

The shape is migrating from:

- **a hierarchical triangle (traditional shape)** – containing a broad base of finance workers reporting upwards to a series of ever narrower management levels
- **to a segregated triangle (last 20 years)** – globalisation and technological advances meant that much of the routine processing of the finance function could be carried out by a shared service centre (i.e. the centralisation of this routine processing into one place). The bottom section of the segregated triangle represents the finance function activity carried out by these shared service centres. (**Note:** This change is discussed in section 5)
- **and finally to the diamond shape (today's digital age)** – the traditional triangular base is being eroded due to automation of many of the basic activities of the finance function.

We will begin by briefly looking at the traditional hierarchical shape of the finance function before looking at how this shape could/has evolve(d) to a diamond shape.

Test your understanding 10

Pick from the following options to complete the sentences below:

Options:

Traditional hierarchy

Legislation

Diamond shape

Globalisation

Boundaryless structure

Technology

Governance

Sentences:

The shape of the finance function has evolved from a

_____ to a _____ in today's digital age.

This has primarily been driven by _____

and _____.

4.2 Traditional hierarchical triangle

In Chapter 1 we learned that the roles of the finance function can be summarised as **enabling**, **shaping how** and **narrating how** the organisation creates and preserves value.

We can understand the traditional hierarchical triangle shape in the context of these roles. In the traditional triangle:

- at the bottom of the triangle, there is a broad base of finance workers carrying out the operational 'enabling' roles of planning, forecasting and resource allocation.

- in the middle of the triangle, there is a narrower set of management level finance workers who are reported to from the level below and who carry out the 'shaping how' roles of performance management and control.

- at the top of the triangle sit a narrower group of senior finance staff. These staff are reported to from below and they concentrate on the 'narrating how' role of financial (corporate) reporting.

4.3 Diamond shape

Evolution into a diamond shape

The traditional hierarchical triangle is evolving into a diamond shape as follows:

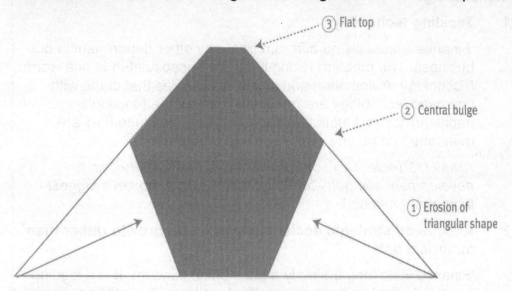

The evolution can be summarised as follows:

1   Technological automation has **eroded the traditional triangular shape** with much of the lower level assembly and processing tasks now being carried out by technology rather than finance professionals.

2   The **central bulge** in the diamond shape is due to many of the higher-value services now being offered by centres of excellence (or shared service centres) where finance professionals will work as part of a multi-disciplinary team, assembled in skills combinations that support the business.

3   The **flat top** of the structure shows a move to a collaborative finance leadership approach – with the chief finance officer (CFO) and other senior finance staff working with and alongside the chief executive officer (CEO).

Illustration 10 – The diamond shape of the finance function

Industry experts have considered the need to design a finance function that is fit for the future. Some useful quotes highlight the importance of the following:

1   Tackling technology

'Finance is actually no different from any other department in our business. The problem facing it can be encapsulated in one word: technology. Automation and all the efficiencies that come with improved technology are removing many of the function's traditional tasks. I think that's a good thing, because they are mundane and no one really wants to do them.'

(Daniel O'Toole, CEO of Retail Merchandising Services, a development company that supports many of the UK's biggest high-street names.)

2   A focus on strategic decision making and growth rather than historical data

'Finance is no longer simply a back-office concern. It is a leading function in the business. It's up front, collating the intelligence and presenting it in a way that is easily understood. In the past it was just about reporting financial performance in the preceding year or quarter, but now things are so different. Today it's about combining financial data with non-financial intelligence to get a much wider perspective on how the business has performed and to predict how it will perform – and it's about using all of this to make sound business decisions.'

(Hari Punchihewa, deputy chief executive and finance director at the University of Derby (UK).)

3   Finance as a business partner

'Management accountants don't really exist now as they once did. They are being replaced with what I would call finance business partners. Accounting was always seen as the boring part of the business, but the new position of finance business partner is much more exciting and creative.'

(Jim Jordan, finance director at the IoD (Institute of Directors – UK).)

The four levels of the diamond shape

This evolution has resulted in a diamond shape. The diamond can be split into four levels. **Level 1 is at the top** and **level 4 is at the bottom** of the diamond.

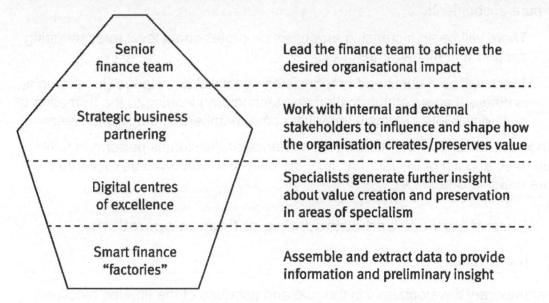

Senior finance team	Lead the finance team to achieve the desired organisational impact
Strategic business partnering	Work with internal and external stakeholders to influence and shape how the organisation creates/preserves value
Digital centres of excellence	Specialists generate further insight about value creation and preservation in areas of specialism
Smart finance "factories"	Assemble and extract data to provide information and preliminary insight

Note: This is an important diagram to learn and to understand for the exam.

Why the shape of the finance function is changing

There are three main reasons why the shape of the finance function is changing:

Reason	Explanation
The changing mandate for finance	The contemporary transformation of the finance function was discussed in section 3. The changes discussed better enable the finance function to focus on level 2 'strategic business partnering' and explain why the diamond shape bulges outwards at this level.
Technology	Technology has impacted the finance function in two main ways: Firstly, it has supported the automation of many of the management information processes and much of the reporting performed at level 4. Secondly, It has increased the need for skills at levels 2 and 3 (as discussed below).
Finance function capability	The changing mandate for finance combined with advancements in technology have changed the competencies required of the finance function. Level 2 is the focal point of these changes and is another reason for the bulge in the finance function shape at this point.

Will the shape of the finance function continue to evolve?

The shape of the finance function will continue to evolve in response to the changing roles of the function, what is clear is that finance will no longer just be for pure accountants.

- There will be an increasing emphasis on professional level roles requiring support and management skills.

- There will be a continued emphasis on specialist knowledge (for example, in different areas of automation and technology) leading to the formation of multi-disciplinary teams who will become members of the finance team.

Important note: The activities that the finance professionals perform to fulfil their roles at each of the four levels of the diamond shape will be explored in more detail in Chapter 4.

5 Shared services and outsourcing of finance operations

5.1 Introduction

Contemporary developments in the role and activities of the finance function have for some organisations meant a structural reconfiguration, with solutions based on, for example:

- greater or less centralisation

- offshoring – the relocation of business activities (such as call centres) from the home country to another country

- shared service provision (as discussed in section 4.1 when we explained the migration of the shape of the finance function from a hierarchical triangle to a segregated triangle)

- business partnering

- outsourcing.

The local variations are endless but the aim is the same – to make the finance function a valued and worthwhile essential of organisational functioning.

Two of these options, outsourcing and shared service provision, are discussed below.

 Outsourcing means contracting out aspects of the work of the organisation previously done in-house, to specialist providers.

 A **shared service centre** may be established for a particular activity of the organisation. The term describes a situation whereby, a usually large, multinational organisation with processing centres in all or several of the countries in which it operates chooses to consolidate these activities at one site, or shared service centre. This is sometimes referred to as 'internal outsourcing'.

5.2 Introduction to outsourcing

The outsourcing of many aspects of business activity is one strategy that has been suggested as a source of adding value and streamlining activities to maintain competitiveness.

It has become **increasingly common over the past two decades.**

In theory, any of the operations that a business performs can be outsourced. However, an organisation will **often outsource its non-core services** to a third party, allowing them to focus on their core competencies which are integral to the organisation's ability to create and to add value.

Non-core activities may include:

- facilities management
- human resource management
- cleaning services
- catering services and
- legal services.

The organisation's core competencies are something that they are able to do that drives competitive advantage and is very difficult for a competitor to emulate. It **may be unwise for an organisation to outsource activities in which they have a core competence** as this could erode competitive advantage.

Illustration 11 – Outsourcing in a clothing retailer

In clothing retail, it may be the case that most firms have outsourced production to Asian manufacturers in order to gain low costs. This outsourcing may be essential just to be a feasible player in the market.

However, the clothing retailers may still retain aspects of the work in which they have a core competence in-house. For example, a particular clothing retailer may have core competencies relating to design and brand management and may retain these activities within the organisation.

Canterell is a bank based in country Z. It is considering outsourcing its IT function. Its current IT systems are considered excellent, which is important, as the banking industry in country Z is highly competitive and innovative.

Which of the following statements regarding this proposal is correct?

A   Canterell will be definitely be able to improve its in house IT expertise as a result

B   Outsourcing could cause Canterell a loss of competitive advantage

C   It will be easy for Canterell to bring IT back in-house if they are not satisfied with the outsource supplier

D   It is not possible to outsource IT

Outsourcing has become increasingly common in organisations. The advantages and disadvantages include:

Advantages of outsourcing

The main reason for outsourcing is that it is cheaper. **Cost advantages** can come from a number of sources:

- A large supplier may benefit from economies of scale in production.

- The firm concerned will benefit from reduced capital expenditure.

- Reduced headcount.

- Research and development expenditure may also be saved.

There can also be **quality advantages**:

- The supplier may have superior skills and expertise. For example, Apple's main reason for outsourcing to China is superior manufacturing capability rather than cost savings.

- Outsourcing may solve the problem of the company having a skills shortage in certain areas.

Other advantages include the following:

- The supplier may have greater production expertise and efficiencies, leading to faster and more flexible supply of components.

- The management of the customer are no longer distracted by fringe areas and so can focus on core business activities.

- The organisation can exercise buyer power over suppliers ensuring favourable terms and conditions.

- The organisation has greater flexibility to switch suppliers based on changing cost/quality considerations.

Disadvantages

- Cost issues – the supplier will want to make a profit margin, suggesting it may be cheaper to do the work in house. In addition, if dealing with a major supplier the organisation may be vulnerable to future price rises.

- Loss of core competence – the service may represent (or contribute to) a core competence for the organisation and therefore outsourcing may lead to a loss of competitive advantage.

- Transaction costs – arise from the effort put into specifying what is required, co-ordinating delivery and monitoring quality. (**Note:** Transaction costs are discussed in more detail later on in the chapter).

- Finality of decision – once a service has been contracted out it may be difficult to take back in-house at a later date, for example due to a loss of in-house expertise.

- Risk of loss of confidential information.

- Risk of continuity of supply if the supplier has problems.

- Difficulty agreeing/enforcing contract terms.

- Damage to employee morale if redundancies occur or if organisational culture is eroded.

Illustration 12 – Outsourcing advantages

Organisations can outsource a wide range of activities and processes.

Robotic process automation (RPA) was discussed earlier on in this chapter. Organisations may want to harness this new technology but do not have the resources or expertise to do so effectively. Therefore, the organisation may outsource this business process to an expert in this field.

This outsourcing will allow the organisation to harness the potential to automate business processes and to enjoy the benefits of RPA including:

- faster processing and improved productivity
- lower costs
- improvements in accuracy and compliance
- a focus on higher value, customer focused activities.

Test your understanding 12

Q Co is considering outsourcing its IT function to a third party IT company on a fixed fee basis. Q does not consider IT to be core function. A junior accountant has produced a list of possible advantages of this to the company.

Which FOUR of the following factors are likely advantages of Q outsourcing its IT function?

A   It will reduce the probability of other organisations gaining access to Q's information

B   It will reduce uncertainty relating to how much the IT function will cost Q each year

C   The third party company may have access to IT skills that Q lacks

D   If the third party fails to perform well, Q can easily bring the IT function back in-house

E   The third party company may have access to more economies of scale for IT, allowing Q to save money on its IT function

F   It will reduce Q's dependence on its suppliers

G   Q is likely to gain competitive advantage over rivals with its IT systems

H   It is likely to allow Q to focus its management time on core activities

Service level agreements

At least some of the potential disadvantages can be controlled though the use of effective service level agreements.

 A **service level agreement** (SLA) is a negotiated agreement between the supplier and the customer and is a legal agreement regarding the level of service to be provided.

Content of service level agreements

- A detailed explanation of exactly what service the supplier is offering to provide.
- The targets/benchmarks to be used and the consequences of failing to meet them.
- Expected response time to technical queries.
- The expected time to recover the operations in the event of a disaster such as a systems crash, terrorist attack, etc.
- The procedure for dealing with complaints.
- The information and reporting procedures to be adopted.
- The procedures for cancelling the contract.

Transaction cost theory

 Transaction costs are the indirect costs (i.e. non-production costs) incurred in performing a particular activity, for example the expenses incurred through outsourcing.

When outsourcing, transaction costs arise from the effort that must be put into specifying what is required and subsequently co-ordinating delivery and monitoring quality.

There are three main types of transaction costs:

- **Search and information costs** – for example, the cost of determining which supplier is cheapest.

- **Bargaining costs** – the cost of agreeing on an acceptable SLA.

- **Policing and enforcement costs** – are the costs of making sure the other party sticks to the terms of the contract, and taking appropriate action (often through the legal system) if this turns out not to be the case.

High transaction costs for outsourcing may suggest an in-house solution whereas low transaction costs for outsourcing would support the argument to outsource.

Test your understanding 13	
Which of the following statements is/are true?	
	True?
High transaction costs will usually lead to a company deciding to outsource	
A robust SLA will prevent the risk of a loss of confidential data	
Transaction costs include bargaining costs	
Transaction costs are incurred when outsourcing is used	
Transaction costs include the cost of production	

Transaction cost theory (Wiliamson and Coase)

Organisations choose between two methods of obtaining control over resources:

- the ownership of assets (hierarchy solutions – decisions over production, supply, and the purchases of inputs are made by managers and imposed through hierarchies) and

- buying-in the use of assets (the market solution – individuals and firms make independent decisions that are guided and co-ordinated by market prices).

The decision is based on a comparison of the transaction costs of the two approaches.

Transactions have three dimensions that determine the costs associated with them:

- uncertainty – the more uncertain the environment the harder it is to write effective long-term contracts and the more unlikely the acquisition of a supplier is

- the frequency with which the transactions recur; and

- asset specificity – the extent to which the transacting firms invest in assets whose value depends on the business relationships remaining intact. The greater the specificity of the assets involved, the greater the likelihood that a transaction will take place within the firm.

These factors translate into 'make-or-buy' decisions: whether it is better to provide a service from within the organisation, with hierarchical co-ordination, or from outside the organisation, with market co-ordination. Williamson and Coase argue that it is the third dimension, the degree of asset specificity, which is the most important determinant of transaction. The more specific the assets are to a transaction then, all other things being equal, the greater will be the associated transaction costs and the more likely that the transaction will be internalised into a hierarchy.

Conversely, when the productive assets are non-specific the process of market contracting is the more efficient because transaction costs will be low.

Asset specificity

An asset is said to be transaction-specific if its value to a given transaction is greater than its value in its best alternative use. The greater the gap between these two values, the greater the degree of specificity of the asset. Williamson and Coase suggested six main types of asset specificity:

- Site specificity – suggests that once sited the assets may be very immobile.

  For example, a car components manufacturer locating a components factory near to a large customer's manufacturing plant.

- Physical asset specificity – when parties make investments in machinery or equipment that are specific to a certain task these will have lower values in alternative uses.

  For example, a supplier of wet cement to building sites may invest in wet cement delivery trucks (a 'hierarchy' solution) since these trucks are so specific to this task that they cannot be sourced via a network.

- Human asset specificity – occurs when workers may have to acquire relationship-specific skills, know-how and information that is more valuable inside a particular transaction than outside it.

  For example, a consultant may have to acquire detailed knowledge of a client's in-house developed systems but this knowledge may not be useful on other clients.

- Brand name capital specificity refers to becoming affiliated with a well-known 'brand name' and thus becoming less free to pursue other opportunities.

  For example, an actor may become 'typecast' in a particular role or show.

- Dedicated asset specificity entails investments in general-purpose plant that are made at the behest of a particular customer.

  For example, the car components manufacturer above invests in dedicated machinery to make bespoke components for just one manufacturer. Should the contract be lost, these components may have to be adapted for sale elsewhere.

- Temporal specificity – arises when the timing of performance is critical, such as with perishable agricultural commodities where a farmer may struggle to find alternative processors at short notice.

5.3   Outsourcing the activities of the finance function

Introduction

Outsourcing of the finance function's activities has become increasingly common in organisations in recent times. The **emphasis has been on reducing costs** but outsourcing has also **enabled the retained finance function to focus on strategic change** by working more closely with the business to provide business partnering to help improve decision making.

Which finance function activities should be outsourced?

A key consideration is which finance activities should be outsourced.

- Transactional processes (such as accounts payable/receivable, travel and entertainment and cash management) tended to be very popular to outsource.

- However, improvements in provider capabilities have also resulted in outsourcing of services such as statutory and regulatory accounting, financial reporting and tax, management accounting, budgeting and forecasting.

Relating this back to the '**information to impact framework**' (discussed in Chapter 2 and section 3 of this chapter) these activities relate largely to the left hand side of the framework and the '**assembly**' and '**analysis**' activities within.

Benefits and drawbacks of outsourcing the finance function's activities

Benefits	Drawbacks
• **Cost reduction** – outsourcing can deliver significant economies of scale through the use of standardised processes and leading-edge technology. • **Radical transformation** – outsourcing can enable broad structural change. Low value, non-core activities can be moved to the external provider allowing the organisation to shift internal resources from operations to innovation, i.e. the 'advisory' and 'application' parts of the 'information to impact framework'. **Note:** A radical transformation and fundamental rethinking of business processes is called business process re-engineering (BPR).	• **Loss of control** – the external provider is relied upon for providing the right level of resource and skill. • The organisation will need to develop expertise and invest time and money in **managing the outsourced services**. • Outsourcing **will cause disruption** and may result in significant resistance to change. • **Risk of intellectual property theft and data breaches.** • **Erosion of internal knowledge and skills.**
• **Access to superior capabilities, expertise and resources** of the specialist provider. • **Business partnering** – the retained finance function can concentrate on their role as business partners, working more closely with the business in decision making.	

5.4 Establishing a shared service centre for the finance function

Introduction

Shared service centres have become a well-established model for organisations to drive efficiencies, improve compliance and controls and enable insight into the business.

The scope of services that are provided include **finance**, HR, IT, procurement, and other business support activities.

As discussed in section 4, the **traditional shape of the finance function was a hierarchical triangle**, with a broad base and few roles at senior levels. Over the **past two decades this shape evolved to a segregated triangle with routine processes** being migrated to and **carried out by shared service centres**.

This change was **driven by two main factors**:

- **Globalisation** – many organisations grew in size and became multinational organisations with operations and processing centres in several countries. The establishment of a shared service centre enabled the consolidation of these activities at one site.

- **Advances in information technology** – enabling automation of many of the lower level tasks carried out by the finance function (as discussed earlier in this chapter).

The **benefits** of establishing a shared service centre for the finance function are as follows:

- Cost reduction – a shared service centre may reduce costs by up to 50% due to factors such as:
    - a reduction in premises and associated costs
    - potentially favourable labour rates, for example if the shared service centre is based in a country with lower wage rates
    - headcount reductions, for example due to the more routine activities benefiting from economies of scale and a reduction in repetition of tasks
    - systems consolidation
    - potential tax savings.

- Opportunity to standardise processes:
    - resulting in a lower potential for errors
    - making the design and update of the control environment easier
    - allowing for consistent reporting.

- An improved level of service – the shared service centre will view the business to be the customer. The more professional supplier/customer relationship should result in marked improvements in the quality of the service provided.

- A better opportunity to compare trends across the organisation.

- Consolidation of systems, to say one type of accountancy software, makes add-ons such as robotics and greater use of automation easier.

However, there are **risks** associated with the establishment of a shared service centre:

- Has the organisation got the resources required to spread the major set up costs?

- Employee issues – these include the potential cost of making staff redundant plus the impact on the morale of the remaining staff due to the changes made.

- Lack of systems integration across the organisation may make migration of diverse systems complicated, costly and time consuming.

- A shared service centre is often established in a multinational organisation which has operations in several countries. The complexities of these countries including different laws, taxes, languages, cultures and reporting requirements may make this difficult.

Tips on establishing a successful shared service centre

- A clear vision of how the shared service centre fits into the overall business model.

- Senior management commitment – senior management need a clear vision and strategy and to support the process.

- Integration with other change initiatives.

- Clear scope with delineation of responsibilities.

- Buy-in of operating units impacted by the change.

- Ensuring that the organisation that remains after service transfer is robust.

- Support from those who have implementation experience to help navigate through the challenges faced.

- A strong customer-focused culture.

- A commitment to continuous improvement.

Test your understanding 14

Which THREE of the following are drawbacks of outsourcing the non-core activities of the finance function?

A   Loss of control

B   Risk of data breaches

C   Erosion of internal knowledge

D   Increased costs

E   Loss of competitive advantage

F   Major set up costs

Alternatives to establishing a shared service centre for the finance function

The benefits must be weighed up against the risks before a decision is taken to establish the shared service centre. It may be that a decision is taken to keep the **finance function's activities in several sites** across the business.

An alternative would be to establish a shared service centre but rather than the services being provided in-house a decision is taken to **outsource the provision of the shared services to a third party** who specialises in the provision of such services.

Illustration 13 – Outsourcing of finance shared services

PwC (UK) is a one of the larger providers of finance shared services. The following is taken from their website and illustrates nicely the future of the finance function and how an outsourcing provider could assist with this future:

'It's 2020 and you're the CFO sat in a finance shared service centre. There's a wall of screens showing the latest profit forecasts for each of your divisions – changing every few minutes. In the corner, there's a Robotic Process Automation (RPA) hub with a few people studiously monitoring the 50 bots deployed across your finance processes. In the general accounting team it's month end – but there's an air of calm as with your cloud based Enterprise Resource planning (ERP) you can close whenever you want within a few minutes. The brightest monitor in the room is at the back, showing the daily Shared Service Centre's (SSC) huddle board with lots of stars and names up in lights.

At PwC we are helping clients take advantage of new digital tools and ways of thinking to move towards this sort of reality. Whether you're just thinking about shared services or outsourcing or have been established for years and are looking to evolve your SSC further to take advantage of the digital revolution, we can help.'

Shared services and the diamond shape of the finance function

The discussion above has focused on the past two decades over which time the shape of the finance function has evolved from a traditional hierarchical triangle to a segregated triangle with routine processes being migrated to and carried out by shared service centres. The scope of the shared service centre's work was very much on the lower level tasks (level 4 tasks) of 'assembling and extracting data and providing limited insight'.

However, as discussed earlier on in this chapter, the shape of the finance function is now evolving to a diamond shape. In the diamond shape the level 3 tasks present within 'specialists generating further insights in their areas of specialism' are now offered by shared service centres. Opportunities for business partnering will also be expanded.

Organisations are demanding a higher level of service, capabilities and understanding within their shared service centres. They will be viewed as centres of excellence formed of the key people that are necessary for areas such as reporting and complex accounting and tax. These people won't all be based in the same location but will utilise collaborative tools such as video calls to create more virtual centres of excellence.

In summary, **shared service centres whether in-house or operated by a service provider (outsourced) have industrialised the provision of routine management and accounting services but now offer scope to expand vertically to offer higher value services.**

6   Chapter summary

```
                    The structure and shape
                     of the finance function
```

Organisational structure
- Mintzberg's effective organisation
- Types of structure
- Centralisation and decentralisation
- Tall and flat organisations
- Contemporary transformation of organisations

Contemporary transformation of the finance function
- Introduction
- Can the finance function cope with this shift?
- The information to impact framework revisited

Shape of the finance function
- Introduction
- Traditional hierarchical shape
- Evolution into a diamond shape

Shared services and outsourcing of finance operations
- Introduction
- Introduction to outsourcing
- Outsourcing the activities of the finance function
- Establishing a shared service centre for the finance function

Test your understanding answers

Test your understanding 1

The correct answer is **C – by definition**.

Test your understanding 2

The correct answer is C

A divisionalised form is characterised by a powerful middle line in which a there are a large number of middle managers who each takes charge of a more or less autonomous division.

Test your understanding 3

The correct answer is **D**

The separate parts of the organisation operate as SBUs in a divisional structure – not a functional structure.

The matrix structure tends to require time-consuming meetings and has significant overlap of authority between managers. This tends to slow the decision-making process down.

Test your understanding 4

The correct answer is **B**

As M has several complex products, a structure that creates a separate division to look after each one seems the most logical. Functional and geographical structures would struggle to cope with the differing needs of the products. The level of work needed to run a large, complex organisation would also probably be beyond the capabilities of an entrepreneurial structure.

Test your understanding 5

The correct answer is **D**

Decentralisation should result in better local decisions being made since autonomy is devolved to local managers.

Test your understanding 6

The correct answer is **B**

The scalar chain relates to the number of levels of management within the organisation.

Test your understanding 7

Narrow

Test your understanding 8

Answer A: Because of advancements in technology the basic activities of the finance function are no longer relevant – FALSE they are still relevant but there has been a shift in emphasis on the importance of each of the activities.

Answer B: Technology allows the contemporary finance function to refocus its energy on value creation – TRUE.

Answer C: Technology has meant that a large amount of the assembly and analysis activities can be automated – TRUE.

Answer D: Technology has meant that a large amount of the advising and applying activities can be automated – FALSE, although some of these activities can be automated the finance function will need to reallocate its resources to these activities.

Test your understanding 9

A, B, D – these are all assembly and analysis activities, which are more heavily impacted by technology and automation.

C and E are advising and applying activities.

Test your understanding 10

The shape of the finance function has evolved from a traditional hierarchy to a diamond shape in today's digital age.

This has primarily been driven by globalisation and technology.

Test your understanding 11

Answer B is the correct answer – outsourcing is likely to cause a loss of competitive advantage as IT is a core competence within this highly competitive and innovative industry. In addition, Canterell will have no way to create its own unique systems.

Outsourcing IT would be likely to mean the closure of their own IT department, which will mean the loss of skilled staff. This will make it difficult to bring IT back in-house in the future (answer C) and will result in a loss of IT expertise (answer A). It is possible to outsource the IT function (answer D) although this decision may not be in the best interest of the company.

Test your understanding 12

The correct answers are **B,C, E and H**

As it is a fixed fee, Q will know how much the IT function will cost each year (answer B). Outsourcers often have a level of expertise that organisations can benefit from if they have skills lacking in-house (answer C). As outsourcers are providing services for many customers they are able to generate economies of scale, often making outsourcing a cheaper option (answer E). Not having to focus on non-core activities mean that management can focus on core activities which often are the source of competitive advantage (answer H).

Test your understanding 13

	True?
High transaction costs will usually lead to a company deciding to outsource	No – opposite
A robust SLA will prevent the risk of a loss of confidential data	Reduce not prevent
Transaction costs include bargaining costs	✓
Transaction costs are incurred when outsourcing is used	✓
Transaction costs include the cost of production	No

83

Test your understanding 14

The correct answers are **A, B and C** – The organisation will become reliant on the external provider and will not have as much control over the function being outsourced (answer A). This leads to the erosion of internal knowledge (answer C) and could increase the risk of data breaches (answer B).

Outsourcing should be a cheaper option thereby reducing costs (answer D). Outsourcing the non-core activities means the remaining activities retained within finance can focus on business partnering enhancing competitive advantage (answer E). Major set up costs are a drawback of setting up a shared service centre not a drawback of outsourcing (answer F).

What each level of the finance function does

Chapter learning objectives

Lead	Component
D2: Explain what each level of the finance function does.	Explain the activities of: (a) Finance operations (b) Specialist areas including financial reporting and financial planning and analysis (FP&A) (c) Strategic partnering for value (d) Strategic leadership of the finance team

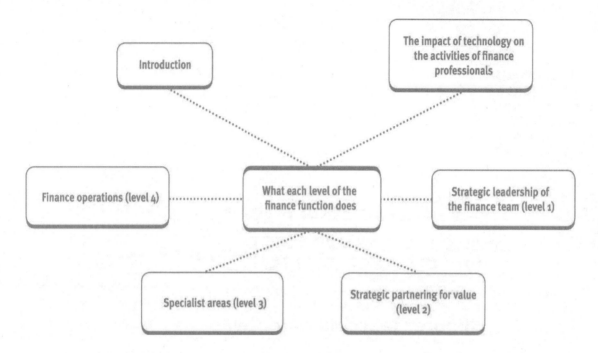

1 Introduction

In Chapter 2 we discussed the basic activities that the finance function performs using the 'information to impact framework'.

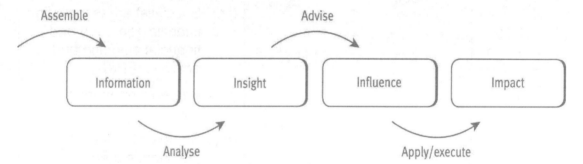

We also **linked these basic activities to the diamond shape of the finance function** (see diagram below).

In this chapter we are going to review each of these activities in more detail, understanding what the role of the finance function is within each of these activities.

We will also briefly discuss how an organisation could use technology to improve the productivity of finance professionals within these areas and we will discuss the threat of automation.

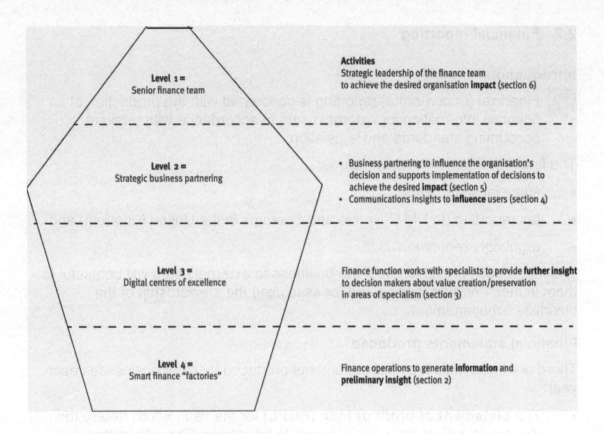

2 Finance operations (level 4)

2.1 Introduction

In this section we are going to look at the basic components of finance operations (i.e. accounting operations) and how these finance operations generate information and preliminary insight. The information and extracted data provided at this level becomes the foundations of the work of finance professionals.

Finance operations consist of the following, often inter-related, components:

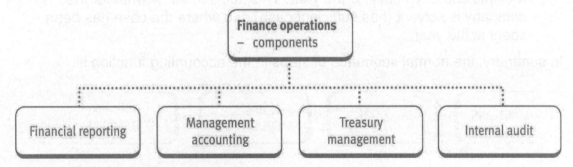

Each of these components will be explored in turn below.

2.2 Financial reporting

Introduction

 Financial (or corporate) reporting is concerned with the production of financial information for external users in accordance with relevant accounting standards and legislation.

The financial information may include:

- financial statements

- tax reporting (to HM Revenue and Customs in the United Kingdom) and

- regulatory reporting.

The information provided about the business to external users will be useful to them in their decision making and for assessing the stewardship of the business's management.

Financial statements produced

There are three main financial statements produced by most businesses each year:

- The **statement of profit or loss (SOPL)** for the year, which details the income as well as the costs incurred in the period. This allows the business to calculate whether it has made a profit (if income exceeds costs) or a loss (if costs exceed income).

- The **statement of financial position (SOFP)** as at the year end, which shows the assets (business resources such as motor vehicles, buildings and cash) and liabilities (money owed to third parties such as banks and suppliers) of the business. This statement also shows the stake that the owners of the business have in the organisation (or their 'capital'). In a company, this is often referred to as 'shareholder's equity'.

- The **statement of cash flows** for the year, which summarises the cash receipts and payments for the year. This helps to show whether the company is solvent (has sufficient cash) and where the cash has been spent in the year.

In summary, the normal sequence of steps in the accounting function is:

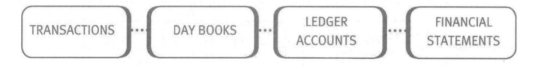

Test your understanding 1

J has been asked to find four pieces of information about FGH Ltd for his manager from the company's statement of profit or loss (SOPL) and statement of financial position (SOFP). He has been asked to find:

(1) The ratio of current assets to current liabilities

(2) Total shareholders' equity

(3) Gross profit as a percentage of turnover

(4) Total rent paid for the year

Which of the following (A, B, C or D) correctly match the information needed with the financial statement each would be found in?

	(1)	(2)	(3)	(4)
A	SOFP	SOFP	SOPL	SOPL
B	SOPL	SOPL	SOFP	SOFP
C	SOFP	SOPL	SOFP	SOPL
D	SOPL	SOFP	SOPL	SOFP

Why do businesses need to prepare financial statements?

The preparation of financial statements is a time-consuming and expensive process. So why do most organisations have a financial reporting component?

The main reason is to satisfy stakeholders who have an interest in the financial performance of the business. These could include:

- **Owners** – interested in how profitable the business is and how well it is being run.

Illustration 1 – Investor ratios

A number of ratios will be of interest to the investor. These include:

Earnings per share (EPS)

EPS is a measure of the profit attributable to each ordinary shareholder.

$$EPS = \frac{\text{Profit after tax (less preference dividends)}}{\text{Weighted average number of ordinary shares in issue}}$$

Price/ earnings (P/E) ratio

$$P/E \text{ ratio} = \frac{\text{Share price}}{\text{EPS}}$$

A high P/E ratio means that investors are paying more for today's earnings in anticipation of future growth.

Dividend yield

$$\text{Dividend yield} = \frac{\text{Dividend per share}}{\text{Current share price}} \times 100$$

- **Managers** – interested in the company's financial situation so that they can plan effectively for the future.

- **Banks** – may wish to see whether the business can afford the repayments on loans and overdrafts.

- **Employees** – interested in the financial position of the company and the impact this will have on their jobs and wages.

- **Suppliers and customers** – may wish to check the financial stability of the business to ensure it will be able to make payments/supply goods as needed.

- **Government** – may wish to check that the business is obeying relevant laws on reporting and taxation.

Companies must send a copy of their financial statements to each of their shareholders at the end of the year. Large and publicly-quoted companies are also required to appoint external auditors each year to give an independent opinion on whether the financial statements have been drawn up properly and whether they give a true and fair view.

2.3 Management accounting

Introduction

 Management accounting is the provision of information to help managers and other internal users in their decision making, performance measurement, planning and control activities.

Management accountants will use financial accounting records as a source of data for their work but they will also use other sources of internal and external data.

While there are no legally required formats for management accounts, there are several key management reports that are common to many businesses. Three of the most common are **cost schedules, budgets** and **variance reports.**

Cost schedules

A **cost schedule** lists the various expenses involved in manufacturing units of a product. This is often shown as a list of the costs incurred when making a unit of each type of product. This may be called a **standard cost card.**

Illustration 2 – Standard cost card

ABC Ltd manufactures toys. One of its products is a wooden train set, which has the following standard costs per unit:

	$
Direct materials (wood and paint)	5.50
Direct labour (time spent cutting and painting)	6.50
Prime cost	12.00
Variable overheads (heat and light)	4.00
Marginal cost	16.00
Fixed overheads (factory rent)	5.00
Total (absorption) cost	21.00

There are several key business decisions that this report can help a business to make:

- **Pricing decisions** – How much should the business sell the products for in order to ensure it makes a profit?

- **Break-even analysis** – Which products are profitable or loss-making? Is a new product worth producing? Can the business sell enough units to cover the costs of making the product?

- **Key factor analysis** – should products be made in-house or should their manufacture be outsourced to somewhere cheaper?

- **Investment appraisal** – should a new machine be bought to replace an old machine? Should the business begin a new project, such as launching a new product?

Budgets

In addition, once the costs per unit have been identified, it should be possible to produce a budget. This shows the total planned revenues and costs for the business for the coming period. It is based on the cost schedules mentioned earlier.

Budgets are useful for several reasons. A useful memory aid is the acronym **CRUMPET**

- **C**o-ordination – the budget provides guidance for managers and ensures they are all working together for the good of the company.

- **R**esponsibility – the budget authorises managers to make expenditure, hire staff and generally follow the plans laid out in the budget.

- **U**tilisation – budgets (especially cash budgets) help managers to get the best out of their business resources in the coming period.

- **M**otivation – the budget can be a useful device for influencing the behaviour of managers and motivating them to perform in line with business objectives.

- **P**lanning – budgets force managers to look ahead. This may help them to identify opportunities for, or threats to, the business and take effective action in advance.

- **E**valuation – budgets are often used as the basis for management appraisal. The manager has performed well if he has met his budgets in the period.

- **T**elling – also called 'communication', budgets ensure that all members of the business understand what is expected from them during the coming period.

One major drawback of budgets is that they are only estimates of what will happen in the coming period. In reality, most businesses will not perfectly achieve the targets set out for them in their budgets.

This means that they will have to prepare a **variance report** at the end of each period, comparing the budget to the actual results and identifying any differences (i.e. variances) between the two.

 The differences between financial reporting and management accounting

	Management accounting	Financial reporting
Why information is mainly produced	For internal use, such as managers and employees.	For external use, such as shareholders, creditors, banks, government.
Purpose of information	To aid planning, controlling and decision making.	To record the financial performance in a period and the financial position at the end of the period.
Legal requirements	None.	Limited companies must produce financial accounts.
Formats	Management decide on the information that they require and the most useful way of presenting it.	Format and content of financial accounts must follow accounting standards and company law.
Nature of information	Financial and non-financial.	Mostly financial.
Time period	Historical and forward-looking.	Mainly a historical record.

Test your understanding 2

Consider the following two statements regarding the management accounting function.

(i)   Variance analysis enables a business to identify why the actual financial results were different to those predicted by the budget.

(ii)   Management accounts follow a set, pre-determined format as laid out in relevant accounting standards.

Which of these statements is/are correct?

A   (i) only

B   (ii) only

C   Both

D   Neither

Variance reports

A variance report compares the budget to the actual results achieved for the budget period and identifies any significant differences, or variances, between the two.

For control purposes, management may need to establish why a particular variance has occurred. Once the reason has been established, a decision can be taken as to what, if any, control measures might be appropriate to:

- prevent adverse variances from occurring again in the future, or

- repeat a favourable variance in the future, or

- bring actual results back on course to achieve the budgeted targets.

The management accountant will assist and interact with other functions in providing solutions to variances.

2.4   Treasury management

Introduction

Treasury management is the management of the funds of the business, namely cash and other working capital items, plus long-term investments, short-term and long-term debt, and equity finance.

The key roles of the treasury function include:

Working capital management	The treasury section will monitor the organisation's cash balance and working capital to ensure that it never runs out of money.
Cash management	Preparation of cash budgets and arrangement of overdrafts where necessary.
Financing	The treasury section will monitor the organisation's investments and borrowings to ensure they gain as much investment income as possible and incur as little interest expense as possible.
Foreign currency	The treasury section will monitor foreign exchange rates and try to manage the organisation's affairs so that it minimises losses due to changes in foreign exchange rates.
Tax	The treasury section will try to manage the organisation's affairs to legally avoid as much tax as possible.

Working capital management

 Working capital is the capital available for conducting the day-to-day operations of an organisation, calculated as the excess of current assets over current liabilities. Thus:

Inventory	X
Trade receivables	X
Cash	X
	___
Total current assets	X
Less: Trade payables	(X)
	___
Working capital balance	X
	___

The treasury function is responsible for deciding on an appropriate level of investment in working capital for the business.

There are advantages in holding either large or small balances of each component of working capital, as shown below.

	Advantage of large balance	Advantage of small balance
Inventory	Customers are happy since they can be immediately provided with goods.	Low holding costs. Less risk of obsolescence costs.
Trade receivables	Customers are happy since they like credit.	Less risk of irrecoverable debts. Good for cash flow.
Cash	Creditors are happy since bills can be paid promptly.	More can be invested elsewhere to earn profits.
Trade payables	Preserves your own cash.	Suppliers are happy and may offer discounts.

Management must decide on the appropriate balance to be struck for each component.

Test your understanding 3

Conservative managers will have a policy of holding a large working capital balance, while aggressive management will hold a low working capital balance.

Which of the following is a consequence of an aggressive management policy?

A   Increased bad and doubtful debts

B   Increased credit periods attract more customers

C   Increased inventory obsolescence

D   Increased risk of inventory outages

Financing

The organisation may need additional funding to allow it to grow and invest in new projects. It may therefore need to raise finance from external sources. There are **two main types of external finance**:

- **Debt** involves borrowing cash from a third party and promising to repay them at a later date. Normally, the company will also have to pay interest on the amount borrowed.

  There are various sources of debt that an organisation can raise funds from, including bank loans and overdrafts, venture capitalists and through selling bonds or debentures.

  The main advantages of raising cash through debt finance are:

  – Interest payments are allowable against tax. Note that dividend payments made to shareholders, by contrast, are **not** an allowable deduction.

  – Raising debt finance does not change the ownership of the organisation.

- Debt tends to be cheaper to service than equity, as it is often secured against the assets of the company and takes priority over equity in the event of the business being liquidated.

- **Equity** involves selling a stake in the business in order to raise cash. For companies, this involves selling shares to either new or existing shareholders.

Raising equity finance has the following advantages:

- There is no minimum level of dividend that must be paid to shareholders. This means that dividends can be suspended if profits are low and the company cannot afford them. Interest payments on debt finance must be paid each year.

- A bank will normally require security on the company's assets before it will offer a loan. Some companies may lack quality assets to offer, making equity more attractive as it does not require security.

The treasury and finance function will weigh up which source of finance best suits the circumstances of the business.

Illustration 3 – Financial gearing

$$\text{Financial gearing} = \frac{\text{Long-term debt}}{\text{Shareholders' funds}} \times 100$$

A high gearing ratio indicates a high level of risk since debt obligations (such as interest payments) must be met, whereas returns to shareholders (such as dividends) are voluntary.

Test your understanding 4

AHG needs to raise $50m to launch a new product. AHG hopes the new product will be a success, but the returns are highly uncertain, with a 30% chance that the launch will be a failure. The product is expected to sell for around 5 years.

AHG is currently trying to decide whether the launch should be financed using a 5 year bank loan, or through raising equity.

Which of the following statements is correct?

A Equity will be cheaper, as dividends are allowable against tax

B AHG should choose equity due to the risky nature of the project

C Equity should be chosen as AHG needs a permanent increase in its finance

D Debt usually does not require security, meaning it may be easier for AHG to raise

Foreign currency

Companies may have borrowings in foreign currencies, or may have customers/suppliers who will pay/expect payment in a foreign currency. The treasury department will try to manage affairs to minimise the company's exposure to foreign exchange losses, i.e. minimise losses.

Managing foreign currency risk

Background

Assume a UK company buys goods costing US$1m from a US company on 1 January 20X1. The goods are due to be paid for on 31 March 20X1.

The exchange rate at 1 January is £1:US$1.5, so the goods will cost £666,667 ($1m/1.5).

However, if the exchange rate changes to, say, £1:US$1.3, then the payment to be made will be £769,231 ($1m/1.3).

Managing the risk

The company can manage this risk by entering into a 'forward exchange contract' at 1 January to fix the rate of exchange at which it can buy $1m at 31 March.

The rate in the forward exchange contract will depend on what the market thinks will happen to exchange rates.

Let us say, for example, that the company can enter into a contract to purchase $1m at the rate of £1:$1.48. The company's cost, in sterling, is then fixed at £675,676 ($1m/1.48).

Tax

One of the roles of the finance and treasury function is to calculate the business tax liability for the organisation and mitigate, or reduce, that liability as far as possible within the law.

Illustration 4 – Tax avoidance, tax evasion and tax mitigation

Tax avoidance is the legal use of the rules of the tax regime to one's own advantage, in order to reduce the amount of tax payable by means that are within the law.

Tax evasion is the use of illegal means to reduce one's tax liability, for example by deliberately misrepresenting the true state of your affairs to the tax authorities.

The directors of a company have a duty to their shareholders to maximise the post-tax profits that are available for distribution as dividends to the shareholders, thus they have a duty to arrange the company's affairs to avoid taxes as far as possible. However, dishonest reporting to the tax authorities (for example, declaring less income than actually earned) would be tax evasion and a criminal offence.

> While the traditional distinction between tax avoidance and tax evasion is clear, recently authorities have introduced the idea of **tax mitigation** to mean conduct that reduces tax liabilities without frustrating the intentions of Parliament, while **tax avoidance** is used to describe schemes which, while they are legal, are designed to defeat the intentions of Parliament. Thus, in the United Kingdom, once a tax avoidance scheme becomes public knowledge, Parliament will nearly always step in to change the law in order to stop the scheme from working.

Note: Operational level candidates should understand the work and scope of the treasury function but are not expected to understand the detail of matters such as foreign exchange contracts. These matters of detail are explored in later levels of the syllabus.

2.5 Internal audit

What is internal audit?

 Internal audit is an independent activity, established by management to examine and evaluate the organisation's risk management processes and systems of control, and to make recommendations for the achievement of company objectives.

The purpose of internal audit

Company directors have a legal requirement to produce true and fair annual financial statements. To help ensure this is done, companies are required to have their published financial statements audited by an external team of experts **(external auditors).**

Directors also need assurance on other financial matters. This assurance is primarily for their own internal use, although in recent years pressure has grown for increasingly more of such work to be made publicly available.

This additional work is carried out by internal auditors, who may be company employees or outside experts from a firm of accountants.

Internal audit is part of the organisational control of a business; it is one of the methods used by management to ensure the efficient and orderly running of the business as a whole, and is part of the overall control environment.

Internal auditors' work has expanded in recent years, and the role of internal audit often now includes:

*   helping to set corporate objectives

*   helping to design and monitor performance measures for these objectives.

Internal audit as part of good corporate governance

A properly functioning internal audit department is part of good corporate governance, as recognised by all national and international corporate governance codes.

Internal audit enables management to perform proper risk assessments (another central theme of corporate governance codes) by means of properly understanding the strengths and weaknesses of all parts of the control systems in the business.

The UK Corporate Governance Code states that companies without an internal audit function should **annually review the need for one**.

Where there is an internal audit function, the board should **annually review its scope of work**, authority and resources.

Ideally, the internal audit function should be staffed with **qualified, experienced staff**, whose work is closely monitored by an audit committee.

The function of internal audit in the context of corporate risk management

Internal audit has a particular interest in evaluating the company's risk management structures. Internal audit can:

- manage the basic data used by management to identify risks

- identify techniques for prioritising and managing risks

- report on the effectiveness of risk management solutions (for example, internal controls).

Scope of internal audit

Internal audit staff are typically expected to carry out a variety of tasks:

- reviewing internal controls and financial reports

- reviewing risk management systems

- carrying out special assignments (e.g. fraud investigations)

- conducting operational reviews (e.g. into efficiency of parts of the business).

The purpose of internal audit can be **summarised** in the table below:

Role	To advise management on whether the organisation has sound systems of internal controls to protect the organisation against loss.
Legal basis	Generally not a legal requirement. However the UK Corporate Governance Code recommends that if a listed company does not have an internal audit department it should annually assess the need for one.

Scope of work	Determined by management. Covers all areas of the organisation, operational as well as financial.
Approach	Increasingly risk-based. Assess risks. Evaluate systems of controls. Test operations of systems. Make recommendations for improvements.
Responsibility	To advise and make recommendations on internal control and corporate governance.

Test your understanding 5

The internal audit is simply a necessary cost that must be incurred by a company and offers few tangible benefits for the organisation.

Is this statement true or false?

A   True

B   False

Test your understanding 6

Internal audit may be carried out by employees of the company being audited, or may be carried out by external accountants who are paid for delivering this service.

Is this statement true or false?

A   True

B   False

Test your understanding 7

In a large company, to who do internal auditors normally report their conclusions?

A   Executive directors

B   Board of directors

C   Shareholders

D   Non-executive directors

The role of internal audit in preventing and detecting fraud

Fraud is an intentional act involving the use of deception to obtain an unjust or illegal advantage – essentially 'theft by deception'. Fraud is a criminal offence, punishable by a fine or imprisonment.

As far as the financial statements are concerned, fraud comprises both the use of deception to obtain an unjust or illegal financial advantage and intentional misrepresentations affecting the financial statements. It is ultimately up to the courts to decide in each instance whether fraud has occurred, for example:

- deliberate falsification of documents/records
- deliberate ignoring of errors requiring correction
- deliberate suppression of relevant information.

There are three prerequisites that are required for fraud to occur:

- **dishonesty** – relates to a lack of integrity or honesty. An honest employee will be unlikely to commit a fraud.
- **opportunity** – the individual must have the opportunity or opening for a fraud to be committed. These opportunities will often be created due to weak internal controls.
- **motivation** – the individual must feel that the rewards that can be earned by the fraud will outweigh the potential costs if they are caught.

All three are usually required – for example an honest employee is unlikely to commit fraud even if given the opportunity and motive

Factors that might indicate an increased risk of fraud and error include (amongst others):

- **management domination by one person, or a small group of people** – dominant individuals often find it easy to circumvent controls and procedures.
- **unnecessarily complex corporate structure** – this makes it harder to trace transactions, meaning it is easier for employees to hide fraud.
- **poor staff morale** – if staff dislike the company they work for, it may give them additional motivation to perpetrate frauds.
- **personnel who do not take leave/holidays** – this may indicate that staff members are unwilling to pass their duties over to other members of staff in case they identify fraudulent activities.
- **lavish lifestyles of employees** – if an employee is clearly living beyond their means, it may indicate they are committing fraud in order to fund it.
- **inadequate segregation of duties** – if tasks are not shared between employees, the risk of fraud rises

- **lack of monitoring of control systems** – for controls to be effective, they need to be monitored on a regular basis

- **unusual transactions** – in cash, or direct to numbered bank accounts

- **payments for services disproportionate to effort** may also be an indication of fraudulent activity.

If management has established a strong system of internal control then the potential for fraud is greatly reduced.

It is up to the directors to decide what internal audit should do, but normally, where there is an effective internal audit department, the internal auditors will be given the responsibility to test the internal control system and to recommend improvements. The better the control system, the less likely it is that fraud will be attempted, or will succeed if it is attempted.

The directors may also ask the internal auditors to carry out a specific investigation into situations where fraud has been discovered, to learn lessons for the future and ensure that such a fraud cannot be repeated.

There is a spectrum of **implications of fraud**, from the immaterial to the critical. These include:

- Loss of shareholder confidence

- Loss of assets

- Financial difficulties

- Collapse of the company

- Fines by tax and other authorities

Once a fraud has been identified, internal audit should be sent to the department to investigate the circumstances and to make recommendations to improve the controls in the area to deter future fraud. Internal audit should report their findings to the audit committee who can monitor whether the recommendations are swiftly implemented by management.

Limitations of internal audit

- Internal auditors have an unavoidable independence problem. They are employed by the management of the company and yet are expected to give an objective opinion on matters for which management are responsible.

- There is an argument that in order to overcome some of the problems of independence (or lack thereof), that internal audit should be completely separate to the finance function. However, although this may be feasible in, say, a large multinational organisation, resource constraints tend to prevent this in smaller organisations. In these organisations, internal audit and the finance function are still inextricably linked.

- Internal audit will only succeed if it is properly staffed and resourced.

- If internal auditors identify fraud, they may be unwilling to disclose it for fear of the repercussions (which could involve the collapse of the company and the loss of their jobs).

These limitations can be reduced if an **audit committee:**

- sets the work agenda for internal audit

- receives internal audit reports

- is able to ensure the internal audit is properly resourced

- has a 'voice' at main board level.

2.6 Recent changes in finance operations

As was touched upon in Chapter 3:

- Over the last two decades **shared service centres** (SSCs), whether in-house or outsourced, have taken control of the management of many of the rules-based finance operations of an organisation.

- More recently the scope of the SSCs work has expanded to handle all of the processes of finance operations from end to end.

- In addition, the quality of service or level of expertise, and the value they can contribute has become more important than being low cost.

Technology (such as robotic process automation, cognitive computing and blockchain) has also had/will have a big impact on finance operations. It has resulted in the creation of '**smart finance factories**' at this level (i.e. level 4) of the diamond shape of the finance function. This will be discussed further in section 6 and the different types of technology (such as those mentioned above) will be fully explored in Chapter 6.

Test your understanding 8
Which of the following statements about changes in finance operations is true?
A A shared service centre is also referred to as outsourcing
B The quality of work produced by an SSC is lower than if it were outsourced
C Establishing an SSC enables a business' processes to be standardised
D Shared service centres can only produce work at the lowest level (level 4) of the finance function

3 Specialist areas (level 3)

3.1 Introduction

In this section we are going to look at the specialist areas that exist within an organisation. The **specialists are experts who provide insight** derived from the information that has been handed over to them (at level 4) in their specialist areas. Their insights create the building blocks of the organisation's value creation. The specialist areas include:

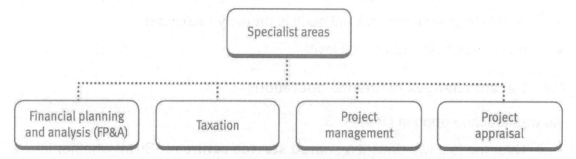

We will briefly introduce each of these specialist areas and will look at **how the finance function works with these specialist areas** to provide further insight to decision makers about value creation/preservation in areas of specialism.

3.2 Financial planning and analysis (FP&A)

Careful financial planning and cash flow management is an important tool in ensuring an organisation is consistently profitable and continues to grow.

FP&A specialists play a crucial role in organisations by performing budgeting, forecasting and data analysis that supports the major organisational decisions of the board.

The specialists utilise both quantitative and qualitative analysis of all the operational aspects of the organisation in order to evaluate its progress towards its goals and to map out future goals and plans.

The specialists consider economic and business trends, review past organisational performance, and attempt to anticipate obstacles and potential problems, all with an eye to forecasting the organisation's future results.

Illustration 5 – Examples of responsibilities of FP&A specialists

- Looking at the effectiveness of the organisation's current investments and comparison to other ways it may utilise its cash flow (for example, other investments or an increased dividend payment).

- Gauging the organisation's overall financial health using key financial ratios (for example, current ratios).

- Identifying which products or product lines are most profitable.

- Working with independent departments to prepare budgets and consolidate them into an overall budget.

3.3 Taxation

Taxation specialists play an important role in an organisation in **minimising risk** and **creating value**. They do this by focusing on two main areas:

- **Tax compliance** – following current legislation, regulation and procedures to **minimise risk**. For example, they will complete and file timely tax returns and produce the required supplementary reports or calculations.

- **Tax planning** – this focuses on ensuring the organisation is working in the most tax efficient manner to reduce the total tax paid and **create value**. Taxation specialists will help the organisation to achieve its goals, playing an important role in:

    - lowering the amount of taxable income

    - reducing the tax rate

    - allowing greater control of when taxes get paid

    - maximising tax relief/tax credits available.

3.4 Project management

 Project management is the integration of all aspects of a project, ensuring that the proper knowledge and resources are available when and where needed, and above all to ensure the expected outcome is produced in a timely, cost effective manner.

Project teams will be put together for the sole purpose of achieving the project goals and objectives.

Projects may run for anything from a few weeks to many years depending on their size and complexity.

Illustration 6 – Project management stages

There are **five stages** to the project management process:

Stage	Explanation
1 Initiation	A project is initiated when a need or organisational objective is identified. The project identified is appraised to ensure it is feasible.
2 Planning	The drawing up of detailed plans. For example, communication of what has to be done, when and by whom, identifying the resources needed and establishing measures of success for the project.
3 Executing	The project team members will perform the tasks they are responsible for and the project manager will provide leadership and co-ordination.

4	Controlling	Projects progress, costs and performance will be tracked against the project plan and any corrective action necessary will be taken.
5	Review and close	Once the project work is finished, the project will be signed off and the team disbanded. A project review meeting will be held.

3.5   Project appraisal

 Project appraisal takes place as part of the first stage (initiation) of the project management process and will involve an assessment and evaluation of the many decisions and potential outcomes of a particular project.

One of the most important project decisions that will need to be appraised is the capital investment decision, since the organisation may commit a substantial proportion of its resources here and this commitment may be long-term or irreversible.

Many different capital investment projects exist including: replacement of assets, cost reduction schemes, new product/service developments and product/service expansions.

To appraise a potential capital project:

- Estimate the costs and benefits from the investment

- Select an appraisal method and use it to assess if the investment is financially worthwhile

- Decide whether or not to go ahead with the project.

There are a number of appraisal methods which are used to assess how financially worthwhile investments are. These include:

- payback

- net present value (NPV)

- internal rate of return (IRR).

Based on the decision rule of the method used, a decision can be made as to whether the investment is financially worthwhile, although there will be other, non-financial considerations which must also be taken into account.

Illustration 7 – An example of an appraisal method: payback

JKL is considering purchasing a new machine. The machine will cost $550,000. The management accountant of JKL has estimated the following additional cash flows will be received over the next 6 years if the new machine is purchased:

Year 1: $40,000

Year 2: $65,000

Year 3: $140,000

Year 4: $175,000

Year 5: $160,000

Year 6: $70,000

JKL has a target payback period of 4 years.

Calculate the payback period for the new machine and advise JKL whether or not to proceed with the investment.

Solution

Note: The investment is shown in year 0.

Work out the **cumulative cash flow** for each year until the cash flow becomes positive. This will highlight when payback has been achieved.

Year	Cash flow	Cumulative cash flow
	$000	$000
0	(550)	(550)
1	40	(510)
2	65	(445)
3	140	(305)
4	175	(130)
5	160	30
6	70	100

You can see that payback is achieved between years 4 and 5. JKL have a target payback period of 4 years. The payback is after this target, so the advice to JKL would be to **not undertake the investment**.

Test your understanding 9

Kazim, Paul, Belinda and Saira all work in a business partnering role, supporting the specialist areas of their organisation.

Match the type of work they do to the specialist area that they support.

- Part of Kazim's role is to manage and minimise the tax risk that the organisation is exposed to. Amongst other things this involves compliance and planning

- Paul is heavily involved in using techniques such as calculating net present values and payback

- Belinda performs budgets and forecasts and data analysis, as well as using key financial ratios

- Saira is in charge of managing resources to achieve a specific objective

A   Financial planning and analysis

B   Taxation

C   Project management

D   Project appraisal

Test your understanding 10

A finance member who is working in the area of project management would typically undertake which FOUR of the following activities?

A   Feasibility study

B   Tax mitigation

C   Resource identification

D   Leadership and co-ordination

E   Net present value analysis

F   Cost control

G   Liquidity ratio calculations and analysis

3.6 How the finance function works with these specialists

The finance function offers expertise in accounting and financial matters.

Their subject matter expertise can be harnessed and developed by different specialist areas.

However, rather than working separately, the finance function works alongside these specialists providing expert support for decisions and projects and helps to formulate strategies so that the business is able to adapt to the ever changing environment.

The finance function is able to question and investigate, to constantly improve the shared understanding of how the business **generates value**.

> **Illustration 8 – How the finance function works with FP&A**
>
> As was discussed in section 3.2, FP&A specialists have a number of responsibilities, such as the calculation of key financial ratios for presentation to decision makers to gauge the organisation's overall financial health. These responsibilities will only be fulfilled by the **provision of accurate information** from the finance function (at level 4 of the diamond shape).
>
> The FP&A specialists will own and be held accountable for the process that generates that data. The finance function can act as an 'expert' from outside of this specialist area ensuring the process is subject to the necessary rigour required. The finance function can **assemble and validate** the analysis presented to decision-makers and is able to provide further insight.

3.7 Recent changes to specialist areas

As was discussed in Chapter 3, the shape of the finance function is now evolving to a diamond shape:

- This has expanded the opportunities for business partnering between the finance function and specialist areas.

- It has also increased the number of tasks present within these specialist areas that are offered by shared service centres. This has enabled experts from different disciplines to work together on the same team to better support the business.

- Technology has been used by the specialist areas, and by the finance function to improve their productivity in working alongside these specialists. (**Note:** Technology will be discussed in greater detail in section 6).

- The use of advanced technology and the creation of shared service centres have resulted in '**digital centres of excellence**' at this level (i.e. level 3) of the diamond shape.

Illustration 9 – Technology developments and FP&A

Technology has had a significant impact on the work carried out by the FP&A specialists and the finance function staff who work alongside them. For example:

- The production of routine management information is being automated.

- Managers across the organisation may have access to user friendly, self-service, dashboards on their desks so they can monitor current performance.

- These self-service tools allow interrogation, so managers are empowered to identify the root cause of problems and address these problems promptly.

- Advanced data visualisation and analytics can provide improved forecasting.

However, rather than posing a **threat** to the work carried out by the FP&A specialists, and the finance function employees who work alongside them, these developments can be seen as an **opportunity**.

Finance professionals can harness the value of the data generated and increase their focus on supporting bigger decisions and projects.

Test your understanding 11

Harry, a finance professional, is concerned that due to advancements in technology his job will be under threat. Moira, Harry's boss, is doing her best to reassure him that there are many advantages of the modern finance function that have been enabled due to the increased use of technology.

Which FOUR of the following could Moira use to explain the benefits to Harry?

A   Technology can improve the productivity of the finance team

B   There are more opportunities for partnering with specialists in the business

C   Technology means the finance team have less work to do and therefore, will have more time to pursue their own interests

D   Automation of routine tasks means the finance team can focus on more value adding analysis for the benefit of the organisation

E   Technology used to support data analytics can provide improved forecasting enabling employees to make better business decisions

F   Advances in technology mean Harry will have no new skills to learn, making his life easier

4 Strategic partnering for value (level 2)

As seen in the diagram in Section 1, level 2 involves:

- communicating insight to influence users (section 4.1)
- business partnering (section 4.2)

4.1 Communicating insight to influence users

As discussed previously:

- Finance operations will **generate information** and **preliminary insight** (level 4)
- The finance function will work with specialists to provide **further insight** to decision makers (level 3)

At the next level (of the diamond shape), the insights that level 3 provide will be passed on to finance professionals working as strategic partners. These strategic partners will:

- interpret and use financial statements along with other data to communicate this insight
- in an appropriate format
- and required frequency
- to internal and external stakeholders such as senior managers, colleagues in other functions (for example, marketing or operations), shareholders and regulators
- to **influence** users of this information in their decision making and implementation and control activities.

The evolving shape of the finance function means that more people will be needed here and the finance function will need to develop the **competencies** required to adequately carry out this activity.

> ### Illustration 10 – Communicating insight to influence users: Budgeting
>
> The finance function's value adding role is often underplayed but they have an important role in communicating insight to influence the effectiveness of the decisions made by the users of the information.
>
> For example, an organisation's budget is often out of date before it is even complete, takes significant time to produce and the numbers can be of questionable value.
>
> However, the process of budgeting sets aside time from day-to-day activities for managers to think about risks to their plans, strategies to develop growth and to reduce costs.
>
> Importantly, **the process can add value even if the output does not**.
>
> The finance function could therefore consider an alternative output that would be more valuable itself, whilst still capturing the value of the process.

Test your understanding 12	
Level 2 of the contemporary shape of the finance function involves Strategic Business Partnering. **Which of the following statements are true and which are false?**	

Statement	True/False?
The finance function will communicate their insights once a month	
The finance function communicates their insights only to internal stakeholders	
Fewer people are required at this level of the finance function than previously	
Insight means the capacity to gain an accurate and deep understanding of someone or something	
New competencies need to be developed by the finance function to be able to effectively generate and communicate insight	

4.2 Business partnering

Strategic business partnering will be an increasingly important activity of the finance function.

The finance function will act as a business partner **influencing** the organisation's decisions to achieve the desired organisational **impact**.

The focus of the finance function's work is shifting from reporting historic performance to challenging management thinking and driving decision making to influence future performance.

The chief financial officer (CFO, i.e. the head of the finance function) works closely with the CEO to support him or her in the running of the organisation. Organisations develop and use finance function professionals as business partners to cascade the CFO's influence throughout the business.

Business partnering services may be provided by:

- individual finance function employees deployed to work alongside departmental mangers

- a multi-disciplinary team in a centre of excellence

- a mix of both with some local support but also an expert team tackling a particular problem or guiding a major initiative.

The expectation for finance to add greater value to the business is growing. Successful finance business partners are seen as leaders that can influence the decisions that a business makes to maximise value.

The CFO must have a team of highly credible finance executives who are capable of acting as a link between finance and the rest of the organisation.

The team's role will include helping to align the work of the analytics teams with business priorities, and helping leaders understand the implications of their data.

Success in this role requires a mix of commercial acumen, analytical skills, an ability to build relationships, to communicate effectively and persuade.

Illustration 11 – The finance business partner: skills needed

Amongst the many skills needed, people skills are critical. The effective finance business partner is adaptable and can deliver information in a digestible way to their particular audience.

This is particularly important when the message is one that the audience may not wish to hear, for example informing the sales function that they have overstated their margin.

Finance business partners must also be able to identify and win over key stakeholders, to build relationships and to persuade stakeholders in order to achieve the organisation's objectives.

Test your understanding 13

Which of the following would be useful as a definition of business partnership? Choose all that apply.

A   Involvement in strategy formulation, implementation and communication

B   Involvement in commercial decision making and negotiations

C   Leading on business analysis

D   Being a sounding board, trusted adviser, critical friend and facilitator of productive business discussions

5   Strategic leadership of the finance team (level 1)

The final activity is strategic leadership of the finance team.

The head of the finance function is the CFO and it is their responsibility to lead the finance team to achieve the desired organisational **impact**:

• leading key initiatives that support the organisation's goals

• executing and funding strategies set by the CEO

• liaising effectively with internal and external stakeholders.

To do this they will need to put a team in place that has the appropriate knowledge, skills and experience to effectively execute all of the finance function activities already discussed in this chapter.

CFOs are increasingly taking a more active leadership role working alongside and with the CEO as a 'co-pilot' in the success of the business.

Illustration 12 – The CFO's changing role: from navigator to co-pilot

CIMA have illustrated well the changing role of the CFO using the analogy of traditional versus modern aviation.

If we think about the cockpit of a large passenger plane (such as the Boeing 707) that flew in the 1950s:

- we would have had a pilot (left), a co-pilot (right) and a small instrument cluster

- plus a wooden chair for the navigator who was an essential part of the crew and who had access to a lot more instruments.

The CFO would have traditionally viewed their role as **navigator** to the business.

If we fast forward to a modern large passenger plane:

- we still have a pilot (left) and co-pilot (right) and they now have a large instrument cluster

- there is no longer a seat (or a need) for the navigator.

The navigator's role has become redundant meaning that the CFO has had to learn to 'fly the plane', using the large cluster of instruments available to them, to act as the **co-pilot** to the CEO.

Today's CFO needs a wider skill set:

- possessing strong analytical and communication skills

- and mastering areas outside of finance such as regulation, risk management, business transformation, supply chain management and IT.

The CFO is increasingly relying on automation of key business processes and is relying more on technology to transform data into actionable insights that can influence and impact the organisation's achievement of its goals.

Test your understanding 14

Which of the options can be best used to correctly fill the blanks in the following sentence?

'It is the responsibility of the CFO to lead the finance team to achieve the desired organisational _____. This involves leading key initiatives to support organisational _____, as well as liaising effectively with internal and external _____.'

	Gap 1	Gap 2	Gap 3
A	profit	efficiencies	stakeholders
B	impact	goals	shareholders
C	mission	norms	reporters
D	impact	goals	stakeholders

6 The impact of technology on the activities of finance professionals

6.1 Introduction

The finance function can view technology as both:

- an **opportunity** and

- a **threat**.

It can be viewed as an **opportunity** and used to improve the efficiency and productivity of the finance professionals in the areas discussed in the previous section of this chapter. It can also free up the finance professional's time to work on more interesting, challenging, value-adding work. This may require the finance function to build new capabilities.

However, automation and new technology can also be viewed as a **threat** to finance professionals since it can be used to reduce or replace many of their traditional roles and activities.

Illustration 13 – Technology and automation of jobs

In 2016, a UK newspaper, the Daily Mail, reported a speech by the Governor of the Bank of England under the headline 'Robots to steal 15 million of your jobs says bank chief'. The article said that the bank '…..predicted that entire professions, such as accountancy, could be pushed to the brink of extinction as developments in computers make roles redundant'.

The World Economic Forum Future of Jobs report (2018) concluded that the top 10 declining roles by 2022 would be:

1   Data entry clerks

2   Accounting, bookkeeping and payroll clerks

3   Administrative and executive secretaries

4   Assembly and factory workers

5   Client information and customer service workers

6   Business services and administration managers

7   Accountants and auditors

8   Material-recording and stock-keeping clerks

9   General and operations managers

10 Postal service clerks

Just as with any other opportunity or threat, the organisation and its finance function must embrace the opportunities that the new technology offers and find a way of eliminating the threat or, even better, turning it into an opportunity.

6.2 Technology and the information to impact framework

Firstly, let's remind ourselves of our discussion from Chapter 2:

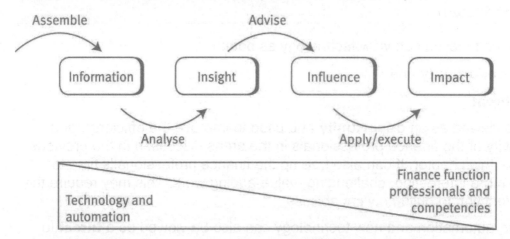

The information to impact framework clearly shows that:

- **Technology and automation** will play an important role in all of the activities of the finance function but will have the largest impact on the 'assembly' and 'analysis' activities.

- This will 'free up' the resource of the **finance function professionals** who can now place greater focus on the 'advising' and 'applying/executing' activities.

- The finance function will need to develop its **competencies**:

    - firstly, so that they are able to **use the up to date technology** and

    - secondly, so that they have the **necessary skills to provide the influence and impact required**.

Expanding on our discussion from Chapter 2, organisations are using technology to support the automation of management information processes and to provide reporting to the rest of the business on a self-service basis:

- This is resulting in a narrowing of the level 4 activities (diamond shape) of finance operations to generate information and preliminary insight.

- It has also increased the need for skills and talent at level 3 (working with specialists to provide further insight) and level 2 (communicating insight to influence users and business partnering to influence and impact the organisation).

Technology and its impact on the finance function will be explored in depth in the next few chapters. However, it is worth noting briefly that there have been two main technological changes that have impacted the finance function:

- New data sources and analysis methods (section 6.3).

- Automation and cognitive computing (section 6.4).

Illustration 14 – Opportunities offered by technology

Finance professionals might anticipate the technological advancements of the 4th Industrial Revolution with fear. However, the use of machines to take over repetitive, time-consuming and redundant tasks, will free the finance professionals to do higher level, value-adding work.

The opportunities offered to the finance function by technology will be explored in later chapters.

Here we will take a look at just a few of the opportunities that are available to an organisation as a whole thanks to this digital transformation:

Accounts payable/receivable – artificial intelligence (AI) powered invoice management systems make invoice processing much more streamlined. They can learn accounting codes that are more appropriate for each invoice.

Supplier management – machines can vet new suppliers by checking their credit scores or tax information and set them up in the system without human involvement.

Procurement – the procurement process for many organisations is filled with paperwork and uses different systems and files that are not compatible with one another. As machines are able to be integrated and the unstructured data is processed, the procurement system will eventually become paperless. Robots are ideally suited to tracking price changes among a number of suppliers.

Expense management – reviewing and approving expenses to ensure they are compliant with the organisation's policies is time consuming. Machines can read receipts, audit expenses and alert humans when a possible infraction has occurred.

AI chatbots – these can be used to efficiently solve common questions or queries from customers including the latest account balances, when certain bills are due, the status on accounts and more.

6.3 New data sources and analysis methods

New data sources and advanced methods for analysing this data are providing opportunities for better informed decision making.

For example, predictive analysis has improved forecasting and reduced the need to rely on the personal judgment of the finance professional.

Analytics has/will extend to areas such as FP&A pulling demand for talent from level 4 of the diamond to level 3.

6.4 Automation and cognitive computing

A 2016 McKinsey report studied which functions could be automated by advancing technology:

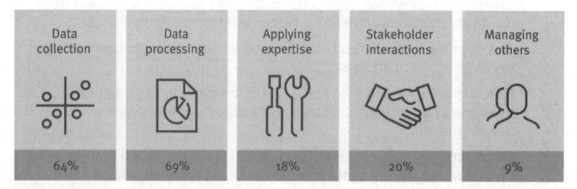

Data collection	Data processing	Applying expertise	Stakeholder interactions	Managing others
64%	69%	18%	20%	9%

Work activities at risk of automation include data collection and data processing.

Less automatable activities include applying expertise, stakeholder interactions and managing others.

The McKinsey illustration can be overlaid across the diamond shape of the finance function:

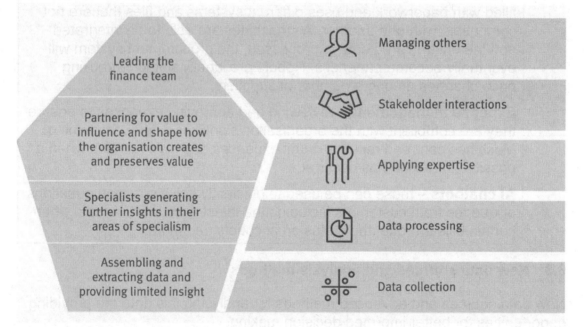

New technology being used includes:

*   Robotic process automation (RPA) providing opportunities to automate many routine, clerical activities.

*   Cognitive computing, such as artificial intelligence (AI), machine learning and natural language programming, providing opportunities to automate, say, advanced data analytics and report writing.

*   Higher up the diamond, new technology will change what finance professionals can do and support roles that require personal interactions and the ability to manage others. These are less likely to be automated.

Test your understanding 15

Which FOUR of the following may be considered to be advantages of automating much of the traditional work of the finance function?

A   Reduced human input, and therefore human error

B   Reduced paperwork, for a more sustainable organisation

C   Faster processing, meaning more real time information is available

D   Improved data integrity

E   Fewer finance staff required, reducing headcount costs

F   Less training required for finance staff, reducing training costs

Test your understanding 16

Stanley, a CIMA student, has been asked by his manager to summarise the various viewpoints of the contemporary finance function.

Complete the table below from the options overleaf.

Level in diamond	Information to impact framework	Activity	Position in finance function	McKinsey's automated functions
Level 1				
Level 2				
Level 3				
Level 4				

- Impact
- Smart finance factory
- Apply
- Data collection
- Advise
- Strategic business partner
- Information
- Stakeholder interactions/ applying expertise
- Influence
- Analyse
- Data processing
- Digital centre of excellence
- Managing others/ stakeholder interactions
- Insight
- Assemble
- Senior finance team

7 Chapter summary

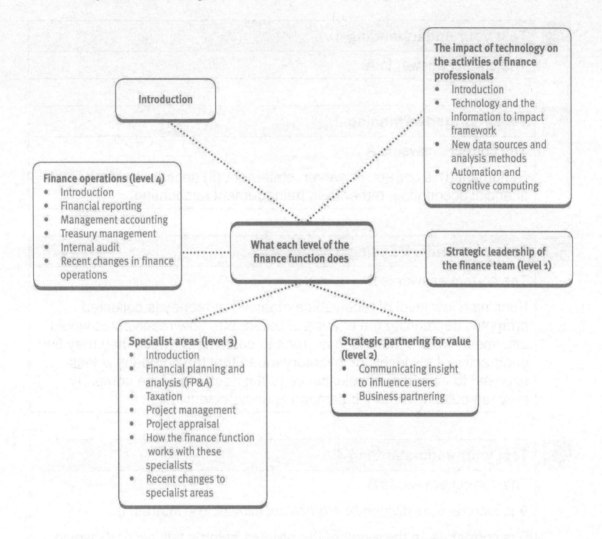

Test your understanding answers

Test your understanding 1

The correct answer is **A**

Test your understanding 2

The correct answer is **A**

Statement (i) is correct. However, statement (ii) describes a feature of financial accounting, rather than management accounting.

Test your understanding 3

The correct answer is **D**

Keeping a low level of receivables means that money is collected promptly, decreasing the chance of bad debts. Low receivables would also mean we are offering less credit to customers, which they may find unattractive. Low levels of inventory mean that the company is less exposed to inventory obsolescence, but it does mean the company may run out of inventory if demand is unexpectedly high.

Test your understanding 4

The correct answer is **B**

A is incorrect, as dividends are not tax allowable – interest is.

B is correct as, in the event of the product being a failure, AHG would not need to make unaffordable repayments to investors if it raises finance from equity.

C is incorrect as AHG only needs the money for 5 years. It could be argued that a 5 year loan would match the term of the project and therefore be more appropriate than equity finance, on which the company will have to pay dividends forever.

D is also incorrect as debt does normally require security from the company. Equity does not.

Test your understanding 5

The correct answer is **B – False**

The benefits of internal audit should exceed the costs. The IIA definition stresses that internal audit is a value-adding activity by helping an organisation to manage its risks and achieve its objectives. If an organisation believes that the costs of internal audit would exceed the benefits, then it shouldn't operate that internal audit function. This is a choice to be made by the directors of a company; there is no requirement to operate an internal audit department.

Test your understanding 6

The correct answer is **A – True**

Internal auditors can either be employees of the company being audited, or may be external experts brought in. Compare this with external auditors who have to be external to the company; employees of the company are not allowed to carry out an external audit of that company.

Test your understanding 7

The correct answer is **D**

Internal audit reports to the management of the company. In a smaller company, internal audit is likely to report directly to the board of directors of the company being audited. In a larger company where there is an audit committee, internal audit is likely to report to the audit committee, which will be made up of non-executive directors.

Test your understanding 8

Answer A is false – a shared service centre may be outsourced (internal outsourcing) but the two terms do not strictly mean the same thing.

Answer B is false – the shared service centre will view the business to be the customer. The more professional supplier/customer relationship should result in marked improvements in the quality of the service provided.

Answer C is true – establishing an SSC enables a business' processes to be standardised.

Answer D is false – in the diamond shape the level 3 tasks present within 'specialists generating further insights in their areas of specialism' are now offered by shared service centres.

Test your understanding 9

Kazim – taxation

Paul – project appraisal

Belinda – financial planning and analysis

Saira – project management

Test your understanding 10

The correct answers are **A, C, D & F**

Tax mitigation (answer B) would be carried out within the specialist area of taxation.

Net present value analysis (answer E) is typically performed by project analysts.

FP&A may use liquidity ratios to gauge the financial health of the organisation (answer G).

Test your understanding 11

The correct answers are **A, B, D & E**

Answer C – the finance team do not have less to do because of changes in technology, but the work they do is of a different nature.

Answer F – there are new skills to learn due to changes in technology and it is important that members within finance are up to date with these changes and have the necessary skills required to adapt.

Test your understanding 12

Statement	True/False?
The finance function will communicate their insights once a month	False – the insights will be communicated as frequently as required.
The finance function communicates their insights only to internal stakeholders	False – the finance function will communicate to both internal and external stakeholders.
Fewer people are required at this level of the finance function than previously	False – the evolving shape of the finance function will mean more people will be required at this level.
Insight means the capacity to gain an accurate and deep understanding of someone or something	True – by definition.
New competencies need to be developed by the finance function to be able to effectively generate and communicate insight	True – new competencies and skills will be required.

Test your understanding 13

The answer is **all of them**. There is no single definition of business partnership. Finance will support the organisation in all of the ways described.

Test your understanding 14

The best answer is **D**

"It is the responsibility of the CFO to lead the finance team to achieve the desired organisational **impact.** This involves leading key initiatives to support organisational **goals,** as well as liaising effectively with internal and external **stakeholders.**"

Test your understanding 15

The four advantages are **A, B, C & D**

Whilst E and F appear to be advantages, it is not necessarily true that fewer staff will be required, merely that the type of work they are performing will be at a different level. Additionally, the transition to the contemporary finance function will require additional training to develop the new competencies required.

Test your understanding 16

Level in diamond	Information to impact framework	Activity	Position in finance function	McKinsey's automated functions
Level 1	Impact	Apply	Senior finance team	Managing others/ stakeholder interactions
Level 2	Influence	Advise	Strategic business partner	Stakeholder interactions/ applying expertise
Level 3	Insight	Analyse	Digital centre of excellence	Data processing
Level 4	information	Assemble	Smart finance factory	Data collection

Technology affecting business and finance

Chapter learning objectives

Lead	Component
B1: Outline and explain the technologies that affect business and finance.	(a) Outline the key features of the fourth industrial revolution.
	(b) Outline and explain the key technologies that define and drive the digital world.

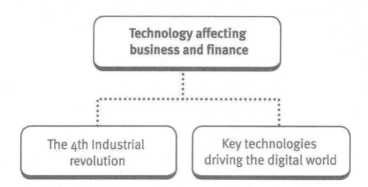

1 Introduction

In this chapter we will look at the technology driven changes facing the business world today. Considering key technologies fuelling what is increasingly being viewed as a new industrial revolution.

2 The 4th Industrial Revolution

2.1 What is an industrial revolution?

An industrial revolution can be generalised as **"a rapid and major change in an economy, driven by a shift in the methods and types of work undertaken"**.

Illustration 1 – Industrial revolutions
The **1st Industrial Revolution** in the 18th and 19th centuries saw a shift from rural, agricultural life to urban, industrialised societies. The growth in steam power and advancements in machinery transformed both agriculture and craft industries, and fundamentally changed the basis of the economy of the time.
The period from 1870-1914 has been labelled the **2nd Industrial Revolution** by historians. Already industrialised societies driven by coal, steam power, iron and textiles were transformed by advancements in the electricity, petroleum and steel industries. This saw the growth of vast corporations and a wave of globalisation.
The **3rd Industrial Revolution** is popularly held as originating in the 1980s. It is known as the **Digital Revolution** and saw a move from mechanical and analogue technology to the digital technology of today. Developments and improvements in communications, computers and the introduction of the internet were some of the key drivers of this period of rapid change.

Technologies such as **cloud computing**, **big data**, **data analytics**, **process automation**, **artificial intelligence**, **data visualisation**, **blockchain**, **internet of things**, **mobile technologies** and **3-D printing** are some of the more commonly known developments predicted to drive the 4th Industrial Revolution.

2.2 Features of the 4th Industrial revolution

Each industrial revolution has impacted upon society in their own specific way. The characteristics predicted to define the **4th Industrial revolution** include:

- **Fusion** – cyber and physical systems will continue to fuse becoming increasingly autonomous

- **Employment** – robotics, automation and digitization are predicted to make many jobs redundant or fundamentally different to today

- **Artificial intelligence and machine learning** – improved computing speed and optimized supply chains, enables products to be customised more easily and more cheaply

- **Machine led manufacturing** – the shift from machines helping workers manufacture, to workers helping machines will accelerate

- **Improved asset management** – Benefits to the natural world through more efficient use of natural assets, a shift to renewables, innovations in recycling, coupled with digitization are anticipated to benefit the natural world.

Illustration 2 – A hypothetical vision of the future

An article from the BBC (October 2018 – Justin Rowlatt) discusses the impact of some of these emerging technologies and predicts how they may revolutionise our lives in the not too distant future.

The article titled **'why you have (*probably*) already bought your last car'** is written to provoke debate and is formed from the ideas of a number of tech analysts who predict within 20 years (so by 2038) we will have stopped owning cars altogether.

This idea is built upon the emergence of self-driving electric vehicles, enabled by tech including AI, internet of things and data analytics amongst others. The article claims that these vehicles will be operated in an '**Uber**' (the ride hailing technology company) style network that will be so cheap the idea of owning a car will become obsolete within a decade.

The idea of this sounds almost unbelievable when viewed through the norms of today, however the rapid emergence of the motor car just over 100 years ago is cited as evidence of how quickly things can change. Once mass production began, city streets changed from almost entirely horse and carriage to cars in the space of a decade.

So how will it all take hold?

The article walks through an example using an Uber style company as its backbone. Uber and their rivals have already transformed the face of urban transport, a driver can be hailed immediately using a smart phone and arrive within minutes, then for a modest fee, say $10, take us from A to B. These services have grown at a rapid pace and despite concerns and media criticism continue unabated.

Now, of the $10 cost, at least 50% is paying the driver a wage. Therefore once **driverless tech** is available and licensed, which many believe could be within 5 years, the cost of your journey has immediately halved to $5. (This timescale is evidenced by every major motor and tech company fighting to take the lead of what will become a vast market worth billions of dollars annually)

The next thing to consider is the development and improvement of **electric powered vehicles**. The cost of purchasing electric cars is currently significantly higher than their fossil-fuelled counterparts. The emergence and growth of companies like Tesla, along with the threat of climate change and dwindling oil reserves, has seen major car companies shift their attentions to electric powered vehicles; they are ploughing billions of dollars in to refining and improving the technology. This level of investment will soon make electric vehicles accessible to the mass market and will ultimately bring the cost down to less than the cost of their fossil fuelled equivalents.

Further to this we must consider the running costs; fuel is one of the biggest costs for any fleet of taxis, a move to electric powered vehicles would see another significant cost removed. Additionally, **electric motors are much simpler** than a conventional engine, with only around 20 moving parts compared to 2,000 or so in the traditional engine. Therefore electric cars are expected to last for at least 500,000 miles delivering a huge increase in the useful life of the asset.

Battery **technology continues to advance** and investments such as Tesla's 'gigafactory' are anticipated to see the efficiency and reliability of batteries improve, the cost and speed of charging will also continue to fall.

Statistics show that the average driver in England drives less than 10,000 miles annually meaning **95% of the time their cars are parked**, which makes for an expensive and somewhat inefficient lump of metal. Especially when compared with an autonomous and intelligently controlled taxi which could be utilised at near full capacity. Then on top of all of these factors, as adoption of this new service takes hold, it will fuel its own growth becoming cheaper and more efficient as more vehicles would be added to the network achieving **significant economies of scale.**

Influential analysts predict with all of these factors combined, the cost of your $10 Uber journey of today could be cut by as much as 90%, so down to just $1! This would be a huge saving on the cost of buying and running your own car.

Additional considerations include **time saved** leading to increased productivity i.e. that 1 hour commute becoming part of your productive working day for instance. Additionally once self-driving technology is perfected the flow of traffic will become much **smoother and safer** as the most unreliable and unpredictable element, the human behind the wheel, is removed. In fact the article goes on to suggest that ultimately humans will be banned from driving altogether due to the threat they pose to the efficient and safe running of the 'self-diving robo-network' of taxis.

If the potential upheaval of all these changes isn't enough, when you consider the array of industries and businesses built around private car ownership and how these could disappear or be radically changed, it makes you realise how far reaching such developments will be to the world of today in terms of **industrial and social upheaval**.

The fact that this sounds like science-fiction, is much like the idea of the light bulb and the motor car would have sounded to people only a handful of generations ago, prior to previous industrial revolutions. Much of the technology discussed above is well on its way so this could well become science fact sooner than we may imagine, and the **4th industrial revolution** will be in full swing.

3 Key technologies driving the digital world

In this section we will we introduce some of the key developments and technologies driving the new wave of innovation and increasingly changing the world around us.

How these technologies are beginning to impact the world of finance and the role of the finance professional will be considered in more detail in later chapters.

3.1 Cloud computing

 Cloud computing is defined as the delivery of on-demand computing resources – everything from applications to data centres – over the internet. (IBM)

The basic idea and application of cloud computing sees users log in to an account in order to access, manage and process files and software via remote servers hosted on the internet. This replaces the traditional method of owning and running software locally on a computer or networked server.

There are two main types of cloud setups:

- **Public cloud** hosted by a third-party company. Specialist companies sell their cloud computing services to anyone over the public internet who wishes to purchase them

- **Private cloud** sees IT services provided over a private infrastructure, typically for the use of a single organisation. They are usually managed internally also.

Illustration 3 – Amazon, cloud computing services
Amazon's market value briefly broke the $1 trillion mark in 2018. A large contributor to this was the continued growth of Amazon Web Services (AWS). They are the market leader in cloud computing, controlling a third of the market in an industry expected to be worth $145bn by 2020. Their customers range from individuals to government agencies. Significantly their AWS business supports operations of other core areas of Amazon's business including e-commerce, Amazon prime video & music and the Amazon home assistant. This is a gateway to the 'internet of things' another marketplace projected to grow significantly in the coming years.

Features of cloud computing

Advantages	Disadvantages
Flexibility and scalability – Cloud computing allows simple and frequent upgrades allowing access to the latest systems developments. A company doesn't become laden with expensive hardware and software that quickly becomes obsolete. This allows organisations to evolve and change, to adapt to new opportunities and working practices	**Organisational change** – Working methods and roles need to be modified to incorporate a move to cloud computing. It may also lead to job losses, primarily in IT support and maintenance roles
Cost efficient – Limited IT maintenance costs and reduced costs of IT hardware, sees capital expenses and fixed costs become operating expenses. Cloud technology also allows pay as you go computing, with charges based on what a company actually needs	**Contract management** –The cloud provider will immediately become a very significant supplier. Managing this relationship, monitoring performance and ensuring contractual obligations will introduce new challenges and costs

Advantages	Disadvantages
Security – Cloud service providers, like any outsourced provider, are specialists. The security and integrity of their systems is fundamental to their business model and will be a strategic priority. Disaster recovery and backups are built in	**Security, privacy & compliance** – Whilst cloud providers will be specialists, they are bigger targets for malicious agents. This can threaten the security of sensitive information. Additionally, compliance with data regulations is put largely in the hands of a third party.
Flexible working – The increase in remote and home working is supported by cloud computing and the ability to access your 'desktop' from any location	**Reliance** – More so than with a standard outsourced arrangement, the reliability of the cloud service provider is essential. Often the entire provision of information systems fundamental to the operation of a business is passed to this third party.
Environment – Less waste from disposal of obsolete technology. More efficient use of scarce resources.	

Test your understanding 1

Which of the following describes a cloud service that can only be accessed by a limited number of authorised people?

A   Management information system

B   Private cloud

C   Public cloud

D   Big data

3.2 Big data

 Big data describes data sets so large and varied they are beyond the capability of traditional data-processing

The key features of big data are described as the **4Vs**:

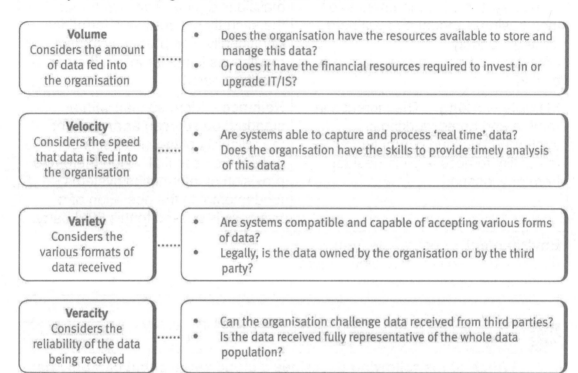

Volume Considers the amount of data fed into the organisation	• Does the organisation have the resources available to store and manage this data? • Or does it have the financial resources required to invest in or upgrade IT/IS?
Velocity Considers the speed that data is fed into the organisation	• Are systems able to capture and process 'real time' data? • Does the organisation have the skills to provide timely analysis of this data?
Variety Considers the various formats of data received	• Are systems compatible and capable of accepting various forms of data? • Legally, is the data owned by the organisation or by the third party?
Veracity Considers the reliability of the data being received	• Can the organisation challenge data received from third parties? • Is the data received fully representative of the whole data population?

Sources of big data

Big data comes in two main forms; structured data is deliberately produced and collected for a specific purpose and therefore exhibits a clear, deliberate structure. For instance, feedback data; when people have been asked to rate a service or product. Unstructured data, this is captured passively without a clear purpose; social media posts and 'likes' are an example of this. Its format is highly variable and non-standard.

The principal sources of these two forms of data are classified as follows:

- **Human-sourced data** – billions of data points are produced every day from social media, text messages, web browsing, emails etc.

- **Machine-generated data** – smart technologies and the internet of things is a growing source of data. Sensors built in to all aspects of modern technology, log and upload data constantly. Home assistants, smart meters, TV boxes and cars are a small selection of items producing machine-generated data.

- **Processed data** – Traditional data, held on databases of businesses and organisations recording customers, transactions and company assets

- **Open data** – Publicly available data stemming from sources such as governments, the public sector and national statistics agencies

Illustration 4 – Big data in everyday life

The sheer volume of data we produce on a daily basis is vast and increasing all the time. It largely goes unnoticed as much of it we produce incidentally as we live our lives. Yet companies are desperate to collect this data as they hope to gain unique insights and information that could deliver a crucial advantage over their rivals.

If you consider a hypothetical morning routine for instance; woken up by your smartphone alarm, you pick it up to silence it before having a look at emails or messages received overnight.

Realising its a little cold you ask your smart home assistant to turn the heating up a few degrees and maybe even turn the lights on. As it's the weekend you decide to turn the TV on, digital of course, constantly firing data back to the service provider. What programme are you watching, how long do you watch for? Which adverts do you watch?

Next up you decide to have a quick browse on social media, a few likes and shares, time spent watching videos and clicking on an interesting advert or two, all adds a little more to this 'gold mine' of data.

So without even leaving bed we have already generated multiple types of data. Not to mention the smart meter that is monitoring the power usage of all this technology and continually harvesting this data.

A quick drive to the shops will see the computer used to control all modern cars collect a wide array of data about the performance and condition of the car, both the car's sat-nav and your smart phone will be communicating data about your location and what the driving conditions are like on the roads you travel down. Monitors in traffic lights and in the roads themselves as well as cameras along the way will also track vehicles passing with data being used for traffic monitoring and surveillance.

You then pull up and park, the car park records your number plate and updates its information on the number of available spaces.

As you enter the shop your footfall is logged, the way we navigate the store, what causes us to stop and pick up certain items, all of this is of huge value to retailers so increasing attention is devoted to trying to capture this data to gain valuable insight.

Our card payment is logged by the provider as we pay for the basket of shopping, the contents of which is recorded and matched to our loyalty card profile which contains all of our shopping history as well as our profile info. This can be used to better understand customers, their habits and how they may be changing, what people want and when they buy it, what was the weather like when these purchases were made? And did this influence your choices?

Data on stock movements will also be generated, which is vital to the supply chain and inventory management systems of stores; these are often almost entirely automated.

So from this simple example, without any deliberate actions or specific intent a surprisingly large amount of different data has been generated by one individual. If you multiply this across billions of different people doing their own morning routine, the result is a truly vast amount of data.

Test your understanding 2

A private educational college is looking at ways they can utilise data in their organisation. The managing director has suggested using the current system that has names of students, their student identity number, and the company they work for.

What kind of data would this be using?

A   Public data

B   Unstructured data

C   Volume of data

D   Structured data

3.3 Data analytics

 Data analytics is the process of collecting, organising and analysing large sets of data (**big data**) to discover patterns and other information which an organisation can use to inform future decisions.

Collection of data
Organisations have access to greater quantities of data available from a number of internal and external sources.

Organisation of data
Once the data has been captured it needs to be organised and stored for future use, often using data warehousing facilities.

Analysis of data
Data mining software uses statistical algorithms to discover correlations and patterns to create useful information.

Uses of data analytics and big data – Understanding the potential value of data and its significance to an organisation presents a real opportunity to gain unique insight. This can be used to improve competitive position and potentially gain competitive advantage over rivals.

Business consultants Mckinsey, summarised the following benefits an organisation can realise from effective data analytics:

- **Fresh insight and understanding** – Seeing underlying patterns through the intelligent use of data can reveal patterns and insight into how a business operates, revealing issues that they may not have known existed

- **Performance improvement** – Data, processed and sorted into relevant management information in real time, can lead to significant operational gains and improved decision making and resource utilisation

- **Market segmentation and customisation** – Refining customer groups into ever more specific segments and understanding the wants and needs of those groups can lead to increased personalisation and customisation of products and services

- **Decision making** – Real time information that is relevant can lead to faster decisions and decisive advantage over competitors

- **Innovation** – Existing products can be improved from understanding the features and elements that customers enjoy and use. This can also lead to the development of whole new products

- **Risk management** – Risk management and control are vital in the effective running of any organisation. The use of data can enhance all stages of the risk management process.

3.4 Process automation

 The technology enabled automation of complex business processes. This can be entire processes or elements therein, aimed at improving consistency, quality and speed whilst delivering cost savings.

Traditional process automation – The traditional idea of process automation is that of a machine carrying out a simple repetitive task, replacing a job that would have been done by hand or in a semi-automated fashion. This type of automation is everywhere and has driven industrialisation, through the ability to produce ever higher volumes of products, with fewer problems and at less cost.

Modern process automation – Increasingly automation and process automation are focusing upon complex business areas, which were previously thought to be beyond the limits of technology.

Big data and the **internet of things** generate huge amounts of data; **data analytics** transforms this into useful information that supports **artificial intelligence** (see next section) and **machine learning**. Essentially process automation is becoming smarter and can make decisions using reasoning, language and learned behaviour.

Illustration 5 – Process automation

Customer contact centres are an area that many businesses are keen to automate. It is a business function deemed to be relatively low skilled in comparison to other business processes, but is an area that customers value so must be handled with care.

This was evidenced by the wave of contact centres being moved overseas to countries with lower labour costs in the 1990s/2000s driven by the aim of achieving cost savings. Customers were however, often dissatisfied with the level of service received resulting in a large number of companies ultimately bringing their contact centres back to the home country.

Companies were still keen to realise cost savings in this area but required a new approach to doing so. Developments in technology have led to significant improvements in process automation, contact centres are now typically heavily automated using the technology in conjunction with humans. The use of automation has been designed to use workers time more efficiently, through redesigning and streamlining processes as well as fully automating simple tasks and processes.

Developments in voice recognition technology and the ability of artificial intelligence allows contact centre calls to be answered robotically, they will typically ask the nature of the call, then place this on the right track. Many calls can be handled fully autonomously for instance making payments or tracing orders. Callers who do require a contact centre operative will then begin the security process, this will then interrogate the system to bring the customer and case information up on the operatives screen before they even speak.

Data capture and analytics are also used to monitor and understand call types, monitoring for new or emerging trends and suspicious or potentially fraudulent activity. This will enable workers to be more prepared and trained specifically to deal with high risk call types.

All of these improvements have led to both cost savings and service improvements through more targeted and efficient use of contact centre workers time, seeing them specifically used on activities where value can be added.

3.5   Artificial intelligence

 Artificial Intelligence (AI) is an area of computer science that emphasises the creation of intelligent machines that work and react like human beings.

A common definition from Kaplan and Haenlein describes AI as a **"system's ability to correctly interpret external data, to learn from such data, and to use those learnings to achieve specific goals and tasks through flexible adaptation"**. This is often considered in the context of human-type robotics but reaches much further than this, and is set to transform the way we live and work.

Some of the more advanced activities and skills artificial intelligence can now master, and therefore present huge opportunity for developers and companies alike, include:

- Voice recognition
- Planning
- Learning
- Problem solving

Illustration 6 – Artificial intelligence

Companies such as **Apple** and **Amazon** have developed and marketed voice recognition systems, either to be built into an existing product (such as Apple with its **Siri** system) or developed new products whose main function is voice recognition (such as Amazon and '**Alexa**').

A further simple example is that of Facebook, and its process of recommending new friends for users to connect with.

There are many, more complex examples of Artificial Intelligence, but a common factor to both the simple and the more involved is machine learning.

Machine learning

Machine learning is a subset of AI where effectively AI computer code is built to mimic how the human brain works. It essentially uses probability based on past experiences through data, events and connections between events. The computer then applies this learning to a given situation to give a fact driven plausible outcome. If the conclusion the computer reaches turns out to be incorrect this will act to add more experience and enhance its understanding further, so in future the same mistake will not be repeated.

Essentially machine learning algorithms detect patterns and learn how to make predictions and recommendations rather than following explicit programming instruction. The algorithms themselves then adapt to new data and experiences to improve their function over time.

Illustration 7 – Artificial Intelligence: 'Move 37'

Go is a highly complex strategy game, believed to originate in China over 2,500 years ago. It is considered to be more complicated and advanced than Chess, with a larger board, more elements meaning each move has many more alternatives to consider.

In 2016 **Google DeepMind (GDM)**, an **AI** technology played a challenge match against Go world champion **Lee Sedol**. The match was won by **GDM** in what many considered to be a significant milestone in AI research and development.

Essentially the program had been built from uploading thousands of previous Go games, which allowed the software to learn moves, patterns and responses to moves, to become a Go expert.

One moment in the match, referred to as **Move 37**, is considered to be a particularly seminal moment in AI development. GDM played its 37th move which to all commentators and indeed Lee Sedol himself, appeared to be completely abstract and in effect a 'bad' move. It turned out to be an innovative new move never seen before. The significance of the move wasn't felt until much later in the game but it turned out to be the pivotal moment, which enabled GDM to win the match.

The fact the computer software, whose 'knowledge' was built upon past games of Go and the moves and permutations encountered, was then able to take this learning and build upon it, doing something completely new was a demonstration of the power of **AI** and **machine learning**.

Interestingly Lee Sedol the human world champion was later able to beat **GDM** by effectively identifying limitations in its coding. He then made moves that were outside of GDM's understanding and the system therefore struggled to respond appropriately. This is a useful illustration of why **AI** and human thinking will need to be used in a mutual and collaborative way to help achieve innovations.

Test your understanding 3

Dollar Co is a chain of banks. It collects data from customers who visit the banks in person, and also from online transactions. For the online banking system, customers need to log in via the website using their login and password. Recently Dollar Co invested in a system that promoted certain products to customers when they were online, based on past transactions and banking history.

What is this is an example of?

A   Traditional process automation

B   Data visualisation

C   Artificial intelligence

D   Virtual reality

3.6 Data visualisation

 Data visualisation allows large volumes of complex data to be displayed in a visually appealing and accessible way that facilitates the understanding and use of the underlying data.

The growing significance of data has seen a rise in the importance of being able to access and understand the data in a clear, concise way. This is where **data visualisation** fits in. The tools of today's market leaders **Tableau** and **Qlik**, go far beyond the simple charts and graphs of Microsoft Excel. Data is displayed in customisable, interactive 3D formats that allow users to manipulate and drill down as required. Central to data visualisation is understanding and ease of use, the leading companies in the field look to make data easier and more accessible for everyone.

Essentially it aims to remove the need for complex extraction, analysis and presentation of data by finance, IT and data scientists. It puts the ability to find data in to the hands of the end user, through intuitive, user friendly interfaces.

The most common use of data visualisation is in creating a dashboard to display the **key performance indicators** of a business in a live format, thus allowing immediate understanding of current performance and potentially prompting action to correct or amend performance accordingly.

An effective data visualisation tool should display these five features:

- **Decision making ability** – Results focused, it should aid decision making

- **Effective infrastructure** – The output is reliant upon sufficient quantity and quality of data

- **Integration capability** – With existing systems and the business overall

- **Prompt discovery of rules and insights** – Live data is vital and delay can render any insight useless

- **Real time collaboration** – Users must interact with each other and the data

3.7 Blockchain

 A **blockchain** has been described as a decentralised, distributed and public digital ledger that is used to record transactions across many computers. This means the record cannot be altered retroactively without the alteration of all subsequent blocks and the consensus of the network.

Alternatively, it has been defined by the **Bank of England** as a technology that allows people who do not know each other to trust a shared record of events.

Benefits of a blockchain

The main benefit of blockchain is security. In the digital era, cyber security is a key risk associated with the use of IT systems and the internet. This is because traditional systems have been 'closed', and so modifications to data have been carried out by just one party. If the system is hacked, there is little control over such modification to prevent it from happening.

A simple illustration is the relationship that individuals have with their banks or credit card companies. If a transaction is carried out with either (for example, you use your credit card to pay for goods or services) there is only one party that records the transaction, your credit card company. How is that company to know that the transaction is valid? If the details appear reasonable, the transactions will be authorised. This allows those who carry out credit card fraud to make their (illegal) gains.

A blockchain provides an effective control mechanism aimed at addressing such cyber security risks. It is a record keeping mechanism that is 'open' or public, as it utilises a distributed ledger; it has been described as a form of collective bookkeeping.

Key features of a blockchain

- In a blockchain system, transactions are recorded by a number of participants using a network which operates via the internet. The same records are maintained by a number of different parties; as a transaction is entered, it is recorded by not just two parties, but instead by all of the parties that make up the overall chain. This can happen because all of the records in the blockchain are publicly available and distributed across everyone that is part of that network.

- When a transaction takes place (for example, between a buyer and a seller) the details of that deal are recorded by everyone – the value, the time, the date and the details of those parties involved. All of the ledgers that make up the blockchain are updated in the same way, and it takes the agreement of all participants in the chain to update their ledgers for the transaction to be accepted.

- The process of verifying the transaction is carried out by computers; it is effectively the computers making up the network that audit the transaction. If all of the computers review the transaction and verify the details are correct, the systems of all participants in the blockchain have updated records. The computers work together to ensure that each transaction is valid before it is added to the blockchain. This decentralised network of computers ensures that a single system cannot add new blocks to the chain.

- When a new block is added to a blockchain, it is linked to the previous block using a cryptographic hash (this turns data into a format that can only be read by authorised users) generated from the contents of the previous block. This ensures that the chain is never broken and that each block is permanently recorded. It is intentionally difficult to alter past transactions in the blockchain because all of the subsequent blocks must be altered first.

It is this control aspect of blockchain technology which addresses the main concern of cyber security. If anyone should attempt to interfere with a transaction, it will be rejected by those network parties making up the blockchain whose role it is to verify the transaction. If just one party disagrees, the transaction will not be recorded.

Typical stages in a blockchain transaction

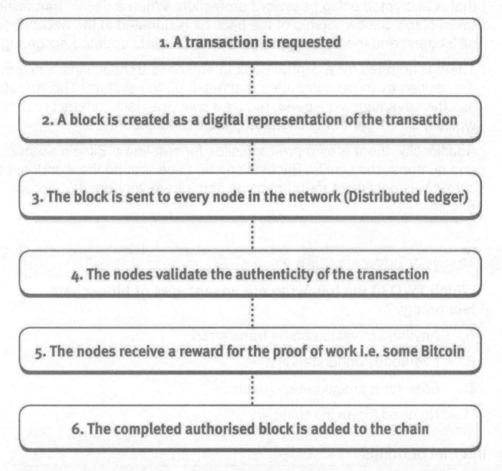

1. A transaction is requested

2. A block is created as a digital representation of the transaction

3. The block is sent to every node in the network (Distributed ledger)

4. The nodes validate the authenticity of the transaction

5. The nodes receive a reward for the proof of work i.e. some Bitcoin

6. The completed authorised block is added to the chain

Illustration 9 – Cryptocurrency

Bitcoin is a digital currency that was introduced in 2009. Other cryptocurrencies exist, such as **Ethereum** and **Litecoin**.

There is no physical version of Bitcoin; all Bitcoin transactions take place over the internet. Unlike traditional currencies, Bitcoin is decentralised, meaning it is not controlled by a single bank or government. Instead, Bitcoin uses a peer-to-peer (P2P) payment network made up of users with Bitcoin accounts.

Bitcoins can be acquired in two different ways: 1) exchanging other currencies for bitcoins; and 2) bitcoin mining.

The first method is by far the most common, and can be done using a Bitcoin exchange such as **Mt.Gox** or **CampBX**. These exchanges allow users to exchange sterling, dollars etc. for bitcoins.

Bitcoin mining involves setting up a computer system to solve maths problems generated by the Bitcoin network. As a bitcoin miner solves these complex problems, bitcoins are credited to the miner. The network is designed to generate increasingly complex math problems which ensure that new bitcoins are generated at a consistent rate.

When a user obtains bitcoins, the balance is stored in a secure 'wallet' that is encrypted using password protection. When a bitcoin transaction takes place, the ownership of the bitcoins is updated in the network on all ledgers, and the balance in the relevant wallets updated accordingly.

There is no need for a central bank to authorise transactions, since they are verified by those computers that make up the system. This therefore has the advantages of speed, reduced cost (transaction fees are small, typically $0.01 per transaction), and increased security.

Additionally, there are no pre-requisites for creating a Bitcoin account, and no transaction limits. Bitcoins can be used around the world, but the currency is only good for purchasing items from vendors that accept Bitcoin.

Test your understanding 4

Which TWO of the following are advantages of blockchain technology?

A   Anything of value can be transferred

B   Everybody understands it

C   Easy for management to override

D   No need for an intermediary

3.8 Internet of things

 The internet of things describes the network of smart devices with inbuilt software and connectivity to the internet allowing them to constantly monitor and exchange data.

What devices are connected to the internet of things (IoT)? Essentially anything with an on/off switch can become a 'smart' device and be connected over the internet. This allows them to talk to us, applications and each other, which is at the core of their functionality.

Common devices currently connected as part of the internet of things include:

- **Smart meters** (contain in-home display screens that show how much energy is used in real-time) and **home control thermostat devices** (allow control of heating, electricity and hot water).

- **Doorbells and security**; these talk to your smart device. A live connection is established if the doorbell is pressed or the motion sensors activated, allowing immediate interaction.

- **Wearable tech** such as smart watches and fitness trackers capture and record an array of data to monitor and record your fitness.

- **Home appliances** such as smart lights, fridges, washing machines, ovens etc... the connectivity built in allows remote access and control of these devices, for instance turning your lights on if you're out at night can be done using a smart phone.

- **Cars;** the computer systems used to control cars are increasingly sophisticated. They track and monitor thousands of parameters on every journey. This capability is central in the continued pursuit of autonomous vehicles.

- **Transport and infrastructure;** smart motorways are a common feature in many countries with traffic sensors monitoring the flow and build-up of traffic and responding to provide extra lanes or activate temporary speed limits.

- **Manufacturing equipment and plant;** monitoring of business assets facilitates efficient utilisation, it allows continual live feedback to track performance and flag maintenance requirements earlier.

The growth in the **internet of things** often termed '**smart technology**' is fuelled by improvements in broadband connectivity and the development of 4G communication networks. As governments look to roll out the next generation 5G networks, connectivity will be improved further. Coupled with the fact that people and businesses are increasingly comfortable with the idea and operation of this **smart technology**, it is anticipated that the **internet of things** will continue grow, becoming increasingly central to how we live and work as new and innovative applications for the technology emerge all the time.

Illustration 10 – Farming

Connected devices are becoming increasingly prevalent in the world of farming. It is an industry that is particularly vulnerable to adversity, through climate and weather effects, disease and pests. Therefore the ability to monitor data on climatic conditions and the health of animals allows farmers to be forewarned of potential problems at an earlier stage. This allows farmers to take preventative action to fix problems or switch to alternative strategies, resulting in increased yields and importantly saving costs, wastage and loss.

A company called Allflex use smart sensors, built into collars which are worn by each animal in the herd. These sensors monitor temperature, health, breathing, activity and nutrition of individual animals and the herd overall. Early warning signs can alert the farmer to potential problems and early preventative action can be taken such as veterinary care or isolating an animal showing markers of infection.

Test your understanding 5

X Co has created a brand of electronic toothbrushes that can sync with a mobile phone to let the user know the appropriate length of time they should be spending brushing their teeth.

This is an example of what?

A   Big data

B   Internet of things

C   3D printing

D   Mobile technologies

3.9 Mobile technologies

Code-division multiple access (CDMA) is the technology that underpins mobile technology. It has developed rapidly over the last decade and increased the capability of mobile technology.

Developments in mobile technology have seen mobile phones progress from basic call and message devices in the late 1980s and 1990s to the **smart phones** and **tablets** we see today. These devices are more like computers than telephones and this is reflected in the prices of the latest models.

The rapid development in the capability of mobile technology has emerged at the same time as huge advances in internet technology and together the two technologies have been perfect partners.

All aspects of modern life are impacted by mobile technology, with major industries being completely transformed or new ones emerging, including:

- **Newspapers** – Physical sales of newspapers are in terminal decline. News is now consumed via mobile devices and is live rather than being a record of yesterday's news. Newspaper companies have attempted to evolve to maintain a presence in this mobile online world.

- **Advertising** – Closely linked with newspapers and other media, advertising is being transformed. Large scale mass advertising is in decline with a growth in smarter, targeted adverts.

- **Music** – CD's were replaced by MP3's which were seen as the future but have in turn have been replaced by music streaming services like **Spotify**

- **Banking** – Increasingly people bank via mobile apps, designed for ease and convenience, the traditional high street branch continues to decline.

- **Socialising** – Social media has transformed how people socialise and communicate with friends using smartphones to post and tag and photograph their every move.

- **TV/Film** – Video streaming services such as **Netflix** and **Amazon Prime** as well as OnDemand TV and video sites like **YouTube** are designed for mobile internet technology and are transforming how we watch TV and films.

3.10 3-D Printing

 3-D printing is part of a process known as **additive manufacturing** where an object is created layer by layer. It allows complex parts and components to be produced much cheaper, faster and in an entirely customisable manner.

How does it work? First a blueprint needs to be made; modelling software is widely available and catering for domestic and industrial scale operations. Alternatively, objects created by others can be accessed on specialist communities.

Once a design is finalised it is ready to be printed. Printers can range from small desktops to industrial arrays. Most 3-D printers use thermoplastic composite type material. The printer follows the precise coordinates laid out by the design, building up the item layer by layer to produce a fully formed single piece 3-D object.

Applications range from producing **prototype parts** for manufacturing to printing human organs and bone using **bio-printing**.

What are the advantages?

- **Speed** – compared with conventional manufacturing such as injection moulds, 3-D printing gives significant time savings from prototype to finished article. Prototypes can be printed and tested in the same day, amendments made and reprinted immediately.

- **Cost effectiveness** – linked to the speed of the process, the labour cost of a conventional prototype process is high as designs need to be made into moulds which will then be tooled for manufacture, before a prototype can be made. Any changes need to follow the same lengthy and costly process.

- **Customisation** – the ability to easily amend designs and tailor them to individual wants is a big draw for 3-D printing over traditional manufacture which is more focused on large volumes of identical products. This is a big selling point that can differentiate a business from its rivals.

- **Less waste** – 3-D printing sees the exact design printed and nothing else so uses raw materials much more efficiently than traditional manufacturing methods which see a lot of offcuts extracting the finished product.

- **Confidentiality** – 3-D printing allows continuous prototyping and manufacturing in-house, thus protecting intellectual property.

4   Chapter summary

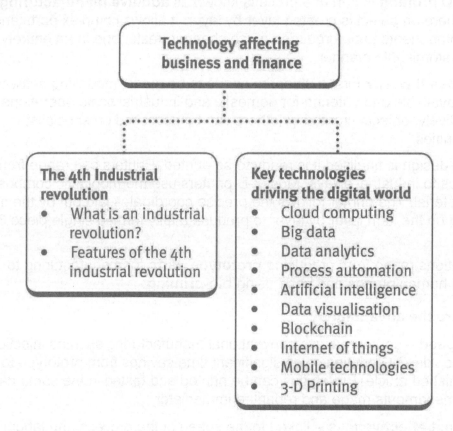

Technology affecting
business and finance

The 4th Industrial revolution
- What is an industrial revolution?
- Features of the 4th industrial revolution

Key technologies driving the digital world
- Cloud computing
- Big data
- Data analytics
- Process automation
- Artificial intelligence
- Data visualisation
- Blockchain
- Internet of things
- Mobile technologies
- 3-D Printing

Test your understanding answers

Test your understanding 1

The correct answer is **B**

Private clouds are on a private infrastructure and managed internally. MIS may be limited in access but is not a cloud service. Public clouds are hosted by 3rd party. Big data is the term for data sets so large that necessitates cloud computing to allow more storage.

Test your understanding 2

The correct answer is **D**

Structured data is usually presented in some order and for particular uses. Public data is open data from governments. Unstructured data comes from a variety of sources, collected passively. Volume of data is a characteristic of big data.

Test your understanding 3

The correct answer is **C**

Artificial intelligence has algorithms that processes data and can use it to make recommendations. Traditional process automation is carrying out a simple repetitive task, which this is not. Data visualisation allows complex data to be viewed in a visually appealing way. Virtual reality is a computer generated experience in a simulated environment.

Test your understanding 4

The correct answer is **A and D**

Anything of value can be transferred, and it removes the need for an intermediary. Not everybody understands blockchain, and there may be some resistance to it. Blockchain technology makes it more difficult to interfere with transactions.

Test your understanding 5

The correct answer is **B**

Internet of things allows everyday objects to be connected to the internet and interact with us. Big data gets generated from products like this. There is no mention that this is done via 3-D printing (though toothbrushes could be!). Mobile technologies involve using them for the transactions, which is not the case here.

How the finance function uses digital technologies

Chapter learning objectives

Lead	Component
B2: Examine how the finance function uses digital technologies to fulfil its roles.	Examine how finance uses the following to guide how it performs its roles: (a) Digital technology (b) Digital mindsets (c) Automation and the future of work (d) Ethics of technology use

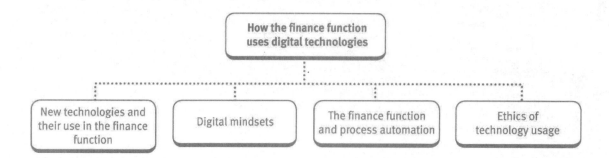

1 Digital technologies and the finance function

1.1 Introduction

In **Chapter 5** we considered the idea of **the 4th industrial revolution**, considering some of the key technology developments driving the changes that will increasingly impact all aspects of modern life.

In this chapter we will look more specifically at how these emerging and developing technologies will affect the finance function of organisations and will shape future finance professionals.

We will consider the innovation and progress this technology can offer as well as investigating some of the ethical, legal and social considerations, through data protection and the idea of overall corporate digital responsibility.

Some of the technologies are anticipated to effectively update existing systems and improve capability; these have been termed **core modernisation tools** and are considered mainstream. Whilst others will deliver new capabilities, pushing the finance function forward, these are referred to as **exponentials** and are still at the early-adopter stage.

Core modernisation tools include:

- Cloud technology

- Data visualisation

Exponentials include:

- Blockchain

- Advanced analytics

Illustration 1 – The changing face of the finance function

Essentially the finance function looks after an organisation's money. They ensure that a company's records are kept up to date, in order to understand, plan and ultimately control the money available within the business.

The finance function must establish sound systems which enable all financial transactions to be recorded. They must also be able to interrogate this data to provide meaningful information that is accurate, complete and timely.

Modern technologies introduced in Chapter 5 are impacting all areas of the finance function including:

- The hardware and software businesses use are being revolutionised with **cloud computing** transforming the way that accounting systems are owned, maintained and operated, leading to time and cost savings and more efficient ways of working.

- The **variety** and **volume** of data that is available to the modern finance professional has grown exponentially and brought about the concepts of **big data** and **data analytics** enabling greater insights into all areas of a business' operations.

- The information generated by the finance function, vital in managing all aspects of business can be brought to life through huge improvements in **data visualisation**.

2 New technologies and their use in the finance function

2.1 Cloud computing

Cloud computing as introduced in **Chapter 5**, involves the provision of shared computing services over the internet. Cloud systems can be **public** (shared) or **private** (closed) depending upon the needs and requirements of users.

Cloud computing and the finance function:

Cloud technology is impacting the provision of computing services within organisations including the finance function. This has wide ranging impacts on the way people and organisations work. The classic idea of office based work around fixed working hours within a physical team is becoming increasingly obsolete and the advent of **cloud computing** is one of the main drivers of this.

Cloud computing has driven the following changes in the structure and working of the finance function:

- **Collaboration** – File sharing and version control issues are minimised. Services such as Google drive for instance allow multiple collaborators to update documents in real time.

- **Flexible working** – Full access to all files and documents anywhere with an internet connection has facilitated increased flexibility to work pattern and arrangements.

- **Increased security** – Cloud service providers understand and acknowledge the security of data, especially financial data is critical to their success.

- **Up to date** – Continually up to date software, helping to ensure compliance with regulations such as GDPR.

- **Easier integration** – Cloud based accounting software can easily link with other cloud based software such as customer relationship management (CRM) allowing an integrated approach to business in a cost effective way when compared with traditional software solutions.

Cloud computing, digital tech and financial reporting – The provision of services via cloud networks has revolutionised many industries. Physical products and the ownership of traditional physical assets like property, plant and equipment are becoming less important in the modern digital world. This has led to a growth in the significance of intangibles, which often aren't recorded on the **statement of financial position**. As a result, it is more difficult to determine the underlying value of digital businesses and to identify their sources of value creation using the traditional routes of financial statement analysis. Using financial statements alone may significantly undervalue such entities as many intangible assets are internally generated and thus can't be recognised. This includes things like intellectual property and staff skills.

Illustration 2 – Cloud services impact on physical goods

Music streaming through services such as **Spotify, Deezer, Apple music** amongst others now dominate the music industry. While the buying of a physical product like a CD from a physical record store like **HMV** or **Virgin** is increasingly a thing of the past.

Other industries like hotels have seen the emergence of new players and business models. **AirBnB** for instance, who act as an online broker, facilitating the short term lets of private accommodation between individuals is one of the largest 'hotel' companies in the world valued at around $30 billion (2019) yet they own no hotels or property.

Similarly companies like **Uber, Lyft** and **Didi,** who offer ride hailing services don't own a single vehicle yet dominate the transport industry and have estimated values beyond that of **AirBnb.**

All these businesses utilise cloud computing technology in the provision of their services and operate in a way that has revolutionised their industries.

They all have in common an absence of physical assets such as stock, property, plant, vehicles and equipment. Therefore, the financial reporting of these entities is a fundamentally different proposition compared to traditional bricks and mortar businesses.

2.2 Big data and data analytics

Computerisation has seen the role of finance professionals evolve over a number of decades from the traditional idea of 'bean counters' to a more strategic value adding position.

Technology has facilitated the ability to sort and analyse data to produce meaningful information far quicker than before, largely through the use of **spreadsheet** and **database** software.

The development and use of ever more sophisticated digital technology means the role of the finance professional continues to evolve. Elements such as **big data** and **data analytics, artificial intelligence** and **data visualisation** present significant opportunities as well as challenges to both businesses and individuals.

Business partnering

Management accountants are embedded within functional departments of the organisation rather than operating from a central accounts department. The object is to provide real-time support and analysis to improve the operational performance of the functional department.

Big data and data analytics will increase the significance of the business partnering role, with the potential for new insights to be gained. It is anticipated accountants will act as the **interface between** data specialists such as **data scientists** (who have a background in statistics and computer science) **and the business**, essentially making the data generated commercially relevant thus transforming it into valuable information.

Other impacts of big data on elements of the finance function:

Management accounting	In management accounting, big data will contribute to the development of more efficient and insightful management control systems and budgeting processes.
Financial accounting	In financial accounting, big data will improve the quality and relevance of accounting information. This can enhance transparency and stakeholder decision making.
Reporting	In reporting, big data can assist with the creation and improvement of accounting standards. This will help to ensure that the accounting profession continues to provide useful information as the dynamic global economy evolves.

Internal audit and big data

Big data and data analytics are expected to enhance the quality and relevance of **internal audit** assignments. Technology advancements in big data and analytics are fundamentally changing how the review of internal controls and systems are carried out.

New technology is driving an expansion beyond sample-based testing to include analysis of entire populations of audit-relevant data, using intelligent analytics to deliver a higher quality of audit evidence and more relevant business insights. Big data and analytics are enabling internal audit to better identify anomalies, fraud and operational business risks and tailor their approach to target more business critical areas.

Test your understanding 1

The impact of big data in organisations will affect which elements of the finance function?

A   Business partnering

B   Management accounting

C   Financial accounting

D   Internal audit

E   All of the above

2.3 Process automation

As discussed in **Chapter 5**, process automation involves the use of technology to automate processes previously carried out by human workers.

Developments in technology are enabling more complex activities to be automated and **process automation** is therefore becoming increasingly significant to the finance function of an organisation.

Repetitive, low skilled manual tasks such as data entry, duplication and processes that add minimal value to the end users of financial information are most likely to be automated by new developments in process automation software. Good examples include the automation of processes associated with the financial close and regulatory reporting and the automation of tasks associated with account reconciliation. This will free up time and resource for higher level value adding activities.

An organisation considering investing in **process automation** technology within the finance function would weigh up the following advantages and disadvantages:

Advantages	Disadvantages
Cost savings – reduction in headcount as routine aspects of finance work automated	**Uncertainty** – process automation changes the way the finance function works and can lead to uncertainty around job security and future prospects
Value adding – staff and management time is freed up to focus on higher level value adding activity	**Relationship management** – for process automation software to be successful, time and resource is required for relationship management with IT support and software providers
Improved accuracy – automated processes will benefit from improved accuracy and efficiency with the removal of human error and working patterns	**Competence** – the automated process is built by IT staff who must also understand in detail the existing process as the automated process is only as effective as the coding that drives it

Advantages	Disadvantages
Positive return – well managed and implemented process automation software will provide positive returns on investment	**Training** – costs of training staff to understand how the new software works and interfaces with their roles can be significant
Adaptability – process automation can be used for existing processes or can form part of an overarching process improvement exercise	**Change management** – as with any significant changes made by an organisation the process must be managed carefully and led effectively for it to be successful

Illustration 3 – Process automation in the finance function

Process automation when considered in the context of a large scale conglomerate organisation such as **Johnson & Johnson** can generate time, cost and resource savings as well as generating significant efficiencies.

Compatibility issues between the multiple systems across **Johnson & Johnson's** many operating locations led the company to investigate the potential benefits process automation could deliver.

An initial project, focused on simplifying their intercompany requests, recharges and postings process to test the capability of process automation and its potential for wider use in the business.

The automated process worked as follows:

- Requests for intercompany transactions are forwarded to an automated inbox instead of going to a member of the finance team.

- They are submitted following a standard and consistent template. This allows the software to open the email and process the details of the transaction.

- The details should be complete due to the standard template used enabling the system to verify the divisions involved, the general ledger codes, authorisation and narrative.

- Any omissions cause the request to be automatically rejected and an email is generated to notify the sender of the reasons.

- Complete requests are then accepted and the details uploaded into the purchase order system automatically.

- The purchase order then needs to be approved.

- This approval triggers the next stage of the system and an invoice is automatically raised by the system in the division that initiated the process.

- All relevant postings are then automatically made in both divisions with sales and receivables on one side and expenses and payables in the other division.

The automation process has improved the consistency, accuracy and timeliness of the intercompany recharge process. Due to the fact that all postings are controlled by the single process there are no longer issues with intercompany balances not agreeing. It also allows for simpler reporting and increased detail with regard to workflows.

The work has freed up finance staff time to focus on more value adding activities and improved the understanding of the core process that has been redeveloped.

Test your understanding 2

Value Co, a chain of supermarkets, is taking action to increase process automation in the finance function for repetitive tasks such as intercompany transactions and reconciliations.

Which of the following is a disadvantage of taking such action?

A   Free up management time

B   Increased risk of human error

C   Less training costs

D   Resistance to change

2.4 Artificial Intelligence (AI)

AI and **machine learning** are anticipated to lead to significant impacts on the future of accountancy. **Process automation** as discussed above, will be enhanced by AI enabling automated reasoning, making automation more flexible and capable of dealing with complexity.

AI enables computers and machines to exhibit higher level, human style learning. A system can interpret data correctly and, over a period of time, continually learn to interpret data better by understanding the differences between its interpretations and the actual outcomes.

Illustration 4 – Artificial Intelligence and forecasting – Salesforce

Saleforce.com, a cloud based provider of CRM systems, has embraced the capability of **AI** to aid their revenue forecasts. The process of forecasting is built on data but with a very significant human input. Research has shown this human input is clouded by emotion and confirmation bias and often amounts to little more than hunches and gut feeling.

By investing in **AI** the data becomes the key driver of forecasting and treats the process of forecasting in a more scientific manner. Using a data driven approach allows for a solid rationale to be visible behind the forecasts that are produced.

For it to be successful the Chief Information Officer of **Salesforce** asserts that data needs to be seen in the day to day operations of a business. This will act to aid understanding and buy-in to the process.

For instance, in a sales driven business, forecasting often involves the assessment of leads and the likelihood these will be realised. Each salesperson's view and assessment of these leads will be impacted by their own opinion and disposition. Introducing a data driven approach to assessing sales leads will be consistent and fact led; it will smooth the human inconsistency, enhance the forecasting and perhaps most significantly, improve the **AI** learning that can be achieved. This is done by the system interrogating and attempting to understand the differences between the forecasts and actuals. The data driving these differences is then 'learned' by the system and will not be replicated in future forecasts. So over time the process of forecasting will become increasingly accurate.

The process of running this change at **Salesforce**, especially the human element, wasn't smooth and took time but the CIO insists the improved forecasting it has resulted in has been more than worth any hardship.

Artificial intelligence and accountancy

Although artificial intelligence techniques such as machine learning are not new, and the pace of change is fast, widespread adoption in business and accounting is still in the relatively early stages.

Increasingly, we are seeing systems that are producing outputs that far exceed the accuracy and consistency of those produced by humans. In the short to medium term, **AI** brings many opportunities for accountants to improve their efficiency, provide more insight and deliver more value to businesses. In the longer term, AI brings opportunities for much more radical change, as systems increasingly carry out decision-making tasks currently done by humans.

AI, no doubt, will contribute to substantial improvements across all areas of accounting, equipping accountants with powerful new capabilities, as well as leading to the automation of many tasks and decisions.

Examples include:

- Using machine learning to code accounting entries and improve on the accuracy of rules-based approaches, enabling **greater automation** of processes
- Improving **fraud detection** through more sophisticated, machine learning models of 'normal' activities and better prediction of fraudulent activities
- Using machine learning based **predictive models** to forecast revenues
- Recommending supplier specific discounts to **optimise cash at hand**
- Extraction of **insights** from real-time data (both financial and non-financial) without information overload.

Despite the opportunities that AI brings, it does not replicate **human intelligence**. The strengths and limits of this different form of intelligence must be recognised, and users need to build an understanding of the best ways for humans and computers to work together.

Illustration 5 – AI and the Serious Fraud Office (SFO)
In the UK, the Serious Fraud Office (SFO) has invested in an **AI** system called **OpenText Axcelerate**. One of the main operations of the system in the SFO's investigations involves interrogating huge volumes of documents. Connections between individuals and groups as well as key words and phrases can be identified and mapped in a way far beyond the capabilities of human workers.
This has not only saved countless man hours spent trawling through and cross referencing documents, it has been proven to actually improve the process, identifying more connections than the average human worker and crucially more complex and opaque connections that would typically not be spotted by the human eye. This has therefore enhanced the investigative power and effectiveness of the fraud agency.

2.5 Data Visualisation

This area of technology is of particular significance to the finance function of an organisation. The provision of information to help support the efficient and effective running of all functions within a business and the business overall is the **fundamental purpose of the finance function**.

Big data and data analytics are now mainstream in business. This growth in data and the need to communicate the information and insights to be found within the data makes **data visualisation** critically important to the finance function. The ability to make data relevant, accessible and easy for all end users is vital.

Key benefits of data visualisation

- **Accessible** – traditional spreadsheets and financial reports can be both difficult to understand and unappealing to look at. Modern data visualisation graphics and dashboards are designed to be user friendly and intuitive

- **Real time** – synchronising real time data with data visualisation tools gives live up to date numbers in a clear, informative style. This allows a quicker response to business changes rather than waiting for weekly or monthly reports

- **Performance optimisation** – the immediacy and clarity of the information being displayed supports better decision making and proactive, efficient utilisation of resources as problems are identified promptly

- **Insight and understanding** – combining data and visualising it in a new way can lead to improved understanding and fresh insights about the cause and effect relationships that underpin performance.

Illustration 6 – Visualisation, key performance indicators

Key performance indicators are a set of metrics used by a business to monitor performance in areas where things must go according to plan for the business to be successful. These critical areas must first be identified, and then suitable metrics established to monitor performance, before finally setting targets to outline the level of desired performance.

The ability to receive real time information about critical areas and feed this back to staff allowing them to understand current performance and respond accordingly can be the difference between success and failure.

The collection and analysis of the data are underpinned by the ideas of **big data**, however, bringing this data to life in an easy to understand and intuitive fashion is the purpose of **data visualisation.**

Companies are increasingly using **dashboards** (a collection of key infographics displayed together) to display key performance indicators to staff in real time and to flag areas requiring improvement in order to hit the pre-determined targets and drive success. This instant feedback allows for action to be taken quickly to highlight and fix potential problems.

For instance, an IT service desk within a business will use key performance indicator dashboards to monitor and display performance for all staff and the department as a whole.

Metrics such as the number of support tickets logged, time taken to open support tickets, time taken to resolve support tickets and customer satisfaction would all be displayed clearly using graphics.

If performance in any of the areas is falling below target levels the graphics will clearly display this, prompting action to resolve the poor performance.

Test your understanding 3

Which TWO of the following are benefits of data visualisation for the finance function?

A   User friendly and intuitive

B   Regular monthly reporting

C   Create fresh insights into the data

D   Wider use of performance metrics

2.6 Blockchain

Blockchain is most widely understood in the context of cryptocurrencies such as **Bitcoin** as illustrated in Chapter 5. The illustration below compares a traditional payment to a payment using cryptocurrency, demonstrating the key differences of the blockchain transaction.

Illustration 7 – Cryptocurrency, how do they work?

First, consider a transaction using a standard currency like pounds or dollars for instance.

- Making a purchase, you present your payment card to the retailer, they then process the payment.

- In doing so the card payment machine essentially asks your bank if you have sufficient funds to make the purchase.

- The bank then checks its ledgers to verify whether you do in fact have the money to make the purchase.

- If so, the bank gives authorisation to the retailer, processes the payment and updates its ledgers. They also charge a small fee for doing so.

- If other intermediaries such as credit card companies or PayPal are added to this process they also take a slice to pay for their input.

Cryptocurrencies such as **Bitcoin** essentially act to remove the bank from the process, they use **blockchain** technology to both authorise the transaction and then also record it, in what is known as a distributed ledger. This replaces the single ledger that is held by a bank, with many separate or distributed ledgers which are all individually held by different people (or essentially computer servers). They all independently verify the transaction and record the movement of cryptocurrency at the same time. The fact that multiple different ledgers all support the same information acts to verify the legitimacy of the transaction. If one of these ledgers tried to record something different, or effectively cheat, this would not agree with the other ledgers and would be refused.

So the process for the transaction using a cryptocurrency would be:

- I would present my payment details to the retailer, detailing my cryptocurrency account

- They would then present this to the distributed ledgers, so effectively would ask all of these different independent ledger holders whether I had sufficient cryptocurrency to make the payment

- If they all agreed that I did, the transaction and the payment would then be authorised and all of the distributed ledgers would update their records to reflect the movement

- **Note:** It is here where an inaccurate entry would be rejected, if someone attempted to change their ledger it would be flagged up as different to all of the other ledgers and would not be processed
- The reward for the ledger holders is that one randomly selected ledger would be given some newly created cryptocurrency for each transaction.

This distributed ledger approach removes the central intermediary i.e. the bank and distributes it in essence to everyone.

Blockchain and the finance function

Blockchain is the most notable example of distributed ledger technology. Its use will impact upon the current operations of the finance function of an organisation. Digital assets recorded and secured by blockchain technology such as cryptocurrencies, present both opportunities and challenges:

Financial reporting – Accounting for cryptocurrency is currently a grey area for standard setters and exactly how they should be classified is subject to ongoing debate. Accounting standards were not designed with such technological developments in mind and therefore do not have an applicable standard. Whether cryptocurrencies should be considered as cash, an intangible asset, a financial instrument or even inventory have all been discussed with elements of each standard working and failing in equal measure.

Cross border payments – these remain complex, expensive and slow. The actions of intermediaries, the fees charged and the exact timescale is often opaque. Blockchain driven solutions such as **RippleNet** are growing in number and use. They aim to make the transfer of money like the transfer of data, easy and seamless by circumventing the traditional centralised intermediaries i.e. banks and payment providers.

Smart contracts – self executing contracts use blockchain technology built upon cryptography, digital signatures and secure computation. Theoretically money, property or any assets can be exchanged in a transparent manner. The document is created and agreed upon and then verified by the distributed ledger. The performance obligations, if met, execute at an agreed time and date and cannot be tampered with, without validation.

Security & traceability – the distributed ledger means all network participants involved in a blockchain hold a copy of the full ledger. Any attempts to amend a single block will become invalid and the peer to peer network will be immediately aware. All blocks are time stamped and secured through cryptography. This may fundamentally impact how finance functions record transactions with third parties.

Examples of how blockchain can enhance the accounting profession include:

- Improving the cash position by better managing resources

- Reducing the costs of maintaining and reconciling ledgers

- Providing absolute certainty over the ownership and history of assets

- Helping accountants gain clarity over available resources

- Freeing up resource to concentrate on value adding activities rather than record keeping.

Test your understanding 4

Lyric Co is a record company that uses music artists to record songs and produces the music itself. Revenues from sales of music come from physical sales in music stores, downloads from websites, and commissions from radio stations. Lyric Co wants the revenues to be distributed in pre-determined measures (i.e. a certain percentage) to the artist and the record company as long as agreed performance requirements are met.

Which of the following areas of technology should they look to use?

A   Artificial intelligence

B   Cryptocurrency

C   Blockchain

D   Digital mindsets

2.7   Internet of things

The **internet of things** considers a network of smart devices with inbuilt sensors and internet connectivity. They collect and transmit data constantly and are an increasingly significant element of **big data**.

The ability to make virtually any asset a business owns and operates a 'smart' asset by building in some relevant sensors and internet connectivity can lead to some very useful data. It should facilitate better business planning, resource allocation and will help to optimise processes, minimise expenditure and give advanced warning of potential issues.

It is thought the finance professionals will work increasingly closely with the IT function of a business as the two functions overlap and require each other's mutual knowledge.

Illustration 8 – Internet of things. Rolls Royce

Rolls-Royce, manufacturer of aircraft engines, has embraced the capabilities of the **internet of things** and **big data** and this has fundamentally changed their business model.

Rolls-Royce engines are manufactured with hundreds of sensors built in throughout the engine unit. These sensors produce constant live data which is fed back to systems engineers at centres across the globe. Any anomalies are immediately flagged and the engineers can make an assessment from the vast array of data available as to the best course of action. Preventative maintenance can be scheduled much earlier than would ordinarily be possible and can be planned for the most convenient and cost effective time and location.

AI is anticipated to replace the human intervention over time as its capability and reliability improves, the stakes are very high when it comes to aircraft engines so there is no room for error.

This new way of monitoring the performance of their engines has facilitated design improvements for new models and has led to an entirely new business model in how Rolls-Royce 'sell' their engines. Customers are now charged per hour of use of an engine and have a package called total care that covers all maintenance and upkeep of the engines.

2.8 Mobile technologies

Mobile technologies are a fundamental aspect of modern life, most notably **smartphones** and **tablet computers**. Their use continues to drive changes in how we live and work, creating both opportunities and threats as new ways of operating and entirely new business models emerge.

The impact of mobile technologies on the finance function remains modest. The focus of this technology and the bulk of investment has been on changing the way we communicate and interact with customers and ensuring we are in tune with customer expectations.

From the finance function perspective the use of mobile technologies has centred on efficient communication within teams. There remains little practical day to day application of smart phones and tablets in the actual functioning of the accountancy operations.

Some areas and efficiencies delivered or facilitated by mobile technologies include:

- **Communication and flexibility** – smart phones and tablets help deliver flexible working and facilitate improved communication between staff
- **Scalability** – mobile tech and cloud tech combined, overcome some of the obstacles traditionally associated with starting and growing a business, most notably the capital costs of setting up systems and IT

- **Less paperwork** – use of mobile technology has reduced duplication and data entry. For instance new app software for logging and recording expenses has reduced manual processing, whilst delivering significant efficiencies and better quality management information

- **Instant data visibility** – accessing and communicating key data through data visualisation tools such as dashboards. Key metrics can be viewed live by all

2.9   3-D printing

3-D printing as discussed in **Chapter 5**, is a process driven by computer-aided design (CAD) and computer-aided manufacturing (CAM) technology that allows almost anything to be printed to exact specifications as defined by the system. It has transformed the way products are prototyped and is anticipated to continue to increase in significance as technology develops and associated costs reduce.

The impact on the finance function is largely from a costing perspective, practically dealing with the changes in operations this technology allows:

- **Less waste** as the material is printed directly so no offcuts or by products

- **No overproduction** as products are made to exact specification as ordered rather than being produced in volume to a forecast demand level

- An increase in **direct costs** as the time spent setting up the systems, the materials used and the parts handling are all distinct to a specific job

- Minimal **tooling and set-up** costs make small production runs and bespoke products cost effective

- **Inventory** holding of finished goods should be zero and with effective supply chain management raw materials should be delivered following the 'just-in-time' principle meaning practically no holding of raw materials.

Test your understanding 5
3-D printing is classed as what type of manufacturing?
A   Just-in-time
B   Subtractive
C   Lean
D   Additive

3 Digital mindsets

3.1 Digital mindsets

 A **digital mindset** is the concept of seeing beyond the individual elements of digital change, to understand the deeper all-pervading ways in which digital technology will ultimately transform every aspect of society and therefore impact an organisation.

A 'helicopter view' is a feature associated with strong visionary leaders. It is the ability to take a step back from an organisation and achieve a clear overview. It's about seeing the bigger picture, not getting stuck in the smaller detail and appreciating how all of the elements of the organisation interconnect.

A digital mindset is an extension of this idea and requires leaders and staff to see beyond the smaller incremental considerations of digital adaptation, instead thinking about the longer term vision for the organisation and how it will appear in a digital world.

The five following qualities, practices and approaches were identified by **Forbes** as being important dimensions of the **digital mindset**:

- **Provide vision** yet **empower others** – clear vision of how a business should evolve and transform in this digital age, whilst supporting the initiatives of employees in translating this vision into tangible action

- **Give up control** yet **'architect' the choices** – empowering employees to adapt the organisation but maintaining sufficient oversight to shape and direct the process

- **Sustain** yet **disrupt** – existing business practices must be sustained and enhanced where possible to ensure profitability. New ideas and concepts will disrupt and challenge the status quo, but must be protected and nurtured for their potential to spark beneficial future change.

- **Rely on data** yet **trust your intuition** – data is a powerful tool in decision making but the digital mind-set is forward looking and change focused so looking beyond the numbers and using vision and intuition are important skills

- **Be sceptical** yet **open-minded** – there are many new technologies and approaches that emerge and could potentially be the 'next big thing' or simply disappear. It is important to maintain a degree of caution yet to also consider and try things to learn lessons and see what fits.

3.2 Implications of a digital mindset on the finance professional

Acknowledging and accepting that technology will increasingly change and disrupt the ways in which society, organisations and therefore the finance function operates will be an important part of a finance professional's skill set.

Change adept organisations have the capability, capacity and readiness to deal with change, through flexible structures, lean processes and forward thinking. A key element of being **change adept** is having staff who share these attributes, so finance professionals must focus on having what Dr Carol Dweck described as a **growth mindset**. This is an appetite to continuously develop and learn. Feedback will be openly given and received and viewed as a tool for growth rather than criticism and confrontation, change will be embraced as a challenge and opportunity not seen as threat.

Illustration 9 – Change as opportunity OR threat

A **digital mindset** talks about seeing the bigger picture and understanding the potential of new technology and the limitations of existing processes and ways of working.

An early illustration of this is the company **Kodak**.

Kodak developed the first digital camera in 1975 but didn't pursue the innovation at the time as they viewed it as a threat to their core business of selling single use photographic film. Eventually digital photography was developed by Kodak's competitors and became mainstream leading to the decline of the traditional film business.

Therefore **Kodak** lost both their core business of photographic film and didn't benefit from being the pioneer of digital photography by seizing the opportunity they discovered and being first to market.

They did eventually enter the digital camera market but were just another name among many. As digital cameras became commodity items and cheap to purchase **Kodak** floundered before filing for Chapter 11 bankruptcy in the US in 2012.

A proactive **digital mindset**, seeing the bigger picture of technology beyond the here and now, would have enabled **Kodak** to embrace the opportunity of this new technology and may have seen a very different story for the business.

4 The finance function and process automation

4.1 Impacts on the finance function of increased automation

Technology and software developments are driving an increase in process automation across the finance function. Routine and transactional areas such as balancing ledger accounts and extracting trial balances and accounting summaries have been automated since computerised accounting packages came on to the market many years ago.

As technology continues to develop, more areas of finance are becoming automated or are likely to become automated.

> **Illustration 10 – New technology impacting finance. Expenses.**
>
> The process of dealing with staff expenses has long been inefficient and unnecessarily complicated. New technology businesses like **Certify** or **Rydoo** allow staff to photograph receipts instantly on their mobile device, this uploads the receipt which is synchronised with their software account. The details are extracted, categorised and where required can be submitted for approval immediately. Exceptions can be flagged and reports can be generated showing line by line detail along with supporting receipts and mileage maps. Approved expenses can then be automatically reimbursed to the employee. The information from all employees is available in instant reports, allowing improved analysis and control.
>
> The process still involves human input but the software enabled automation of the compilation and submission of expenses, as well as the removal of manual receipts and the need for physical verification saves staff time and improves the efficiency of the process whilst also significantly improving the management information available.

4.2 Skills required by the future finance professional

Accountants and **finance professionals** in the future will see basic routine, transactional work reduced with a shift to higher-level skills. The following skills are anticipated to be fundamental to future accountants:

- **Analytical skills** – much of the data produced will come from automated processes and data specialists. Accountants will add value through analysing this data in the business context for meaning and insight

- **Business acumen** – having a wide understanding of all aspects of a business and the environment they are in is crucial to effective decision-making and the ability to provide insight to other functions

- **Judgement** – making decisions, evaluating data sources and applying knowledge to make sound judgements will be a key higher-level skill

- **People skills** – interpersonal skills including the ability to communicate, empathise and understand people will be increasingly important as accountants occupy more central business partnering roles, rather than just producing accounts and reports for others

- **Leadership** – accountants have a unique central position in organisations. This is necessary to be able to understand and question the numbers and information they are given. This provides them a wider understanding of the entire business and sees accountants increasingly occupying senior executive positions in companies.

Illustration 11 – Automation. Where machines will replace humans.

A 2017 **McKinsey** report investigated occupational activities where machines would be most likely to replace humans.

The report summarised that roles involving routine repetitive programmable tasks such as **data collection, data processing and repetitive physical activities are most at risk.**

The following is a summary of the extent to which various role types were believed to be automatable:

Data collection – 64%

Data processing – 69%

Applying expertise – 18%

Stakeholder interactions – 20%

Managing others – 9%

As these numbers illustrate some relatively basic areas associated with today's finance professional are likely to disappear, at least partially. Other areas with higher level skills are likely to become much more significant.

4.3 The automation paradox

Increased **automation** of routine tasks takes them out of human control. This can result in the loss of these skills on a practical level, as the automated process takes over and is relied upon.

However atypical events can undermine an automated process as they are built by humans using code and algorithms that cannot accommodate all possible permutations. In this situation, where manual control is required, the deskilling of humans can see organisations unable to cope and therefore slow to respond.

Retaining expertise and ensuring knowledge and understanding of the basic functions of accounting systems and how they operate will be a challenge for the modern finance professional.

For example, the basic process of manually maintaining ledger accounts and balancing them off is fundamental to every bookkeeping course yet it is a task seldom undertaken by accountants today. Modern accounting systems perform multiple checks and balances automatically. Yet this underpinning knowledge is essential to ensure a full understanding of how the system functions and means an accountant can step in should the system fail.

5 Ethics of technology usage

5.1 Legal considerations of technology use

Technology – as discussed in Chapter 5, data is a central aspect of the technology developments driving the 4th industrial revolution.

The amount of personal data available to and used by organisations means that the privacy, sensitivity and security of this data are very significant considerations in modern business.

A business must ensure it is compliant with all legislation but there are also considerations from an ethical and social responsibility point of view in terms of what is right and wrong in the eyes of the public.

Data protection – General Data Protection Regulation (GDPR) was introduced throughout the EU in 2018. It is legislation which details the following principles about data:

- Used fairly, lawfully and transparently
- Used for specified, explicit purposes
- Used in a way that is adequate, relevant and limited to only what is necessary
- Accurate and, where required, kept up to date
- Kept for no longer than is necessary
- Handled in a way that ensures appropriate security. Including protection against unlawful or unauthorised processing, access, loss, destruction or damage.

Data controllers within organisations have to ensure adequate safeguards and controls to implement these data principles.

Background to GDPR

This new legislation was designed to overhaul the previous data protection act from 1995. This was written at a time when the internet was in its infancy, smartphones didn't exist and some of the largest and most influential companies in the world such as Facebook, Google and Amazon were barely even conceived.

The way data is used in 2018 and beyond required new laws that were fit for purpose and designed with the modern landscape in mind and are therefore able to safeguard the privacy and rights of individuals today.

Illustration 12 – Facebook and the Cambridge Analytica scandal

Facebook received a £500,000 fine for its role in the Cambridge Analytica scandal. The fine was the maximum available under the data protection legislation in place at the time (prior to the introduction of GDPR legislation).

Facebook was found to have breached data protection legislation by allowing third party app developers access to user's data without sufficiently clear and informed consent. They also failed to make suitable checks on apps and developers using the platform.

What was the Cambridge Analytica scandal?

A third party app designed as a personality quiz collected the data of 87 million Facebook users without their knowledge or explicit consent. This data was then sold on to third parties, one of whom was Cambridge Analytica.

They then used this data to profile voters in the US election based on personality and psychology before targeting advertising which took advantage of this information.

Around 1 million UK users' data was obtained in the scandal.

Test your understanding 6

GDPR legislation in the EU attempts to ensure that organisations follow the principles about data.

Which TWO of the following are contained in those principles?

A   Data is kept up to date

B   Data is kept for longer than is necessary

C   Data is used for implicit purposes

D   Data is protected against unlawful access

E   Data should always be in hard copy format

5.2   Ethical and social considerations of technology use

Ethics was introduced in Chapter 1. Let's begin by recapping what is meant by ethics:

Ethics is a system of moral principles that affect how people and organisations make decisions. It involves acting in a way deemed acceptable by society.

Ethical and social considerations – Compliance with legislation such as the **GDPR** laws noted above is something that all companies should achieve. However, the question of whether this is sufficient opens up ethical considerations as to what companies should do and how they should act.

When considering the way in which an organisation handles technology and data, **ethical and social considerations are important** for the following reasons:

- A company that handles technology and data in an ethical way will give investors confidence

- Customer confidence in data security is vital in the digital age and is an important element of brand confidence

- Consumers feel safer dealing with companies that are proactive and responsible in their use of data

- Employees are attracted to companies that exhibit a strong ethical stance when it comes to how they use technology and data

- Ethical handling of technology and data helps ensure long-term sustainability of an organisation through stakeholder confidence and trust

- It demonstrates a proactive approach and an awareness of the risks associated with data and technology

Illustration 13 – Microsoft AI ethical principles

Microsoft is one of a number of high profile technology companies to lay down a voluntary set of ethical principles surrounding its use of **artificial intelligence** (AI). AI is an area of technology that presents some of the most challenging ethical questions.

Microsoft's AI principles:

Fairness – AI systems should treat all people fairly

Reliability & safety – AI systems should perform reliably and safely

Privacy & security – AI systems should be secure and respect privacy

Inclusiveness – AI systems should empower everyone and engage people

Transparency – AI systems should be understandable

Accountability – AI systems should have algorithmic accountability

5.3 Corporate digital responsibility

Corporate digital responsibility or **CDR** is a relatively new concept which extends the idea and ethos of **corporate social responsibility** (**CSR**) to the digital world.

It is a voluntary commitment by organisations to go beyond mere compliance with legislation, when it comes to how they handle technology and data. It considers the broader ethical values of organisations driving forward the advancement of technology to do so in a manner that is fundamentally leading toward a positive future.

CDR involves a commitment to protecting both customers and employees and ensuring that new technologies and data are used both productively and wisely.

The development of a **CDR strategy** is increasingly common in modern business and would include the following **5 key areas**:

- **Digital stewardship**, using data in a responsible and secure way that is in line with customer's and employee's expectations of what is reasonable

- **Customer expectations** around data use and the need for transparency are increasing. The ability to opt in and be rewarded for sharing data empowers the consumer

- **Giving back** means that companies can share data in a benevolent way to help society. For example, a bank with knowledge of financial information could help to inform a customer's choices to improve their financial management, even if it meant a loss of overdraft or credit card fees. Additionally, a pharmaceutical company sharing clinical trial data with university researchers for no gain

- **Data value** is becoming increasingly apparent to customers as well as businesses, so the need to reward and incentivise customers to give more data will become the norm

- **Digital inclusion** is about ensuring all members of society have the skills, tools and ability to access the online digital world, and are not left behind through lack of education or opportunity. Businesses need to be proactive to help and support users and reduce barriers and obstacles.

Test your understanding 7

X Co is a traffic data management company, involved in town planning and transport logistics. They heavily invest in software to look at real time data on the impact of cycle lanes, new roads, types of cars etc. on traffic times in city centres. This wealth of knowledge has been built up for years, and recently X Co has looked at the possibility of sharing this information with hospitals and the emergency services, free of charge. This is to help the emergency services get to incidents quicker.

What is this project a specific example of?

A   Corporate digital responsibility

B   Corporate social responsibly

C   Lobbying

D   Artificial intelligence

6   Chapter summary

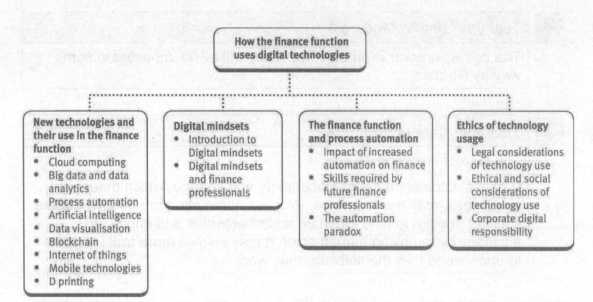

How the finance function uses digital technologies

New technologies and their use in the finance function
- Cloud computing
- Big data and data analytics
- Process automation
- Artificial intelligence
- Data visualisation
- Blockchain
- Internet of things
- Mobile technologies
- D printing

Digital mindsets
- Introduction to Digital mindsets
- Digital mindsets and finance professionals

The finance function and process automation
- Impact of increased automation on finance
- Skills required by future finance professionals
- The automation paradox

Ethics of technology usage
- Legal considerations of technology use
- Ethical and social considerations of technology use
- Corporate digital responsibility

Test your understanding answers

Test your understanding 1

The correct answer is **all options**. They will all be impacted in some way by big data.

Test your understanding 2

The correct answer is **D**

Process automation brings uncertainty and change, which means employees, may resist change. Process automation brings advantages such as freeing up time for value added activities and improving accuracy by removing human error. It may involve more training costs to understand how the software may work.

Test your understanding 3

The correct answer is **A and C**

Data visualisation uses graphics and dashboard to be user friendly and intuitive. It also allows better understanding and fresh views on the data. Data visualisation can use real time data, to avoid monthly reporting. It does not necessarily involve a wider use of performance metrics, data visualisation just shows them in different ways.

Test your understanding 4

The correct answer is **C**

Blockchain would allow smart contracts to be used, which are self-executing and can't be tampered with. Artificial intelligence wouldn't be needed to make decisions. Cryptocurrency uses blockchain to underpin the digital transactions. Digital mindsets look at how technology may impact society.

Test your understanding 5

The correct answer is **D**

Additive manufacturing is creating additional layers to build up a structure, like 3-D printing. Subtractive manufacturing removes layers e.g. cutting sections. Just in Time generates raw material orders to coordinate with demand to reduce production cycles. Lean manufacturing concentrates on waste reduction.

Test your understanding 6

The correct answer is **A and D**

GDPR wants data to be kept up to date and protected. It also requires data to only be kept for as long as necessary and that it is used for explicit, specified purposes. Data can be stored in a variety of formats.

Test your understanding 7

The correct answer is **A**

Corporate digital responsibility (CDR) goes beyond legislation when handling technology and data. Corporate social responsibility looks at maximising positive impacts on society and minimising negative, and may incorporate CDR. Lobbying tries to influence the policies of government officials. Artificial intelligence is the creation of intelligent machines that work and react like humans.

Data and the finance function

Chapter learning objectives

Lead	Component
C1: Describe the ways in which data is used by the finance function.	Identify the ways in which the finance function uses data: (a) In a general sense (b) Specifically in each of the primary activities of finance

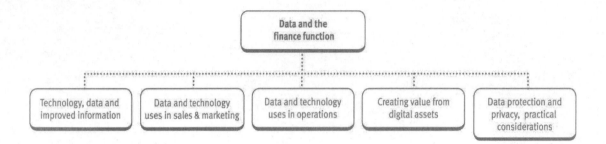

1 Introduction

We have introduced some of the key developments in technology which are transforming the world in which we work and live.

In this chapter we will look more closely at the growing importance of data and how this is both a key driver of new technologies, whilst also being a product of these same technologies.

We will also look at how data is used by the finance function to help the business across their various functions, for example to increase sales, generate new and innovative products, control costs and drive operational efficiencies. This relates back to our previous discussion (Chapter 2, Section 2) on the basic primary activities of the finance function in that they will:

- Assemble information

- Analyse it for insights

- Advise to influence

- Apply for impact

2 Technology, data and improved information

2.1 The importance of information to decision makers

Decision making is a vital task in any business and takes place at 3 different levels in an organisation; strategic, tactical and operational.

Strategic – Long term, complex decisions made by directors and senior management. Decisions at this level impact the overall strategic direction of an organisation.

Tactical – Decisions are medium term and involve putting the strategic plan into action. This may involve selecting what products to stock in the current season or whether to open new branches.

Operational – Day to day decisions at junior levels of management concerned with the practical running of the business in line with plans set higher up the organisation.

Information

Firstly, let's recap what is meant by information from Chapter 2, Section 2.

Information is data, processed in such a way that it has meaning to the person who receives it; this can then be used to improve the quality of decision making.

Accountants and the finance function are tasked with providing high quality information to support the successful operation of a business. The more **insight** this **information** can provide the more valuable it is to an organisation.

Some of the technological developments discussed in the previous chapters, are providing and utilising data on a new level, which if harnessed correctly can provide high value **information,** facilitating enhanced decision making across all levels of an organisation.

Some of the benefits of enhanced information include:

- Greater customer insights

- Potential for new sources of competitive advantage

- New business models and revenue streams

- Operational efficiencies offering significant cost savings as well as improved products and service for customers

- Quicker more reactive decision making

- Early warning of potential problems

- Customised products specific to a customer needs

Test your understanding 1
Which of the following is the definition of information?
A   A large store of data obtained from a wide variety of sources that can be used for decision making.
B   Raw and unprocessed numbers, facts or symbols that may contain valuable information if analysed effectively
C   A structured set of data held in a computer
D   Data processed in a way that it has a meaning to the person who receives it

2.2 Technology and data

As discussed in Chapter 2, Section 2:

 Data is raw and unprocessed numbers, facts or symbols that may contain potentially valuable information if analysed effectively.

Big data, data analytics and insight

Big data and **data analytics** are providing new **insights** and understanding of all aspects of the world around us. Accessing these insights is an opportunity for businesses but also a sizeable challenge and a potential threat should a business fall behind its rivals.

The main sources of **big data** are the technologies seen in the previous two chapters, the most significant being the **internet, mobile technologies** and the **internet of things.** These technologies facilitate software, applications (apps) and websites which generate vast amounts of data every second of every day.

> ## Illustration 1 – The scale of big data
>
> **Internet** – There are 5.5 billion internet searches every day and in 2020 almost 2 billion people made online purchases, with each individual search and transaction providing multiple data points
>
> **Mobile technologies** – Smartphones have sound sensors, image sensors, touch sensors, an accelerometer, a light sensor, a proximity sensor and positional sensors for GPS. These are all used in the functioning of the smartphone but also produce enormous amounts of data continuously
>
> **Internet of things** – there are expected to be 200 billion 'connected' devices in 2020, all with multiple sensors generating constant data about how devices are used and performing
>
> **Applications, software and websites** – Facebook has over 2.4 billion users, with 1.6 billion active mobile users daily on the site. Users of the site generate 4 million likes every minute.

2.3 Improving information for decision makers

Decision makers at all levels of an organisation rely on good quality information to help inform and guide them. Whether it is an aged receivables report used by a credit controller or an investment proposal being considered at board level, the information used will be built from data.

In order to improve the information for decision makers, an organisation needs to improve the data being used to generate the information.

Internet of things, social media and the **internet** itself are three significant sources of data for organisations. Collecting this data and using it in a deliberate manner is hugely beneficial to decision makers for the following reasons.

- **Enhanced data transparency** – Improved systems for handling data allows new meaning to be found in data which may have previously been unviable to process. Technological developments allow data to be more easily integrated with other data sources across the business, generating greater insight.

- **Enhanced performance** – Real time monitoring of data, summarised into key metrics can enable corrective action to be taken immediately to improve controllable changes in performance.

- **Market segmentation and customisation** – Data can enable new market segments to be identified, which may previously have been lost within a broader market segment. Once identified, this segment can be more actively targeted with a customised message.

- **Improved decision-making** – Better understanding and insight into consumer behaviour through detailed data analysis can facilitate improved decision-making. For instance choosing which products to stock not just based on sales volumes but due to related purchases they encourage and the type of customer they attract are insights driven by deeper data driven understanding.

- **New products and services** – Understanding the various drivers that prompt customers to purchase a specific product or service over another can provide valuable insight into the development of new products or service offerings.

- **Operational gains** – Detailed insight into a business's operations can highlight potential efficiencies, cost savings and service improvements that can give a company an advantage over their rivals.

3 Data and technology uses in sales & marketing

3.1 Sales and marketing

 Marketing is the management process that identifies, anticipates and supplies customer needs efficiently and profitably.

Marketing is considered in detail in **Chapter 10**. In this section we are considering how the use of **technology and data** can help both the marketing and sales functions within a business.

Data use in marketing and sales – Big data and the use of smart technology, which collects relevant data, summarises it and presents the key findings, are driving real changes in the way businesses choose what to sell, the price to charge, when to sell it and when to discount.

The use of data is providing real, fact based insight into customer's and competitor's actions and thereby acting to remove a lot of the 'guesswork' from the business critical decisions made in the marketing and sales departments.

Pricing – Is a critical decision. Price too low and a business misses out on potential revenue, price too high and sales volumes will be low, followed by heavy discounting which can reflect badly on brand image. Live market data allows a company to compare and benchmark prices across an entire industry, as well as seeing the rate of sales. This data indicates the right price point for a given product so the first price of a product can be set optimally.

Products – The days of retailers buying huge quantities of products in advance of distinct seasons are a thing of the past. Retailers test the market and constantly monitor what products and trends are selling both for themselves and their competitors. Short lead times allow products to be sourced almost immediately.

Segmentation – Analysis of buying patterns and social media trends and interactions can refine and identify new market segments by grouping similar data-points. This can be an opportunity enabling more targeted marketing; it may also provide data to show a segment isn't as significant as first thought and may not be viable.

Promotions – Data from past product launches and company promotions for an entire industry combined with the subsequent sales performance of those products provides huge insight into what promotions work best and when. This can reduce the guesswork by supporting companies with real data.

Customer relationship management (CRM) – Data on customers provides a profile which, together with their past buying trends, can make advertising and communications more personalised and tailored to meet their specific 'wants'. For instance knowing a customer likes a bargain means offering them a discount on specific items which may lead to a sale.

Targeting – By analysing market trends and seeing products, colours and designs that are on-trend and selling out elsewhere, a business can then push specific items to the front page of their website or a priority position in store and incorporate it in their advertising, targeted at specific consumers.

> ### Illustration 2 – Data use in marketing and sales. Edited
>
> **Edited** is a technology company that provides real-time **data analytics** software for retailers and fashion brands.
>
> The software utilises **AI** and **SpiderBots** or **web crawlers** (these are automated programs which browse the web methodically extracting target data, such as pricing, styles, colours etc.)
>
> The **Edited** software pulls together key industry wide metrics for the types of products being sold, those selling fast, the key colours and fashion trends and crucially pricing data. This information is available instantly and provides retailers with data on what products they should be designing or ordering, the pricing architecture of products and what products should be discounted and by how much.
>
> All of this information is publically available but the process of searching for and sorting this data would traditionally be a laborious and time consuming task and by the time the data was available or usable it would be old. **Edited** cuts out the leg work and provides live data in a visually appealing and accessible way using **data visualisations** to highlight the key data points required.
>
> The software is used by retailers such as **John Lewis, Topshop, Ted Baker, Boohoo** to name just a few.

Test your understanding 2

Trolley Co is a supermarket. It analyses weather patterns and forecasts for the upcoming weeks, and links it to its product portfolio.

In terms of marketing, which area would this help the most?

A   Price

B   Place

C   Segmentation

D   Promotion

Illustration 3 – Data use and CRM

By harnessing technology and building a profile on customers, even small independent restaurants are incorporating data driven **customer relationship management (CRM)** in driving repeat custom.

Rather than taking a booking and it being a one-time only transaction, a restaurant will collect data such as an email address and/or phone number when taking this booking. This will then be used to create a new customer profile.

In addition they will look at what the type of booking it is i.e. couple, group, family as well as the time and date of the booking. They may even try to find out if it is a special occasion which could also be used for future marketing.

The **data** collection continues as once the profile is established what food you order and the drinks you have will also be added to the profile giving them an insight into what you like and what in future may prompt you to return.

Then with all this data collected if the restaurant notices that you are a fairly regular customer and you haven't visited for some time a marketing email can be generated; this can be tailored to hit the specific data held in your profile. For instance if every time you visit you order the same starter the email may contain a picture of this dish to whet your appetite as well as offering a complimentary starter on your next visit. This may well be enough to convince you to make that next booking.

4   Data and technology uses in operations

4.1   Using data to enhance operations

Data and technology provide insights, and opportunity for businesses to drive sales growth and identify new revenue streams, but it is also playing a major role for businesses in changing and improving their internal operations and processes.

This can lead to multiple benefits for a business, these include:

- **Cost saving** – As with any efficiency gains, insights gained from the use of technology can generate significant cost savings through alleviating bottlenecks, reducing waste and reducing downtime.

- **Improved service** – Operational improvements and live data in operational processes can lead to significant service improvement and information availability for customers. Modern logistics companies allow live tracking of all deliveries through the use of data and connectivity.

- **Supply chain** – Big data is enabling increasingly complex supply chain networks through knowledge sharing and collaboration. Data sharing enables suppliers and customers to collaborate in order to modify either components or end products in the most cost effective manner.

- **Preventative maintenance** – Using an **internet of things** based approach, embedding sensors and connectivity in machines and assets facilitates continual monitoring of performance. Deviations from expected performance give early warning of potential problems and preventative maintenance can be scheduled at a convenient time and before an asset breaks down.

- **Forecasting** – Companies can use big data analytics to map the behaviour of customers, using sophisticated forecasting and predictive modelling techniques in order to schedule production processes for efficient utilisation and order fulfilment.

Illustration 4 – Data use in manufacturing

A case study from consulting firm **McKinsey** looked at the manufacturing processes of a leading pharmaceutical company.

The company manufactured vaccines and blood components, in which the need for purity is critical. Over 200 variables were monitored to inform on the level of purity, these would vary between batches impacting the ultimate yield of saleable vaccine or blood products achieved each time.

By analysing the huge amounts of data generated in the manufacturing process, 9 key parameters were identified. These were found to have a direct causal impact on the yield achieved in the process. The company was able to then target improvements and consistency in these 9 specific areas to achieve increased standardisation and optimise these parameters, ultimately increasing the saleable yield. Output data from the process is now tracked and monitored against target levels.

The yield from the vaccine production process increased by 50% which led to savings for the business of over $7.5 million dollars per annum

Illustration 5 – Data use in operations. DHL

DHL have invested heavily in an **internet of things** based tracking and monitoring system using embedded sensors in their various machinery and assets. This allows the business to track a huge range of metrics including vehicle behaviour and performance, the actual packages they are processing and environmental performance through sensors in their warehouses and vehicles. All of this data is collected and harnessed to generate real time monitoring and process improvement as well as providing a huge array of data the business can mine to identify further insight that may drive future performance improvement.

This system at **DHL** is still in its infancy but is already generating efficiencies, cost savings and service improvements. The long term picture promises vast improvements in the scale and capability of such systems to companies like DHL, and by adopting this technology DHL hope to be ahead of the curve in realising the benefits the **internet of things** and the **big data** it generates, can offer.

Test your understanding 3

Core Co is a mining company. It extracts minerals from the ground using drills. Core buys drills that have software contained within them that records when each drill became operational; the hours used each day and the drill performance.

Which of the following would be the main benefit to Core Co of this software?

A   Immediate cost savings

B   Improved customer retention

C   Preventative maintenance

D   Reduction of accidents

5   Creating value from digital assets

5.1 Digital assets

Assets held by a business in digital form that do not have physical substance. This typically includes images, animations, audio, video and PDF files.

The volume of **digital assets** is rising rapidly in line with the increase in **internet** usage, **connectivity** and **mobile technologies**. These are the media upon which digital asset content is consumed and are now central to everyday life. Digital assets have become a significant part of modern businesses and must be managed in a deliberate and coordinated manner in order to leverage them to their maximum.

5.2 Digital asset management systems

A **digital asset management (DAM) system** is designed to coordinate the digital assets of a business, ensuring they are held centrally in an accessible, secure and logically designed repository. This supports the efficient running of the business, by facilitating availability and use of these increasingly important assets.

The **finance function** of a business would be involved in the process of building a **business case for investing** in a digital asset management system, coordinating the search for a suitable provider of a DAM system and managing the change in working practices to incorporate the system. This would need to be managed as a standalone project, outside of day to day activities.

Features of **DAM** system include:

- DAM systems are essentially a database specifically designed to manage digital assets

- Single central location for digital asset storage and access

- Often facilitated by cloud based software, supporting security and allowing access from any location

- Access levels built into the system, allow access only to those with authorisation

- Assets categorised by format with associated metadata describing the content to facilitate search functionality

Illustration 6 – DAM system. American Kennel Club

The **American Kennel Club** (AKC) invested in a DAM system from the specialist provider **Canto**.

The organisation is the authority on purebred dogs in the US, they maintain a registry of pedigrees and organise numerous dog shows. AKC hold a vast catalogue of digital assets, including photos, videos and certified documentation which is all held electronically. Organising these assets for efficient use was a significant challenge and countless hours of staff time were being spent scouring through a variety of locations on the network and hard drives trying to locate images or documents needed for promotional material, newsletters, their website and social media accounts.

The organisation recognised the need for a solution to this problem and looked into DAM systems. **Canto** was the provider they ultimately opted for; they provided a cloud-based centralised library of digital assets tailored to their exact requirements. Assets are logged in the DAM system with numerous tags or metadata, which provides detailed information about the asset to facilitate easy searches, built on a user friendly platform with intuitive design. This had made the use of these assets more efficient and saved hundreds of staff hours searching for or duplicating content.

Benefits of a **digital asset management systems** include:

- Strengthen relationships across teams by facilitating the sharing of assets and content

- Improve service to customers and partners through easy asset sharing using web portals

- A standardised approach to metadata as prescribed by a DAM system eliminates wasted time spent searching for files and digital assets and prevents duplication and re-creation of content.

- Cost and space saving through use of cloud technology designed specifically for the purpose of managing digital assets

- Version control, watermarking and embargo dates allow increased security and protect assets from improper or untimely use

- Provides valuable data on the usage and access of digital assets that can provide insight and direct the production and type of digital assets that generate value

- Copyrighting and contact information can automatically be attached to every digital asset held. This provides consistency in publication and clarity to external users.

Test your understanding 4

Y Ltd is a newspaper and magazine publisher, established over 100 years ago. In that time, they have collected millions of photos to accompany their news stories. The Board have decided they need to make more efficient use of the photo bank.

Which of the following would be needed to utilise the photo bank?

A   Augmented reality

B   3-D printing

C   Non-market strategy

D   Digital asset management system

6   Data protection and privacy, practical considerations

6.1   Data protection and privacy

In **Chapter 6** we introduced the ethical considerations of technology use, looking at legal elements such as **GDPR** and the ethical and social side of things through **corporate digital responsibility (CDR)**. Here we will consider some of the practical considerations of data protection for a business.

Data protection can be defined as the process of safeguarding important information from corruption, compromise or loss.

Businesses as a minimum must ensure they are compliant with data protection legislation such as **GDPR** in order to avoid potential fines and legal recourse. Ideally a business should go above and beyond the requirements of **GDPR** by having a strong moral and ethical stance on how and why they handle data. This is covered by the concept of **CDR** covered in **Chapter 6.**

As a starting point to assess the adequacy of a business's data security, the **UK information commissioner's office (ICO)** outlined the following key questions a business must address. Any questions that a business fails to answer should be immediately flagged as a critical weakness, with immediate action taken to correct the issues identified.

Key questions to assess data security capabilities

- Do you have a record of what personal data you hold? Do you know what you use it for?

- Do people know you have their personal data and know how you use it?

- Do you only collect the personal data you need?

- Do you only keep personal data for as long as it is needed?

- Do you keep personal data accurate and up to date?

- Do you keep personal data secure?

- Do you have a way for people to exercise their rights regarding the personal data you hold about them?

- Do you and your staff know your data protection responsibilities?

Test your understanding 5
Which of the following is not one of the 5 key areas of an effective approach to corporate digital responsibility?
A   Digital stewardship
B   Digital inclusion
C   Digital sustainability
D   Data value

6.2   Features of sound data management

Traditionally data in organisations was not viewed with strategic significance both from a risk perspective i.e. **GDPR** and legislation, and as an opportunity i.e. **big data**. It would often be found under the umbrella of IT due to the obvious crossovers.

However, as data has grown in significance organisations are changing their approach to how data and data management fits within their overall organisation. The following are some of the features of modern organisational structures and their approach to data:

- **Chief Data Officer (CDO)** – This is an increasingly common executive role in larger organisations. The CDO holds overall responsibility for governance and protection of data as well as strategies to optimise the use of data as an asset

- **Data strategy** – Is now a deliberate and integrated part of overall corporate strategy. The **SAS institute**, a specialist in data analytics, identified the five following key building blocks of data strategy:

    - **Identify** – What data does a business have and require? What is its structure, origin and location?

    - **Store** – What structure and storage approach will enable easy sharing and access to data whilst ensuring it is adequately protected?

    - **Provision** – An overarching data strategy should ensure data is packaged to allow easy use throughout the organisation. Rules, guidelines and access levels will be essential.

    - **Process** – Current and existing data should be designed for easy clear and consistent processing. Unifying separate data stores to maximise the processing potential.

    - **Govern** – Establish clear, consistent user friendly policies on the use and storage of data to ensure correct use and minimise risk of data breaches.

- **Culture** – Promoting the significance of data at all levels of the organisation is essential. This must be led from the top of the business to show intent and commitment.

- **Training** – Additional to the areas such as health and safety and cyber security, data awareness training is increasingly mandatory to ensure compliance with legislation.

7   Chapter summary

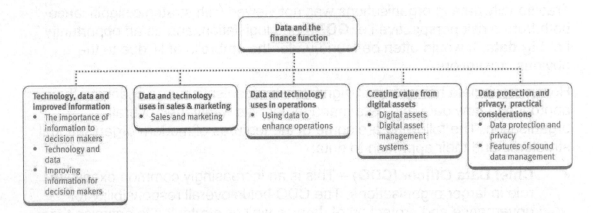

Test your understanding answers

Test your understanding 1

The correct answer is **D**

Information can be used by people for decision making, therefore must have some meaning. A large store of data is called a data warehouse. Raw and unprocessed numbers and facts is the definition of data itself. A structured set of data in a computer is a database.

Test your understanding 2

The correct answer is **D**

Weather patterns can dictate what products sell well at certain times and temperatures. This information can be used to promote specific goods, with in-store promotions such as end of aisle displays. Price is what the ultimately the products get sold for and how you set it. Place looks at the length and breadth of distribution channels. Segmentation is dividing populations up into homogenous groups so you can treat them the same for marketing purposes

Test your understanding 3

The correct answer is **C**

Software/sensors can give ideas of when assets have reached their useful lives, or need to be replaced or improved. This may cost more initially, but leads to savings further down the line. Customers would not necessarily see the impact of this. Accidents may still occur due to the nature of the work.

Test your understanding 4

The correct answer is **D**

Digital asset management looks at all assets held in a digital format. Augmented reality is an interactive experience where a real world scenario is augmented by computer generated perceptual information. 3-D printing is an additive manufacturing process. Non-Market strategy looks at stakeholders outside of the normal commercial interests, such as governments.

Test your understanding 5

The correct answer is **C**

The other two areas of effective CDR not listed are Giving back and Customer expectations. Digital sustainability is not a real concept and is a blend of elements of CDR and CSR.

8

Data to create and preserve value for organisations

Chapter learning objectives

Lead	Component
C2: Explain the competencies required to use data to create and preserve value for organisations.	Explain the competencies that finance professionals need in: (a) Data strategy and planning (b) Data engineering, extraction and mining (c) Data modelling, manipulation and analysis (d) Data insight and communication

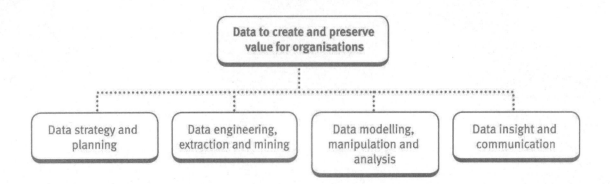

1   Introduction

Having considered data, and how it plays an increasingly significant role in modern business, this chapter looks at more technical elements of **data management** and how these impact the finance function.

We will consider the main stakeholders of the finance function, considering some of their data needs, before taking a closer look at the data strategy of a business as introduced in **Chapter 7**.

To underpin this discussion, we also need to consider the **competencies** required by finance professionals in the digital world in order for them to **use data to create and preserve value for the organisation**. Finance professionals will require competencies in:

- Data strategy and planning

- Data engineering, extraction and mining

- Data modelling, manipulation and analysis

- Data insight and communication

These four areas are discussed in Sections 2-5.

The skills required by the **future** finance professional were briefly discussed in Chapter 6, Section 4.2.

The CGMA (Chartered Global Management Accountant) 2019 competency framework outlines the skills needed by finance professionals in **current and future** roles. They can be grouped into five types of competency, all underpinned by **ethics, integrity and professionalism**.

Competency	Explanation
Technical skills	The finance professional will be required to **apply accounting and finance skills**. As discussed previously, activities such as data collection and processing are increasingly automated. However, the finance function will still be required to act as a 'guardian' of the automated finance process; for example, retaining the skills required when faced with an unusual situation that requires a switch to manual control.

Note: The next three competencies below are less susceptible to automation (this relates back to the diagram in Chapter 4, Section 6.2).	
Business skills	Finance professionals will increasingly require good **knowledge of data sources**, **analytical skills** and **judgement**.
People skills	Finance professionals will be required to work alongside other parts of the organisation, collaborating to generate insight to improve performance. They will need to focus on **building empathy** and **interactions** with stakeholders.
Leadership skills	These will centre on **team building**, **coaching** and **mentoring**, **driving performance** and **change management**, and the **ability to motivate and inspire**.
Digital skills	Includes, for example, **understanding information and data** in a digital environment, **data strategy and planning**, planning/use of **data analytics** and applying existing/developing new **data visualisation** tools. As well as being a standalone skill, digital skills also permeate through the other four skill areas.

Technological advancements are constantly changing the skills and knowledge organisations value in the finance professional. Therefore, the need for a **growth mindset** and **continued learning** is paramount.

2 Data strategy and planning

2.1 Data requirements and stakeholders

A **stakeholder** can be defined in many ways (a definition was given in Chapter 1) but is often summarised as being anybody who can affect or be affected by an organisation's actions. In this section, we are more specifically interested in the stakeholders of the finance function of an organisation. So who would this typically include?

- Other departments and managers – The finance function of an organisation conducts the budgeting process and provides important management information and performance data to all functions of an organisation

- External stakeholders – Users of the financial statements include shareholders, lenders and investors. Auditors, customers and suppliers would be other significant external stakeholders of the finance department

- Employees – Staff in the finance department will clearly be a very significant stakeholder in the department and will need to be considered in all future strategies

- Directors – Key metrics and performance reports for the board are an important component of the finance department's work

Having considered the finance functions main stakeholders, the next consideration is what type of **feedback** we might receive from them and how could this impact the future **data needs** of the organisation. This would be an important element of informing an overall **data strategy**. Some examples are given in the table below:

Stakeholder	Feedback	Data needs
Sales	Selling prices, sales volumes, customer feedback	Live data on competitors' pricing and market trends. Metrics on key customer feedback about products and services received.
Production	Order levels, lead times, approved suppliers and unit cost information	Data collection and recording could be designed to support the collecting of cost data to enable more accurate understanding of costs and drivers of costs. Live systems such as smart shelves can automatically reorder stock.
HR	Staff performance and development, the level of training planned and achieved. Appraisal process	Data system requirements would need to incorporate appraisal systems, productivity analysis as well as collecting data on internal progressions and training days. An integrated office management system could be considered.
Shareholders	Requirement for more information about impacts and future prospects of a business, over the standard annual report	A move to integrated reporting could see a shift in data needs and reporting. For instance, data about carbon footprint and water usage could be collected to report under the natural capital section of an integrated report.
Employees	Hands on users of systems and processes within finance	Unique position to flag inefficiencies in the system and potentially suggest improvements and test solutions.
Managers and directors	Seek insight and clarity from information provided by finance	Investment in improved systems to facilitate the use of data in an organisation incorporating effective data visualisations to summarise key metrics.

3 Data engineering, extraction and mining

3.1 Extraction, transformation and loading (ETL)

 Extraction, transformation and loading (**ETL**) are the three stages in transferring data. They are combined into a single tool to automatically bring data from various sources into a destination system.

- **Extraction** – This is the process of harvesting data from source databases and locations. There will typically be multiple data sources used in the extraction process. Data profiling in the extraction stage is vital to validate the source data and to make sure it is consistent and manageable and will allow successful transformation.

- **Transformation** – The source data will be transformed into a format suitable for the destination database and its ultimate intended use. This is done using code and rules, designed to interrogate the source data before converting it to a new format as per the code instructions.

- **Loading** – This is the process of the newly cleaned and prepared data being uploaded into the destination database ready for use. This will often be a **data warehouse**.

- **Data profiling** – Is an important element in an ETL process. Prior to extraction the data needs to be analysed to understand its content, formats and structure. This then informs the data conditions built into the rules and code used in the extraction and transformation process.

- **Data warehouse** – A data warehouse is a store for data that has been loaded in the ETL process. The data will be held in a systematic and logical way ready for further interrogation and analysis by the **business intelligence** function

ETL systems are a vital component of the **business intelligence** (**BI**) process. BI and ETL developers coordinate to pull together relevant data from multiple sources into one place. This can then be used by the BI function for further interrogation.

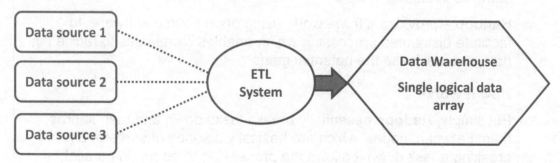

3.2 Business intelligence (BI)

 Business intelligence (BI) is the technology driven process of analysing business data to create insightful and actionable information to help improve the operations or products of a business.

As discussed, **ETL** systems are an important element of **BI**, providing the data in clean and ready-to-use format. BI systems are built to access and analyse this data further and present the findings using **data visualisation** techniques as well as traditional summaries and reports. BI software has evolved to become more user friendly and intuitive allowing users throughout an organisation to access data that may be of value without IT or finance assistance being required.

Big data, ETL and BI

Traditional **ETL** systems are not a new development and have been around since the 1970s. The modern digital world means these **ETL** or data integration systems are faced with fresh challenges. The main trends include:

- **Rate of growth** – data volumes are growing at unprecedented levels

- **Types and sources** – traditional database integration is a thing of the past. Data for the modern business comes in all shapes and sizes and from an array of sources both internal and external; social media, connected devices, live streaming etc.

- **New technologies** – ETL software is still a fundamental element of BI but new solutions such as **Hadoop** and **GoogleBigQuery** are designed for the modern landscape of big data. They use innovative techniques in order to handle the challenges presented by the volume, variety and velocity of big data.

Illustration 1 – Hadoop and modern data requirements

Hadoop is a name synonymous with **big data** and is an example of **BI** software in the digital age.

Hadoop – provides a framework, using open source software, to facilitate distributed processing which enables companies to tackle big data and maximise the potential gains.

How it works

Put simply, **Hadoop** essentially breaks tasks down and then shares them between 'nodes' which are basically a series of servers. By breaking a task down it allows the processing to be run in parallel, making a task much faster, it also has inbuilt failsafes so if one node fails, its work will be picked up and processed elsewhere.

For instance if I had a task that was going to take me 20 days to complete but it needed to be done quicker, the obvious route would be to break the work down into blocks and get others to help. I would then reassemble the blocks of work and present the finished task.

Another advantage is that should one of the workers get ill (or fail from a computing perspective) their block of work could be shared between the other workers without any significant impact on the ultimate outcome.

Components of Hadoop

HDFS (Hadoop Distribute File System) – This is the part of the system responsible for breaking down a task into chunks of work and distributing them. HDFS operates following a similar logic to that on your personal computer, but scales this up to operate and arrange files across many machines.

MapReduce framework – Having broken the data into chunks, the MapReduce element of Hadoop then coordinates the actual distributed processing of this data to achieve an outcome.

So for instance if we were trying to interrogate a large data set looking for key words, the **HDFS** would take the large volume of data, break it into manageable chunks and spread this across multiple nodes. The **MapReduce** element would then find the instances of these key words in each chunk (mapping) and then summarise the outcome (reduce) to say how many instances we had overall.

Test your understanding 1

Which THREE of the following are reasons why traditional ETL systems may no longer be valid for an organisation today?

A   Increased rate of data growth

B   Wider sources of data

C   More balanced composition of the Board

D   Increased use of Corporate Social Responsibility

E   Introduction of new big data technologies

F   Restrictions in employee skillset

4   Data modelling, manipulation and analysis

4.1   Data modelling and the finance function

 A **data model** considers the data of an organisation in a systematic way that allows it to be stored and retrieved in an efficient and effective manner.

The process of data modelling involves laying out an organisation's data requirements in a way that can be easily and deliberately converted to computer code. The modelling process requires a clear and systematic plan of the key data being stored and how this should be organised to allow it to be retrieved, interrogated, linked and grouped.

The advantages of data modelling include:

- **Foundation** for handling data, it facilitates the effective use of that data throughout the organisation

- Enforces **business rules** and helps achieve regulatory compliance by ensuring data is complete and secure

- **Consistency** of naming conventions and values ultimately underpin a systematic and reliable database

- The **quality** of data is enhanced. Data modelling provides an organisation with a well-planned approach to its data, ensuring completeness and facilitating high quality data warehouses.

Three levels of a data modelling process

Conceptual – Business oriented and practical, considering the business data and its requirements

Logical – This level begins to develop a technical map of rules and data structures, defining how data will be held and used

Physical – This considers how the defined system requirements will be implemented using a specific database management system (DBMS)

4.2 Data manipulation

 Data manipulation is the process of changing data to make it easier to read. It involves adding, deleting, querying and modifying data in a datastore using a **data manipulation language** or **DML.**

Data held in a database is held according to the parameters of the **data model** used to design it. This data can then be searched and interrogated using **data manipulation language** (**DML**) which essentially gives instructions to a database in a consistent and structured fashion.

From a finance perspective, the query function of **DML** is the most relevant feature, allowing users to ask the database questions about the data held. This is done in order to gather information required by management for things like analysis, reporting and decision-making.

Test your understanding 2
What are the THREE levels of the data modelling process?
A   Rational, Time variant, Logical
B   Conceptual, Irrational, Variety
C   Conceptual, Logical, Physical
D   Extraction, Transformation, Loading

5 Data insight and communication

5.1 Managing big data – the finance function

The role of providing management information in business has long been the remit of the finance function. **Big data** has seen the pool of data available to compile this management information increase exponentially. The finance function still plays an integral role in understanding and managing the data and information of a business.

Data strategy – the use of data is of fundamental importance to most modern businesses. In line with the concept of developing a **digital mindset**; digital technology and data must be considered at a strategic level within a business. Data is central to the overall strategic thinking of business and must be incorporated in strategic planning. An overall **data strategy** is a common element of overall corporate strategy and is defined by the Harvard Business Review as follows:

 Data strategy is a coherent approach for organising, governing, analysing and deploying an organisation's information assets.

As introduced in **Chapter 7**, developing a data strategy is a key part of the modern business landscape and an effective data strategy should consist of the 5 elements, **identify, store, provision, process** and **govern** as covered earlier. The strategy should provide a coherent, organisation wide approach, moving away from isolated data projects being conducted throughout the business in a haphazard fashion.

A key element of any data strategy from a value adding perspective is how to effectively capture and utilise big data.

To maximise the benefits it can deliver, a system must be designed that can cope with the attributes of big data as outlined by the **4Vs** in **Chapter 5**:

- **Volume** – As discussed the volume of data available from modern technologies is vast; the capability to handle and process the sheer quantity of data, which will continue to grow, must be a key consideration in any data strategy.

- **Velocity** – The stream of data coming in to organisations is constant, transactions, web clicks, 'likes' on social media etc… occur in their millions every minute of every day. Data systems must have the capability to process this live data, providing up to date information as well as storing it for further use.

- **Variety** – Data comes from a range of sources both internal and external and in an array of formats. Traditional data use was largely internal and structured, but the growth in external sources such as social media and web cookies sees data in a range of unstructured formats. Systems must have the capability to handle this increasingly rich source of data.

- **Veracity** – This considers how trustworthy data is and is crucial to effective use of data. Systems must ensure data can be validated to reduce uncertainty to tolerable levels. Combining data with other sources can act as a check of data authenticity. For instance GPS location data in cities suffers high levels of interference, this data could be validated by comparison to other data such as purchase data, accelerometer data or social media updates.

Overall, an effective data strategy must address the challenges of big data considering how data is collected, held and incorporated across the business to maximise its value adding potential

5.2 Data visualisations and the finance function

As introduced in **Chapter 5, data visualisation** is an enabling technology that complements data analytics by facilitating user friendly and accessible presentation of key data through the following:

- **Information** – Providing information for stakeholders in and outside the business is core to the finance function's responsibilities, therefore data visualisation is a very important concept for the finance professional

- **Users** – Many users of the data finance departments produce do not have a finance background so it is important to avoid data heavy presentations and technical jargon. Instead the focus is on highlighting the key pieces of data the audience need and presenting these in an engaging and informative way

- **Simplicity** – Effective visualisations should be intuitive and involve practically no training for the end user

Prior to producing a data visualisation it is useful to consider some simple questions in order to improve its effectiveness:

- **Who are the audience?** Who are we producing the data for and what level of detail they require are key considerations. It is also useful to consider the technical ability of the audience too.

- **How do they want the data?** Is it for our sales force? If so the data should be mobile friendly, summarised and quick to read, with the potential to drill down where required. Generally the level of detail, the interface, medium and interactivity should all be considered.

- **What outcome do we want?** Ultimately what do they want to take from the data and how should it help enhance performance.

Illustration 2 – Data visualisation. Edited.

This is an example of a data visualisation from **Edited** the retail data analytics technology company discussed in **Chapter 7**. It demonstrates a summary of the stock movements, replenishment rates and price discounting across a range of retailers in the same sector of the market. The visualised data summarises a vast amount of data into a visually appealing and useful infographic that highlights just the key information needed by users.

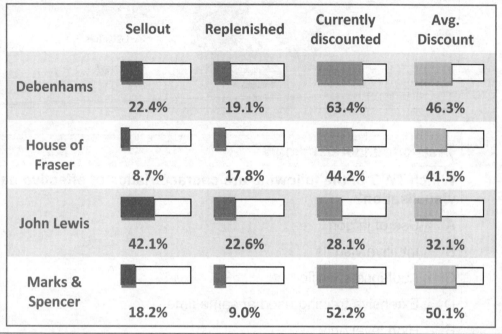

	Sellout	Replenished	Currently discounted	Avg. Discount
Debenhams	22.4%	19.1%	63.4%	46.3%
House of Fraser	8.7%	17.8%	44.2%	41.5%
John Lewis	42.1%	22.6%	28.1%	32.1%
Marks & Spencer	18.2%	9.0%	52.2%	50.1%

Illustration 3 – Data visualisation. Accounts receivable (AR)

The **visualisation** below is an extract from an accounts receivable report; this simple pie chart gives the user a clear indication of the ageing of the receivables balances in a clear and concise way. The heavy detail of multiple pages of individual credit customers along with the breakdown of their balances is not needed by most users and this infographic directs users to the key headline information.

Here the figures of AR turnover and the AR turnover ratio are displayed clearly at the top and can be easily compared against budget to get an indication of performance.

A visualisation like this would typically allow users to drilldown into the detail behind the numbers; for instance, by selecting the 90+ days segment of the pie chart, the user would access the customers and balances that make up this figure and further questions could then be asked upon these. This is the idea of layering data and making visualisations intuitive and simple to navigate.

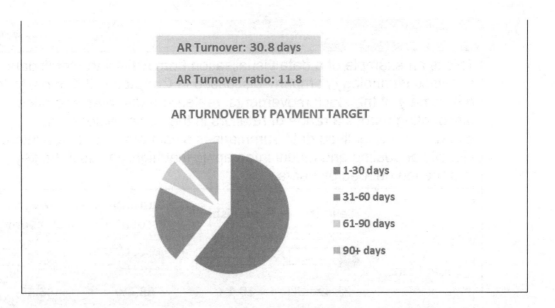

AR Turnover: 30.8 days

AR Turnover ratio: 11.8

AR TURNOVER BY PAYMENT TARGET

- 1-30 days
- 31-60 days
- 61-90 days
- 90+ days

Test your understanding 3

Which TWO of the following are characteristics of effective data visualisation?

A   Use of jargon

B   Intuitive visuals

C   Audience specific

D   Extensive training used at same time

E   High level only

F   Paper format only

5.3   Business focused data

Data scientists are individuals with the ability to extract meaning from and interpret data, which requires both tools and methods from statistics and machine learning.

Data science is a very new field. It is an amalgam of data experts with a background in mathematics, statistics, programming and computer science. Organisations looking to capitalise on **big data** using **data analytics** are increasingly employing specialist data scientists.

In this data driven world it is important to maintain a coherent commercial, business focus to the work being undertaken by data scientists. This is where **management accountants** are ideally situated to take the lead, partnering with data scientists to ensure the work they undertake is deliberate and targeted with clear objectives to ultimately support or enhance the business. Management accountants should also act to translate insights gained back to the wider business in a practical and commercial way.

Essentially **management accountants will act as an interface between the business functions and the data specialists**; they are uniquely positioned to do so for the following reasons:

- All activities have a financial consequence so the finance function is central to an organisation with a unique understanding of the overall business picture.

- The information produced is already trusted, typically audited and grounded in factual accounting reality.

- The management accounting function and the information produced provide the basis of performance management across the business.

- Finance is based on rational and measurable information. Finance professionals have credibility and ethical guidelines which underpin their objectivity and rigour in decision making.

6   Chapter summary

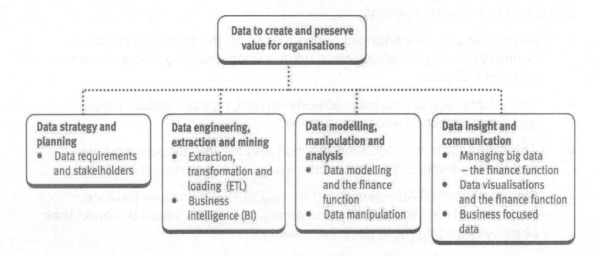

Test your understanding answers

Test your understanding 1

The correct answer is **A, B, E**

Growth of data, sources of data and new data technologies all mean traditional ETL programs may not be as valid today. The composition of the Board should not influence this, as the board have a duty to safeguard assets and manage risk, whatever era they are in. Employee skillsets will change, but won't be the reason the systems are no longer valid.

Test your understanding 2

The correct answer is **C**

The three levels are Conceptual, Logical, and Physical. Extraction, transformation and Loading (ETL) are stages in transferring data into a single destination.

Test your understanding 3

The correct answer is **B, C**

Data visualisation should allow the audience to intuitively see results, and be focused at the right level for the audience. It should not use excessive jargon, need much training to understand. It can drill down into further depth if required, and be across several mediums, including paper copies.

How the finance function interacts with operations

Chapter learning objectives

Lead	Component
E1: Describe how the finance function interacts with operations.	Describe: (a) Main role of operations (b) Areas of interface with finance (c) Key performance indicators

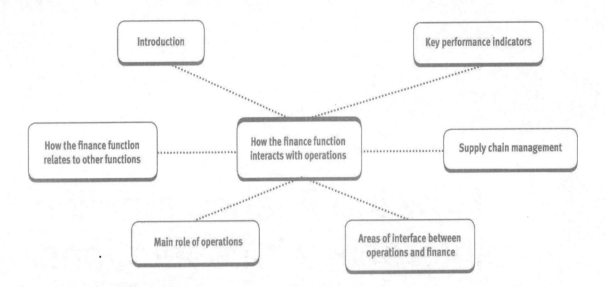

1 Introduction

Chapters 9 to 12 will cover syllabus area E 'Finance Interacting with the Organisation'. We will bring together previous sections and link them to other areas of the organisation, describing how the finance function plays its role by interacting with the rest of the organisation.

The functions that need to be performed in a business depend on many variables, such as what industry it is in, how geographically spread it is, and what its plans are for the future. Most commonly, however, these **functions** are identified generically as follows:

- Operations
- Sales and marketing
- Human resources (HR)
- Information technology (IT)
- Finance

In today's interconnected organisations, finance will need to work collaboratively as business partners with other functional areas to achieve the objectives of finance, these other areas and crucially the objectives of the whole organisation.

In syllabus area E we will look at the main role of the first four of these five functions before understanding the areas of each function that interface with finance and, finally, understanding how the finance function helps to manage these functions.

Operations will be covered in this chapter.

2   How the finance function relates to the other functions

This area will be explored in more detail in each of Chapters 9 to 12 but a short introduction is useful at this point.

The finance function's role in managing the financial resources of the organisation and providing information to help economic decision making will be integral to the effectiveness of the other function (in this case the operations function).

The finance function will:

- Assemble and extract data to provide **information** to the other function and **insight** about value creation/preservation

- Work with the other function (an internal stakeholder) and other stakeholders to **influence** and shape how this function creates and preserves value

- The CFO will work with the head of each function (for example, the chief operating officer (COO)) to achieve the desired organisational **impact** for this function.

3   Main role of operations

3.1   Definitions

 Operations are those activities concerned with the acquisition of raw materials, their conversion into finished products and the supply of that finished product to the customer.

Contemporary thinking has broadened the definition to 'what the company does' to include service operations as well as manufacturing operations.

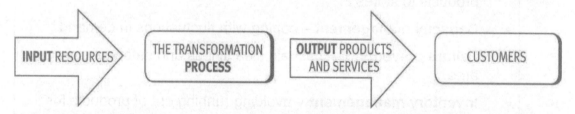

INPUT RESOURCES → THE TRANSFORMATION PROCESS → OUTPUT PRODUCTS AND SERVICES → CUSTOMERS

 Illustration 1 – Examples of operations

Organisation	Operations function	Operation
McDonalds	Kitchen and serving staff	Selling fast food
Vauxhall	Production line	Making cars
Dell	Production line, internet	Making and selling computers
Real Madrid	Football coaches, training facilities	Playing football

Operations management is the activities involved in designing, producing and delivering products and services that satisfy the customer's requirements.

Illustration 2 – Operations management in IKEA

IKEA is the most successful furniture retailer ever. With over 400 stores in 25 countries, it has managed to develop its own special way of selling furniture. **Innovations in its operations** dramatically reduced its selling costs. These included the idea of selling furniture as self-assembly flat packs (resulting in reduced production and transport costs) and its 'showroom-warehouse' concept which required customers to pick the furniture up themselves from the warehouse (which reduced retailing costs). Both of these operating principles are still the basis of IKEA's retail operations process today.

IKEA's **operations managers** are involved in a number of activities. These include:

- **Process design** – arranging the store's layout to give smooth and effective flow of customers

- **Product design** – designing stylish products that can be flat-packed efficiently

- **Job design** – making sure that all staff can contribute to the company's success

- **Supply network design** – locating stores of an appropriate size in the most effective place

- **Supply chain management** – arranging for the delivery of products to stores

- **Capacity management** – coping with fluctuations in demand

- **Failure prevention** – maintain cleanliness and safety of storage area

- **Inventory management** – avoiding running out of products for sale

- **Quality management** – monitoring and enhancing quality of service to customers

- **Operations improvement** – continually examining and improving operations practice.

These activities are only a small part of IKEA's total operations management effort but they do give an indication of how operations management can contribute to business success.

Processes – All operations consist of a collection of processes. These are the building blocks of operations and connect with one another to form a network. The processes transform the input resources into output products/services.

Illustration 3 – Some operations described in terms of their processes

Operation	Inputs	Processes	Outputs
Airline	Aircraft Pilots and air crew Ground crew Passengers and freight	Check passengers in Board passengers Fly passengers and freight around the world Care for passengers	Transported passengers and freight
Department store	Goods for sale Sales staff Information systems Customers	Source and store goods Display goods Give sales advice Sell goods	Customers and goods 'assembled' together
Police	Police officers Information systems Public (law-abiding and criminals)	Crime prevention Crime detection Information gathering Detaining suspects	Lawful society, public with a feeling of security
Frozen food manufacturer	Fresh food Operators Process technology Cold storage facilities	Source raw materials Prepare foods Pack and freeze food	Frozen food

3.2 The different characteristics of operations processes

Although all operations processes are similar in that they all transform inputs into outputs, they do differ in a number of ways, four of which, known as the **4 Vs**, are particularly important. Each of these impact the way in which an operation will be organised and managed.

Volume of inputs and outputs

Operations differ in the volume of inputs they process. High-volume operations are likely to be more capital-intensive than low-volume operations, and there is likely to be a greater specialisation of labour skills.

> ### Illustration 4 – The volume dimensions at McDonalds
>
> McDonald's serves millions of burgers around the world every day. Volume has important implications for the way McDonald's operations are organised. The first thing you notice is the **repeatability** of the tasks people are doing and the **systemisation** of the work where standard procedures are set down specifying how each part of the job should be carried out. Also, because tasks are systemised and repeated, it is worthwhile developing specialised fryers and ovens. All this gives low unit costs.

Variety of inputs and outputs

Some operations handle a wide range of different inputs, or produce a wide range of output products or services. Others are much more restricted in the range of inputs they handle or outputs they produce.

Variation in demand

With some operations demand might vary significantly from one season of the year to another or from one time of the day to another, with some periods of peak demand and some periods of low demand. Other operations might handle a fairly constant volume of demand at all times.

Visibility to customers

Visibility refers to the extent to which an organisation is visible to its customers. When an operation is highly visible, the employees will have to show good communication skills and interpersonal skills in dealing with customers.

All four dimensions have implications for the cost of creating the products or services. Put simply, high volume, low variety, low variation and low customer contact (visibility) all help keep processing costs down.

(**Note**: These should not be confused with the 4Vs of big data).

Test your understanding 1

Company A is an online retailer specialising in basic household cleaning products, it has a limited product range and sells many of its goods in bulk to cleaning companies.

Company B sells seasonal organic food stuffs from its local retail outlet. Its staff are expected to provide cooking and recipe guidance to its customers.

Using the 4 Vs, which company would be expected to have the lower processing costs?

3.3 Porter's value chain

The value chain model is based around **activities** rather than traditional functional departments (such as operations or finance).

It considers the organisation's activities that create value and drive costs and therefore the organisation should focus on improving those activities. **Many of the activities relate to the operations function**.

The activities are split into **primary** ones (the customer interacts with these and can 'see' the value being created) and **secondary** (or support) activities which are necessary to support the primary activities. Each activity is looked at to see if they give a cost advantage or a quality advantage.

Margin, i.e. profit will be achieved if the customer is willing to pay more for the product/service than the sum of the costs of all the activities in the value chain.

Infrastructure				
Human Resource Management				
Technology				
Procurement				
Inbound logistics	Operations	Outbound logistics	Marketing and sales	After Sales Service

Margin

Value chain activities

Primary activities – directly concerned with the creation or delivery of a product/service.

Activity	Description	Example
Inbound logistics	Receiving, storing and handling raw material inputs.	A just-in-time stock system could give a cost advantage.
Operations	Transformation of raw materials into finished goods and services.	Using skilled employees could give a quality advantage.
Outbound logistics	Storing, distributing and delivering finished goods and services.	Outsourcing activities could give a cost advantage.
Marketing and sales	The mechanism by which the customer is made aware of the product or service.	Sponsorship of a sports celebrity could enhance the image of a product.
After sales service	All activities that occur after the point of sale, such as customer enquiries, returns and repairs/maintenance.	A friendly approach to returns gives it a perceived quality advantage.

Operations management is concerned with all of these primary activities apart from marketing and sales.

Support activities – help improve the efficiency and effectiveness of the primary activities.

Activity	Description	Example
Infrastructure	How the firm is organised.	A firm could have a very 'lean' structure at head office in contrast to competitors with more staff and more bureaucracy.
Human resource management	How people contribute to competitive advantage. Includes activities such as recruitment, selection, training and development and reward policies.	Employing expert buyers could enable a supermarket to purchase better wines than competitors.

Activity	Description	Example
Technology	How the firm uses technology.	The latest computer-controlled machinery gives greater flexibility to tailor products to customer specifications.
Procurement	Purchasing, but not just limited to materials.	Buying a building out of town could give a cost advantage over High Street competitors.

Operations management is directly concerned with procurement and some elements of firm infrastructure and technology development.

Illustration 5 – Value chain

One particular clothes manufacturer may spend large amounts on:

- Buying good quality raw materials (inbound logistics)

- Hand-finishing garments (operations)

- Building a successful brand image (marketing)

- Running its own fleet of delivery trucks in order to deliver finished clothes quickly to customers (outbound logistics).

All of these should add value to the product, allowing the company to charge a premium for its clothes.

Another clothes manufacturer may:

- Reduce the cost of its raw materials by buying in cheaper supplies from abroad (inbound logistics)

- Making all its clothes by machinery running 24 hours a day (operations)

- Delaying distribution until delivery trucks can be filled with garments for a particular request (outbound logistics).

All of these should allow the company to be able to gain economies of scale and be able to sell clothes at a cheaper price than its rivals.

Linkages connect the interdependent elements of the value chain together. For example, better quality production could reduce the need for after-sales service.

Test your understanding 2

Which of the following is a value-added activity?

A   Painting a car, if the organisation manufactures cars

B   The board of directors who decide on the financial structure and technicalities of a business

C   Purchasing of materials

D   A staff development programme

Test your understanding 3

BB makes and sells freshly baked bread. It has recently developed an automated inventory control system for its finished loaves, which significantly reduces wastage.

Which of the following value chain activities will BB's automated inventory system directly improve?

A   Inbound logistics

B   Operations

C   Outbound logistics

D   Marketing

E   Procurement

3.4 Process design

Process design is the method by which individual specialists seek to understand business processes and ensure that these processes are designed to be as efficient and effective as possible. The design of processes will go hand in hand with the design of new products and services.

Before any changes in processes are undertaken it is necessary to understand the organisation's mission, goals and customer needs and to carry out a detailed analysis of existing processes. Process maps can assist in such an examination.

A **process map** provides a visual representation of the steps and decisions by which a product or transaction is processed.

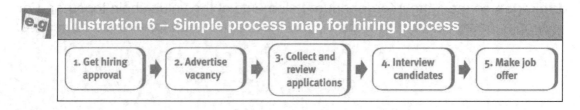

Illustration 6 – Simple process map for hiring process

1. Get hiring approval → 2. Advertise vacancy → 3. Collect and review applications → 4. Interview candidates → 5. Make job offer

Advantages of process maps

- **Management understanding** – allows a better understanding of the basic processes that are undertaken, so providing management with a convenient overview demonstrating responsibilities and key stages in the operations.

- **Role understanding** – allows workers to understand what their job is and how their work fits into the whole process (and therefore the importance of undertaking their role effectively). Process mapping also allows consideration of role reallocation.

- **Standardisation** – highlights where opportunities exist to standardise processes.

- **Highlights inefficiencies** – visually highlights areas where inefficiencies are present through analysis of queues, value and location, so pinpointing areas of waste. This provides an agenda to tackle duplication of effort, the requirement to complete unnecessary paperwork, and misdirected queries that hold up production, etc.

- **Supports corporate initiatives** – mapping can be used as a tool as part of a corporate initiative such as customer satisfaction improvement programmes.

Example of a process map

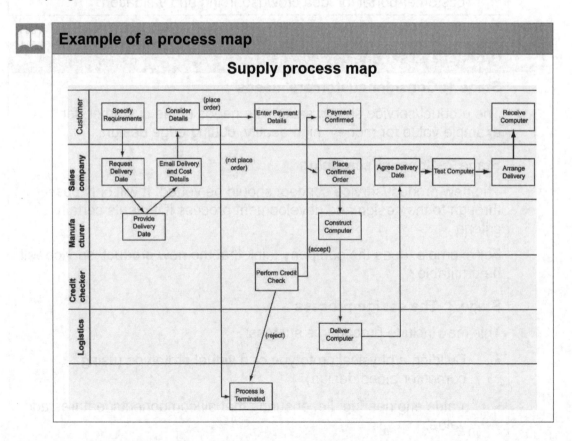

Supply process map

3.5 Product and service development

Companies need to continually look for new or improved products or services, to achieve or maintain competitive advantage in their market.

The stages of product/service development are as follows:

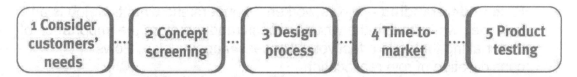

Illustration 7 – Considering customers' needs

The design of a new product/service should begin by understanding the needs of the customer. There are a number of ways to do this, for example:

- Customer relationship management (CRM) systems will allow this either directly via customer surveys or more softly via prudent logging of customer sentiment.

- More radical solutions, e.g. Lego created Lego Ideas – a customer portal for idea crowdsourcing and validation.

Product and service development

Stage 1: Consider customers' needs

The product/service should satisfy the needs of the customer, for example value for money, high quality, cutting edge design.

Stage 2: Concept screening

The new product/service concept should be vetted. It will only pass through to the design and development process if it meets certain criteria.

For example, does the company think that the new product/ service will be profitable?

Stage 3: The design process

This may include procedures such as:

- Building a physical prototype or a virtual prototype (using computer aided design)

- Value engineering, i.e. ensuring that all components/features add value.

> **Stage 4: Time-to-market**
>
> A short time-to-market is desirable since:
>
> - New products/services may be released ahead of competitors
> - Development costs may be lower.
>
> **Stage 5: Product testing**
>
> The new product should be tested before it is released to the market:
>
> - Does it work properly?
> - Do customers like it?

4 Areas of interface between operations and finance

4.1 Introduction

Operations management will be an important contributor to effective and efficient purchasing, production and delivery of customer specific goods and services.

The operations function and the finance function should work in partnership to ensure this efficiency and effectiveness is optimised.

In this section we will examine how specific parts of an organisation's operations (i.e. purchasing, production and service provision) interact with the organisation's finance function. The **focus here will be on the operational level** tasks performed by the finance function.

Section 5 will explain how relationships in the supply chain can be managed and the interface with the finance function will be examined at a more **strategic level** here.

4.2 Purchasing (procurement)

Purchasing is an important part of the operations function. It is responsible for placing and following up orders. It co-ordinates with the finance function as follows:

Establishing credit terms	The finance function will work with purchasing to liaise with suppliers to obtain a credit account and to negotiate credit terms which are acceptable.
Prices	The finance function can advise purchasing on the maximum price that should be paid to maintain margins.
Payment	Payments may be approved by purchasing but are made by the finance function.
Data capture, for example, orders	Order details will be input by purchasing and details passed to the finance function.

Inventory	Purchasing will consult with the inventory section of the finance function to determine the quantity of items already in stock and therefore the quantity required.
Budgeting	The finance function will consult with purchasing on the likely costs in preparing budgets.

Illustration 8 – Purchasing

XYZ Limited is a company manufacturing handbags.

Describe how purchasing liaises with the finance function when buying some leather to make handbags from DEF Limited, a new supplier.

Establishing credit terms	Purchasing will advise the finance function that the preferred supplier is DEF. The finance function contacts the credit controller at DEF and provides the information required to set up a credit account.
Prices	The finance function obtains the cost estimate for the handbag being produced. It discusses with purchasing how much can be paid for the leather in order to maintain margins.
Payment	The payment for the leather is approved by purchasing and then made by the finance function.
Data capture, for example, orders	Order details for the leather will be input by purchasing and details passed to the finance function to check that the price on the invoice is correct.
Inventory	Before placing the order, purchasing will consult with the inventory section to determine how much suitable leather is already in stock.

Test your understanding 4

Which of the following is an example of co-ordination between purchasing and the finance function?

A   Establishing credit terms

B   Determining sales prices

C   Allocating costs

D   Calculating pay rises

4.3 Production

Production is a core part of the operations function. It plans and oversees the production of goods. It liaises with the finance function as follows:

Cost measurement, allocation, absorption	Production measures quantities of materials and time used; the management accountant gives a monetary value to them. Costs are then allocated and absorbed to calculate production costs based on advice given by production.
Budgeting	Production will decide how many items of what type are to be produced. The cost of producing these will be determined by the finance function and production together, and incorporated into the overall budget.
Cost v quality	Production and the finance function will discuss the features that can be included in products and the raw materials that should be used. They should agree which better quality materials and features justify the extra cost, and discuss how to maximise quality and profit.
Production process	Finance can assist production in identifying inefficiencies in the production process (such as bottlenecks) and suggesting improvements.
Inventory	Production will liaise with the inventory section of the finance function to ensure that there are sufficient raw materials in inventory for the production that is planned.

Illustration 9 – Production

XYZ Limited is a company manufacturing handbags. The company has commissioned a designer to design a new style of handbag and discussions are taking place about the materials to be used and the quantity to be produced.

Describe how the finance function and production would liaise over this.

Cost measurement, allocation, absorption	Production would estimate the quantity of raw materials required and (in conjunction with purchasing) estimate their cost. Together with the finance function overheads will be allocated to determine the full cost of the handbag.
Budgeting	Production, the finance function and marketing will discuss how many bags are likely to be sold at what price and determine how many should be produced. A budget can then be produced.

Cost v quality	Production, the finance function (and marketing) will discuss the various grades of leather and the material that could be used, their costs, and the extra price that could be charged for better quality material. They will decide on the best combination of cost/quality/profit.
Production process	The finance function and production will work together to ensure that the newly designed production process is of optimum efficiency and avoids issues such as bottlenecks.
Inventory	Production will discuss with the inventory section of the finance function the materials required. Some existing materials may be usable for the new product or entirely new materials may need to be acquired.

4.4 Service provision

Characteristics of services

Services are said to have four main characteristics.

- **Intangibility** – services are activities undertaken by the organisation on behalf of its customers and therefore cannot be packaged for the customer to take away with them. They often have few, if any, physical aspects.

- **Inseparability** – services are often created by the organisation at the same time as they are consumed by the customer. The service cannot therefore be easily distinguished from the person or organisation providing the service.

- **Perishability** – services cannot be stored for later.

- **Variability** – each service is unique and cannot usually be repeated in exactly the same way, making offering a standardised service to customers very difficult.

These characteristics must be considered when seeking to manage the performance of the service.

The relationship between service provision and the finance function

A business very often provides services to customers, at the same time as a sale or afterwards. For example, a computer retailer may charge an extra fee to help customers set up their system, or a car dealer may provide car servicing.

This service provision will form an important part of the operations function.

There are several issues about which the service departments may need the input of the finance function.

Charge-out rates	This is the hourly rate which the company charges clients. It should be higher than the salary, as it should include a share of overheads, for example training, and any profit the company wishes to make. However, if the charge-out rate is too high customers will not use the service.
Estimating costs	Problems arise in determining the amount of overhead to be included in the charge-out rate. Also, if the service takes longer to provide than expected, the company may not be able to pass on the extra cost.
Problems measuring benefits	Market conditions may mean that the charge-out rate contains a very low profit element. The company may question whether it is worth carrying out these services. The problem is that the benefits are intangible and not easy to measure, but nevertheless real. A company with effective service provision has happier customers, and happy customers are more likely to buy from the company in future, therefore leading to lower selling costs. But it is very difficult to measure these benefits.

Test your understanding 5

Which of the following is a likely advantage of providing a good service?

A   Greater customer satisfaction

B   Higher payroll costs

C   Higher inventory turnover

D   Economies of scale

Test your understanding 6

'Most services provided by an organisation will be created at the same time as they are consumed.'

Which feature of services is being described?

A   Intangibility

B   Inseparability

C   Perishability

D   Variability

5 Supply chain management

5.1 Introduction

 A **supply chain** consists of a network of organisations. Together they provide and process the necessary raw materials firstly into work in progress and then into finished goods for distribution and sale to the end customer.

| RAW MATERIALS SUPPLIER | MANUFACTURER | WHOLESALER AND RETAILER | CUSTOMER |

The transformation of the product along the supply chain includes activities such as:

- production planning
- purchasing
- materials management
- distribution
- customer service
- forecasting.

> **More complex supply chains**
>
> The situation is usually more complex than is shown in the diagram above. Most businesses have several suppliers and several customers. Some businesses may compete for customers and have common suppliers. There may be several supply chains serving one group of customers and they may form complex webs.

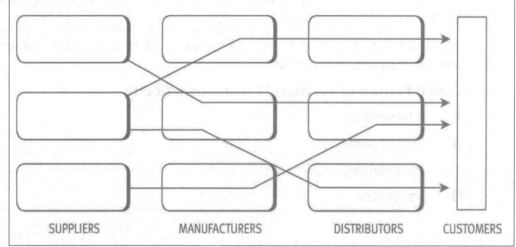

SUPPLIERS   MANUFACTURERS   DISTRIBUTORS   CUSTOMERS

Supply chain management (SCM) involves the co-ordination of activities from the supplier(s) of raw materials at one end of the supply chain to the customer at the other end.

The idea behind supply chain management is that co-ordinating the activities of the different businesses in the supply chain can save costs while also adding value.

Technology can play a key part in effective SCM.

Illustration 10 – Use of blockchain in supply chain transparency
Start-up tech firm Provenance has developed technology which tracks the journey of organic food from farm to shop shelf. It is hoped that shoppers will be able to tap their smartphones on food, such as organic bacon, and instantly retrieve the product's complete supply chain journey. The pilot uses blockchain technology. This means the information of a product's journey and exactly what it means to be certified organic is now instantaneously accessible to shoppers with their smart phones, no app required. The technology will be available both on product packaging and on the shop shelf.

Traditionally, businesses within the supply chain operated independently. However, organisations are recognising that there are benefits associated with establishing links between different businesses in the supply chain. The objective of SCM is to achieve synergies that benefit every player along the chain.

In this section we will understand:

- how the relationships within the supply chain can be managed and

- the interface between SCM and the finance function.

5.2   The strategic supply wheel – Cousins

Traditionally, supply was viewed as an **operational issue**. Purchasing was seen as an administrative task with the emphasis being on price negotiations with suppliers. There was little awareness that supply could affect the firm's strategic goals or that it should be viewed as a key part of strategic planning.

Successful organisations in **today's competitive environment** have recognised that supply should be viewed as a **strategic issue**. The organisation's supply strategy should be aligned with the overall corporate goals and strategy and is integral to the organisation's competitive strategy.

Cousins' model emphasises the importance of viewing supply as central to the organisation and its effectiveness.

Cousins' thinking is based on the notion that an organisation's supply strategy should involve a number of key areas described as 'spokes' in the wheel. As such, the model can help an organisation concentrate on key areas for attention and action.

The wheel depicts the corporate supply strategy at the hub of the wheel and underlines the need for an integrated approach to supply strategy involving balancing all five 'spokes'.

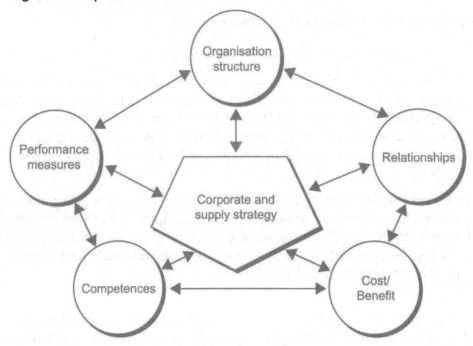

Spoke of wheel	Explanation
Organisation structure	The choice of structure (centralised, decentralised or a mix of these) impacts control and interaction. It should enhance rather than hinder supply strategy.
Relationships with suppliers	Relationships can be: • competitive (contractual) – based on price deals, or • collaborative (relational) – a more positive relationship based on a joint quest to reduce costs and a sharing of technology and innovations to improve quality.
Cost/benefit	Supply decisions should be based on benefits as well as costs. Cost/benefit analysis should be at the heart of any strategic decision.
Competences	Do the skills exist to achieve the chosen strategy? For example, the development of long term supplier relations may lead to a need to retrain key personnel.
Performance measures	Necessary for monitoring and controlling the strategy chosen. Measures should extend beyond price and be aligned with the strategy.

Test your understanding 7

Which of the following statements about supply chain management (SCM) are true and which are false?

Statement	True/False?
The co-ordination of activities from the supplier(s) of raw materials at one end of the supply chain to the customer at the other end is known as supply chain management	
Cost savings are the only advantage of SCM	
The objective of SCM is to achieve synergies that benefit the customers at the end of the supply chain.	
Cousins' supply wheel is a model used to look at the traditional supply function	
Cousins' supply wheel has five spokes	

5.3 Relationship with suppliers

As mentioned above, Cousins identified two broad approaches to supplier relationships:

- competitive (also known as contractual) and
- collaborative (also known as relational).

Competitive (contractual)

In the past, the supply chain was typically defined by competitive relationships.

- The purchasing function sought out the lowest-price suppliers, often through a process of tendering, the use of 'power' and the constant switching of supply sources to prevent getting too close to any individual source.

- Supplier contracts featured heavy penalty clauses and were drawn up in a spirit of general mistrust of all external providers.

- The knowledge and skills of the supplier could not be exploited effectively. Information was deliberately withheld in case the supplier used it to gain power during price negotiations.

Hence, no single supplier ever knew enough about the ultimate customer to suggest ways of improving the cost-effectiveness and quality of the trading relationship.

Collaborative (relational)

Over the last 15-20 years there has been an increased recognition that successful management of suppliers is based upon collaboration and offers benefits to an organisation's suppliers as well as to the organisation itself. By working together and forming relationships, organisations can make a much better job of satisfying the requirements of their end market, and thus both can increase their market share.

- Organisations seek to enter into partnerships with key customers and suppliers so as to better understand how to provide value and customer service.

- Organisations' product design processes include discussions that involve both customers and suppliers. By opening up design departments and supply problems to selected suppliers, a synergy results, generating new ideas, solutions, and new innovative products.

- To enhance the nature of collaboration, the organisation may reward suppliers with long-term sole sourcing agreements in return for a greater level of support to the business and a commitment to on-going improvements of materials, deliveries and relationships.

- The nature of the collaboration needs to shift to reflect the constant change in the environment (see illustration below).

Illustration 11 – Recent changes in UK supply chain relationships

Partnerships within the supply chain must continue to adapt to reflect the unprecedented level of change in the external environment.

For example, a number of recent changes are impacting supply chain collaboration in the United Kingdom (UK). These changes include:

- a volatile political and economic climate

- increased urbanisation in the UK

- a dramatic change in consumer behaviour, for example with a preference for convenience, online shopping and smaller but more frequent shopping

- the growth in automation

- a shift towards digitisation.

The supply chain needs to address these changes, viewing them as an opportunity to reinvent itself and improve the effectiveness of collaboration across the supply chain:

- Changing technology combined with more accurate data is allowing for greater collaboration. For example, distribution is planned more effectively to minimise empty miles and waste.

- Today's consumers, driven by urbanisation, have moved away from the traditional large weekly shop in out-of-town retail parks and are seeking smaller urban stores and online shopping. The supply chain has collaborated to introduce new distribution models and retailing formats (such as meal delivery subscriptions and 'click and collect') in a cost effective manner.

5.4 Material requirement planning

One important aspect of supply chain management is to ensure that materials are ready when they are needed. A number of systems can be used to assist with this requirement.

 MRP is a computerised system for planning the requirements for raw materials, work-in-progress and finished items.

MRP is designed to answer three questions:

- **What** is needed?
- **How** much is needed?
- **When** is it needed?

Functions include:

- Identifying firm orders and forecasting future orders with confidence.
- Using orders to determine quantities of material required.
- Determining the timing of the material requirement.
- Calculating purchase orders based on stock levels.
- Automatically placing purchase orders.
- Scheduling materials for future production.

 Benefits of MRP

- Improved forecasting.
- Improved ability to meet orders leading to increased customer satisfaction.
- Reduced stock holding.
- The MRP schedule can be amended quickly if demand estimates change since the system is computerised.
- System can warn of purchasing or production problems due to bottlenecks or delays in the supply chain.
- A close relationship tends to be built with suppliers (it is consistent with just-in-time – see discussion in section 5.6).

However, MRP will not be suitable if it is not possible to predict sales in advance.

The following technology has been developed from MRP:

- **Manufacturing resource planning (MRPII)** – goes several steps beyond MRP and includes:
    - production planning
    - machine capacity scheduling
    - demand forecasting and analysis
    - quality tracking tools
    - employee attendance and
    - productivity tracking.

- **Enterprise resource planning (ERP)** – the next evolution of an MRP system. It integrates information from many aspects of operations (for example, manufacturing, inventory management, invoicing and management accounting) and support functions (such as human resource management and marketing) into one single system.

Benefits of ERP

Benefits of ERP to the organisation include:

- Identification and planning of the use of resources across the organisation to ensure customers' needs are fulfilled

- The free flow of information across all functions and improved communication between departments

- Aids management decision making due to decision support features

- Can be extended to incorporate supply chain management (SCM) and customer relationship management (CRM) software, thus helping to manage connections outside the organisation.

Test your understanding 8

Which THREE of the following are possible advantages of a collaborative relationship with suppliers?

A   Increased market share

B   Development of innovative products

C   Better understanding of how to satisfy customer needs

D   Improved quality is guaranteed

E   The relationships will be harder to manage

F   Relationship management will be more time consuming

5.5 Quality management

Introduction to quality

In today's competitive global business environment, quality is one of the key ways in which a business can differentiate its product or service, improve performance and gain competitive advantage. Quality can form a key part of a strategic supply chain management.

Quality can be defined in a number of ways:

- Is the product/service free from errors and does it adhere to design specifications?

- Is the product/service fit for use?

- Does the product/service meet customers' needs?

What is quality?

In order to control and improve quality, it must first be defined. Most dictionaries define quality as 'the degree of excellence' but this leaves one having to define what is meant by 'excellence'. Who defines what is excellent and by what standards is it measured? In response to this problem, a number of different definitions of quality have been developed.

In an industrial context, quality is defined in a functional way. Here, quality means that a product is made free from errors and according to its design specifications, within an acceptable production tolerance level.

Such an approach also emphasises that every unit produced should meet the design specifications, so the idea of consistency becomes important. Note that consistency is a key aspect of quality standards such as the ISO 9000 series.

This still leaves a problem, however. How should standards and specifications be set? Who decides what an 'acceptable' tolerance level should be?

An alternative approach to defining quality is thus to focus on the user.

- Japanese companies found the definition of quality as 'the degree of conformance to a standard' too narrow and consequently started to use a new definition of quality as 'user satisfaction'.

- Juran defines quality as 'fitness for use' (1988).

In these definitions, customer requirements and customer satisfaction are the main factors. If an organisation can meet the requirements of its customers, customers will presumably be satisfied. The ability to define accurately the needs related to design, performance, price, safety, delivery, and other business activities and processes will place an organisation ahead of its competitors in the market.

Taking these definitions together, Ken Holmes (Total Quality Management) has defined quality as 'the totality of features and characteristics of a product or service which bears on its ability to meet stated or implied needs'.

Quality is also normally seen in relation to price, and customers judge the quality of a product in relation to the price they have to pay. Customers will accept a product of lower design quality provided that the price is lower than the price of a better quality alternative.

Illustration 12 – Pret A Manger's focus on quality

Described by the press as having 'revolutionised the concept of sandwich making and eating', Pret A Manger (Pret) opened their first store in the mid-1980s, in London. Now they have over 500 shops in the UK and other locations such as New York, Hong Kong and Tokyo.

They say that their secret is to continually focus on quality – not just of their food but in every aspect of their operations practice. They go to extraordinary lengths to avoid the chemicals and preservatives common in many other 'fast' foods which are often used by retailers to extend the shelf life of their products. Pret hopes to maintain the edge by selling food that simply can't be beaten for freshness. At the end of each day, they give whatever they haven't sold to charity to help feed those who might otherwise go hungry.

Pret rejected the idea of a huge centralised sandwich factory even though it could significantly reduce costs. Instead, each shop has its own kitchen where fresh ingredients are delivered first thing every morning, and food is prepared throughout the day.

Pret have also worked hard to build great teams – taking reward schemes and career opportunities very seriously.

Customer feedback is also regarded as being particularly important at Pret. Examining customers' comments for feedback is a key part of weekly management meetings, and of the daily team briefs in each shop.

Test your understanding 9

Explain the reasons why quality may be important to an organisation.

The growth of global companies has resulted in dramatic improvements in the quality of products and services. Much of this impetus can be attributed to the efforts of **Japanese manufacturing companies.**

Key writers on quality	

There are a number of key writers on quality.

Writer	Main contribution
W. Edward Deming	Believed: • managers should set up and then **continuously improve** the systems in which people work • managers should work with employees to gain feedback from those who do the job • workers should be trained in quality to identify what needs changing and how. Deming was credited with the creation of TQM in Japan and developed 14 points for quality improvement.
Joseph M. Juran	• Drew on the Pareto principle and stated that **85% of quality problems are due to the systems that employees work within rather than the employees themselves**. • Therefore, the need to develop key projects for dealing with quality problems rather than concentrating on employee motivation is key. • He argued that quality should focus on the role of the customer. He believed that anyone affected by the product is considered a customer, so introduced the idea of internal as well as external customers.
Phillip P. Crosby	• Introduced the concept of '**zero defects**'. • Believed that prevention is key and that the importance of quality is measured by the cost of not having quality. • He argued for worker participation and the need to motivate individuals to do something about quality.

Methods of quality measurement

- There are four main types of quality-related costs. The organisation needs to identify these costs.

- Monitoring the costs of quality is central to the operation of any quality improvement programme.

- Targets should be set for each of the quality-related costs.

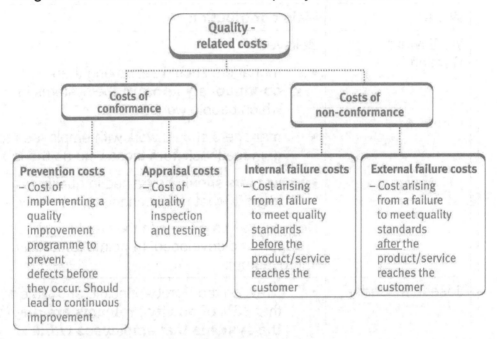

 Illustration 13 – Examples of quality-related costs

Category	Examples
Prevention costs	• Cost of designing products and services with built in quality • Cost of training employees in the best way to do their job • Cost of equipment testing to ensure it conforms to quality standards required
Appraisal costs	• Inspection and testing, for example of purchased material or a service
Internal failure costs	• Cost of scrapped material due to poor quality • Cost of re-working parts • Re-inspection costs • Lower selling prices for sub-quality products
External failure costs	• Cost of recalling and correcting products • Cost of lost goodwill

Test your understanding 10

Which TWO of the following are examples of prevention costs of quality?

A   Inspection of raw materials

B   Routine repairs and maintenance of machinery

C   Returns of faulty products

D   Machine breakdown repairs

E   Training costs of operational staff

5.6 Operational improvements

Introduction

There are a number of techniques that an organisation may use to improve the effectiveness of the supply chain and the management of relationships within the supply chain. These include:

- Statistical process control

- Total quality management (TQM)

- Kaizen

- Six sigma

- Lean thinking

- Just-in-time and

- Reverse logistics.

It is worth noting these techniques all have a **quality** focus and that the techniques are often be used alongside one another.

Each of the techniques will be introduced below.

Statistical process control

Statistical process control (SPC) is a method for measuring and controlling quality during a process.

Quality data is obtained in real-time and plotted on a graph with a pre-determined target and control limits.

Data that falls within the control limits indicates that everything is operating as expected – any variation within the control limits is due to natural variation that is expected as part of a process.

If data falls outside of the control limits, the variation should be investigated and corrective action taken before a defect occurs.

Illustration 14 – Statistical process control and Mars Bars

Statistical process control may be used when a large number of similar items, such as Mars Bars, are being produced. Every process is subject to variability, for example it is not possible to put exactly the same amount of ingredients in each Mars Bar.

A target weight is set for a Mars Bar (51g) and control limits assigned (1g above and below the target). The weight of the Mars Bars produced will be plotted on a chart and any points outside of the control limits (i.e. below 50g and above 52g) should be investigated and corrective action taken.

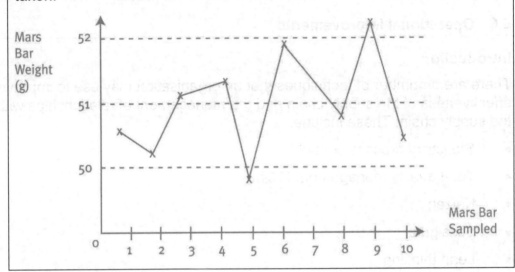

Total quality management

Total quality management (TQM) is a philosophy of quality management that originated in Japan in the 1950s.

TQM is the continuous improvement in quality, productivity and effectiveness obtained by establishing management responsibility for processes as well as outputs. In this, every process has an identified process owner and every person in an entity operates within a process and contributes to its improvement.

Fundamental features of TQM include:

- **Prevention of errors before they occur** – the aim of TQM is to 'get things right first time'. TQM will result in an increase in prevention costs but internal and external failure costs will fall.

- **Continual improvement** – quality management is not a one-off process, but is the continuous examination and improvement of processes.

- **Real participation by all** – the 'total' in TQM means that everyone in the value chain is involved in the process, including:

  Employees – they are expected to seek out, identify and correct quality problems. Teamwork will be vital. Employees should be empowered to decide how best to do their work and should be responsible for achieving targets.

  Suppliers – quality and reliability of suppliers will play a vital role.

  Customers – the goal is to identify and meet the needs of the customer.

- **Commitment of senior management** – management must be fully committed and encourage everyone else to become quality conscious.

Illustration 15 – TQM success and failure

A TQM success story

Corning Inc is the world leader in speciality glass and ceramics. This is partly due to the implementation of a TQM approach. In 1983 the CEO announced a $1.6 billion investment in TQM. After several years of intensive training and a decade of applying the TQM approach, all of Corning's employees had bought into the quality concept. They knew the lingo – continuous improvement, empowerment, customer focus, management by prevention and they witnessed the impact of the firm's techniques as profits soared.

An example of TQM failure

British Telecom launched a total quality program in the late 1980s. This resulted in the company getting bogged down in its quality processes and bureaucracy. The company failed to focus on its customers and later decided to dismantle its TQM program. This was at great cost to the company and they have failed to make a full recovery.

Implementation of a TQM approach

The implementation of a TQM approach may involve the following steps

> **Step 1: Senior management consultancy –** Managers must be committed to the programme and should undergo quality training

> **Step 2: Establish a quality steering committee –** The committee will guide the company through the process of implementing TQM

> **Step 3: Presentations and training –** The steering committee should communicate the benefits of the change programme to employees in order to gain buy-in

> **Step 4: Establish quality circles –** This will involve employees in the process of quality improvement

> **Step 5: Documentation –** The actions carried out should be clearly documented

> **Step 6: Monitor progress –** Actual results should be monitored against the standard set

 Test your understanding 11

Discuss some of the common reasons for the failure of TQM programmes.

Kaizen

What is Kaizen?

Kaizen is a Japanese term for the philosophy of continuous improvement in performance via small, incremental steps.

Characteristics

- Kaizen involves setting standards and then continually improving these standards to achieve long-term sustainable improvements.

- The focus is on eliminating waste, improving processes and systems and improving productivity.

- Kaizen involves all areas of the business.

- Employees often work in teams and are empowered to make changes. Rather than viewing employees as the source of high costs, Kaizen views the employees as a source of ideas on how to reduce costs. A change of culture will be required, encouraging employees to suggest ideas to reduce costs.

- Kaizen allows the organisation to respond quickly to changes in the competitive environment.

Illustration 16 – Kaizen

Many Japanese companies have introduced a Kaizen approach:

- In companies such as Toyota and Canon, a total of 60–70 suggestions per employee are written down and shared every year.

- It is not unusual for over 90% of those suggestions to be implemented.

Illustration 17 – British cycling

British cycling's revolution through small, incremental improvements

When Sir David Brailsford became performance director of British cycling, he believed that if it were possible to make a 1% improvement in a whole host of areas, the cumulative gains would end up being hugely significant. He was on the look-out for all the weaknesses in the team's assumptions and saw these as opportunities to adapt and make marginal gains. For example:

- By experimenting in a wind tunnel he noted that the bike was not sufficiently aerodynamic. Then by analysing the mechanics area in the team truck, he discovered that dust was accumulating on the floor, undermining bike maintenance. So he had the floor painted pristine white, in order to spot any impurities.

- The team started using antibacterial hand gel to cut down on any infections.

- The team bus was redesigned to improve comfort and recuperation.

Many critiqued the approach and saw David Brailsford as a laughing stock. However, the last two Olympics have seen the team win an unprecedented host of gold medals and, never having previously secured a win in over 100 years, British riders have won the Tour de France a number of times since 2012.

 Continuous improvement explained

Continuous improvement is the continual examination and improvement of existing processes and is very different from approaches such as business process re-engineering (BPR), which seeks to make radical one-off changes to improve an organisation's operations and processes. The concepts underlying continuous improvement are:

- The organisation should always seek perfection. Since perfection is never achieved, there must always be scope for improving on the current methods.

- The search for perfection should be ingrained into the culture and mind-set of all employees. Improvements should be sought all the time.

- Individual improvements identified by the work force will be small rather than far-reaching.

Six sigma

- Six sigma is a **quality management programme** that was pioneered in the 1980s by Motorola.

- The aim of the approach is to achieve a reduction in the number of faults that go beyond an accepted tolerance limit through the use of statistical techniques.

- The sigma stands for standard deviation. For reasons that need not be explained here, it can be demonstrated that, **if the error rate lies beyond the sixth sigma of probability, there will be fewer than 3.4 defects in every one million.**

- This is the tolerance level set. It is almost perfection since customers will have a reason to complain fewer than four times in a million.

Illustration 18 – The six sigma approach

A hospital is using the six sigma process to improve patient waiting times. An investigation of the views of patients has revealed that:

- Patients do not want to be called before their appointment time as they do not want to feel that they have to be at the hospital early to avoid missing an appointment

- The maximum length of time they are prepared to wait after the appointment time is 30 minutes.

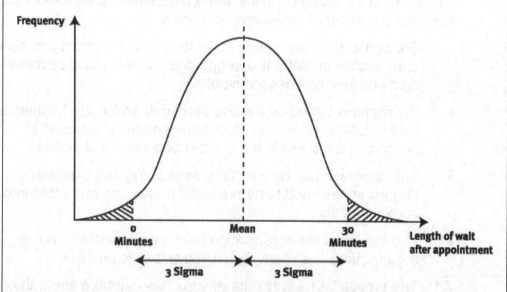

The aim of the six sigma programme will be to ensure that no more than 3.4 waits in every million occurrences exceed 30 minutes or are less than 0 minutes.

Further aspects of six sigma

Key requirements for successful six sigma implementation

There are a number of key requirements for the implementation of six sigma.

- Six sigma should be focused on the customer and based on the level of performance acceptable to the customer.

- Six sigma targets for a process should be related to the main drivers of performance.

- To maximise savings, six sigma needs to be part of a wider performance management programme which is linked to the strategy of the organisation. It should not be just about doing things better but about doing things differently.

- Senior managers within the organisation have a key role in driving the process.

- Training and education about the process throughout the organisation are essential for success.

- Six sigma sets a tight target, but accepts some failure – the target is not zero defects.

Some criticisms and limitations of six sigma

Literature on six sigma contains some criticisms of the process and identifies a number of limitations as follows:

- Six sigma has been criticised for its focus on current processes and reliance on data. It is suggested that this could become too rigid and limit process innovation.

- Six sigma is based on the use of models which are by their nature simplifications of real life. Judgement needs to be used in applying the models in the context of business objectives.

- The approach can be very time consuming and expensive. Organisations need to be prepared to put time and effort into its implementation.

- The culture of the organisation must be supportive – not all organisations are ready for such a scientific process.

- The process is heavily data-driven. This can be a strength but can become over-bureaucratic.

- Six sigma can give all parts of the organisation a common language for process improvement, but it is important to ensure that this does not become jargon but is expressed in terms specific to the organisation and its business.

- There is an underlying assumption in six sigma that the existing business processes meet customers' expectations. It does not ask whether it is the right process.

Lean thinking

As the name suggests, **lean** is a philosophy that aims to **systematically eliminate waste** through the identification and elimination of all non-value adding activities.

Illustration 19 – Lean production at Toyota

60 years ago, the cars that Toyota was making were uncompetitive in both cost and quality terms. In a bid to catch up with its American competitors, it developed lean production. Lean production helped Toyota to become what it is now – the biggest car manufacturer in the world.

Wastes to be eliminated include:

- **Inventory** – holding or purchasing unnecessary raw materials, work-in-progress and finished goods

- **Waiting** – time delays/idle time when value is not added to the product

- **Defective units** – production of a part that is scrapped or requires rework

- **Effort or motion** – actions of people/equipment that do not add value

- **Transportation** – delays in transportation or unnecessary handling due to poor planning or factory layout

- **Over-processing** – unnecessary steps that do not add value

- **Over-production** – produce more than customers have ordered.

Characteristics of lean

Characteristics of lean include:

- **Improved production scheduling** – production is initiated by customer demand rather than ability and capacity to produce, i.e. production is demand-pull, not supply-push.

- **Small batch production or continuous production** – production is based on customer demand, resulting in highly flexible and responsive processes.

- **Economies of scope** – lean production is only achieved where 'economies of scope' make it economical to produce small batches of a variety of products with the same machines. This is in stark contrast with traditional manufacturing and its emphasis on economies of scale.

- **Continuous improvement** – the company continually finds ways to reduce process times:

  - A multi-skilled, trained workforce provides flexibility. Employees should be involved in and engaged with the lean philosophy.

  - The machines, tools and people used to make an item are located close together.

  - Quality at source reduces re-working.

  - A clean and orderly workplace.

- **Zero inventory** – just-in-time purchasing (this is discussed below) eliminates waste.

- **Zero waiting time** – JIT production (this is discussed below) means that the work performed at each stage of the process is dictated solely by the demand for materials for the next stage, thus reducing lead time.

Illustration 20 – Lean management in the NHS

Toyota pioneered the concept of a 'lean' operating system and it has now been implemented in countless manufacturing companies. Lean techniques can also be applied to service organisations.

With service operations, a lean approach often focuses on improving the customer experience.

Within the NHS (National Health Service) in England, lean thinking is being used to improve performance. Its use is based on a number of core principles:

Patient perspective

Under lean, value is defined solely from the customer's (normally the patient) perspective. Anything that helps treat the patient is value-adding, anything else is waste.

Pull

To create value, the NHS aims to provide services in line with demand.

The lean supply chain

The main objective of a lean supply chain is to completely remove waste in order to achieve competitive advantage through a reduction in costs and an improvement in quality. Other benefits are:

- reduced inventories (and thus increased cash flows and profits)

- shorter lead times, and thus faster deliveries to customers

- few bottlenecks, so better utilisation of resources, and further improvements in profit

- few quality problems, so less re-work, lower costs of quality failures, and happier customers.

However, disadvantages include the potential for large, powerful customers to dominate the supply chain and an over-emphasis on cost reduction rather than quality improvement.

Criticisms and limitations of lean manufacturing

- **High initial outlay** – It might involve a large amount of initial expenditure to switch from 'traditional' production systems to a system based on cellular manufacturing. All the tools and equipment needed to manufacture a product need to be re-located to the same area of the factory floor. Employees need to be trained in multiple skills.

- **Requires a change in culture** – Lean manufacturing, like TQM, is a philosophy or culture of working, and it might be difficult for management and employees to acquire this culture. Employees might not be prepared to give the necessary commitment.

- **Part adoption** – It might be tempting for companies to select some elements of lean manufacturing (such as production based on cellular manufacturing), but not to adopt others (such as empowering employees to make on-the-spot decisions).

- **Cost may exceed benefit** – In practice, the expected benefits of lean manufacturing (lower costs and shorter cycle times) have not always materialised, or might not have been as large as expected.

Illustration 21

Comparison of Toyota to a non-lean car manufacturer

	Non-lean manufacturer	Lean pioneer – Toyota
Production	Mass production requiring: • time to set up machinery and • skilled engineers	Produce smaller batches leading to: • quick set up • flexibility • production line staff trained to do set ups
Human resources	Cyclical nature of industry resulting in: • staff layoffs • unmotivated staff	• Job for life • Defined career path • Empowered staff

	Non-lean manufacturer	Lean pioneer – Toyota
Employee roles	• Assembly worker • Foreman • Housekeeper • Engineer	Eliminates non-value adding activities so all workers trained on all aspects hence no indirect wages
Production problems	• Couldn't stop the production line • 20–25% defects	• Stops the production line and then the team works to solve issues quickly • Zero defects
Suppliers	Chosen on cost	• Use supplier expertise • Fair price • JIT
Sales	• Sell through dealers • Narrow product range	• Sell direct to customers • Customer feedback valued • Flexibility resulting in wide product range

 Lean synchronisation aims to meet demand instantaneously with perfect quality and no waste.

Lean synchronisation overlaps to a large degree with the general concept of lean (elimination of waste) and just-in-time (which emphasises the idea of producing items only when they are needed).

Just-in-time

Most inventory management systems assume that it is necessary to hold some inventory. An alternative view is that inventory is wasteful and adds no value to operations.

 Just-in-time (JIT) is a system whose objective it is to produce or procure products or components as they are required by the customer or for use, rather than for inventory. This means that inventory levels of raw materials, work-in-progress and finished goods can be kept to a minimum.

JIT purchasing and JIT production

JIT applies to both production within an organisation and to purchasing from external suppliers:

- **JIT purchasing** is a method of purchasing that involves ordering materials only when customers place an order. When the goods are received, they go straight into production.

- **JIT production** is a production system that is driven by demand for the finished products (a 'pull' system), whereby each component on a production line is produced only when needed for the next stage.

Illustration 22 – JIT at Toyota

Toyota pioneered the JIT manufacturing system, in which suppliers send parts daily – or several times a day – and are notified electronically when the assembly line is running out.

More than 400 trucks a day come in and out of Toyota's Georgetown plant in the USA, with a separate logistics company organising the shipment from Toyota's 300 suppliers – most located in neighbouring states within half a day's drive of the plant.

Toyota aims to build long-term relationships with its suppliers, many of whom it has a stake in, and says it now produces 80% of its parts within North America.

Requirements for successful operation of a JIT system

- **High quality and reliability** – disruptions create hold ups in the entire system and must be avoided. The emphasis is on getting the work 'right first time':
  - Highly skilled and well trained staff should be used.
  - Machinery must be fully maintained.
  - Long-term links should be established with suppliers in order to ensure a reliable and high quality service.

- **Elimination of non-value added activities** – value is only being added whilst a product is being processed. For example, value is not added whilst storing the products and therefore inventory levels should be minimised.

- **Speed of throughput** – the speed of production should match the rate at which customers demand the product. Production runs should be shorter with smaller stocks of finished goods.

- **Flexibility** – a flexible production system is needed in order to be able to respond immediately to customer orders:

    – The system should be capable of switching from making one product to making another.

    – The workforce should be dedicated and have the appropriate skills JIT is an organisational culture and the concept should be adopted by everyone.

    – Management should allow the work teams to use their initiative and to deal with problems as they arise.

- **Lower costs** – another objective of JIT is to reduce costs by:

    – Raising quality and eliminating waste.

    – Achieving faster throughput.

    – Minimising inventory levels.

Test your understanding 12

Explain the advantages and disadvantages to an organisation of operating a JIT system.

JIT and supplier relations

As mentioned previously, many of the steps taken to improve the supply chain (and hence profitability) involve **improving the relationship between the manufacturer and its suppliers**.

This will be of particular importance in a company operating a JIT system.

The advantages to a JIT company of developing close supplier relationships are as follows:

- **No rejects/returns** – a strong relationship should help to improve the quality of supplies. This should minimise production delays since there will be less inspection, fewer returns and less reworking of goods.

- **On-time deliveries** – the development of close working relationships should help to guarantee on-time deliveries of supplies.

- **Low inventory** – suppliers can be relied upon for frequent deliveries of small quantities of material to the company, ensuring that each delivery is just enough to meet the immediate production schedule.

- **Close proximity** – the supplier/portfolio of suppliers will be located close to the manufacturing plant. This will reduce delivery times and costs.

Reverse logistics

 Reverse logistics is the return of unwanted or surplus goods, materials or equipment back to the organisation for reuse, recycling or disposal.

The emergence of internet selling (some internet retailers estimate returns of 50%) and shorter product life cycles has led to many organisations focusing on their reverse logistics capability.

The main reasons for returns are as follows:

- The **customer is not satisfied** with the product and takes advantage of the organisation's return policy

- **Installation or usage problems** – a common problem if installation or usage is complicated, for example with IT equipment

- **Warranty claims** for defective products or parts

- Some manufacturers allow the **return of unsold stock** by retailers, for example this is common practice in the book industry

- **Manufacturer recall** program due to faults.

Attacking the returns challenge is a critical area of supply chain management. Steps should be taken to:

- **Minimise returns**, for example through the production of good quality products or parts, which meet customer requirements and have clear guidelines for installation and usage

- **Ensure the possible reuse or recycling of material**. This is closely linked to corporate social responsibility but should contribute to increased profitability.

Techniques include:

- Root cause analysis to understand the reasons for returns

- Creation of profit centres around the returns process to focus organisations on maximising the price that they will get for any returns

- Separation of the supply chain into separate forward and reverse logistics

- Centralising the returns centre to improve the speed and efficiency of handling returns

- Outsourcing the returns process to a competent and dedicated provider

- The use of technology such as enterprise resource planning (ERP) which supports reverse logistics processes.

The use of these techniques should reduce costs, improve customer service and increase revenue.

Test your understanding 13

Match the following techniques to their explanation.

Technique	Explanation
Statistical Process Control	The philosophy of continuous improvement via small, incremental steps
Just in Time	The return of unwanted or surplus goods, materials or equipment back to the organisation
Total Quality Management	An approach to achieve a reduction in the number of faults that go beyond an accepted tolerance limit
Six sigma	A method for measuring and controlling quality during a process.
Lean thinking	A system whose objective it is to produce or procure products or components as they are required by the customer or for use, rather than for inventory.
Reverse logistics	A philosophy that aims to systematically eliminate waste
Kaizen	The continuous improvement in quality, productivity and effectiveness obtained by establishing management responsibility for processes as well as outputs

Test your understanding 14

Lean thinking identifies seven wastes to be eliminated. **These include which FIVE of the following?**

A   Over-processing

B   Over-production

C   Over-thinking

D   Over-selling

E   Transportation

F   Effort or motion

G   Human resources

H   Inventory

Illustration 23 – Reverse logistics at Estee Lauder

A good example of a complete reverse logistics program is a project by cosmetics manufacturer Estee Lauder. The firm used to dump $60 million of its products into landfills each year, destroying more than a third of the name brand cosmetics returned by retailers.

Estee Lauder made a small investment of $1.3 million to build its reverse logistics system and apparently recovered its investment in the first year.

Estee Lauder has reduced its production and inventory levels through its increased ability to put returned goods back on the market and the availability of better data on the reasons for returns. In the first year Estee Lauder was able to evaluate 24 per cent more returned products, redistribute 150 per cent more of its returns, reduce the destroyed products from 37 per cent to 27 per cent and save about $0.5 million on labour costs.

5.7 SCM interface with finance

Introduction

- Organisations with strong links between their finance function and supply chain teams are more likely to have effective supply chain management.

- A **collaborative relationship** between the CFO and the leader of the supply chain (either directly or through their teams) is advantageous for organisational growth and competitive advantage:

  - The role of the leader of the supply chain has become more prominent in recent years. As discussed earlier in this chapter, the focus of SCM has moved away from cost reductions to creating a supply chain strategy that is aligned to the broader corporate goals of the organisation and is efficient in enabling the organisation to respond to new opportunities.

  - Meanwhile, the role of the finance function has been transformed (as discussed in Chapter 2). The finance function now collaborates more closely with other internal functions; not just from a monitoring, reporting and risk management perspective, but also as supporters and enablers of performance.

  - The result is that CFOs and supply chain leaders are working increasingly together to understand, analyse and address supply chain issues. CFOs are drawing on their skills and unique view of the organisation to provide insight to deliver more informed decision-making.

Illustration 24 – Supplier decision management

When it comes to supplier decision management, the operations function will make the decision regarding which supplier(s) to choose but the finance function would help with some aspects of the supplier relationship (mainly the financial side).

Opportunities for business partnering

The finance function has a unique end-to-end view of the organisation and is considered a trusted advisor. As a result, there are a number of areas where the CFO (and their team) has an opportunity to enhance performance through business partnering with the supply chain. These include:

- Stronger alignment between the supply chain and the broader strategy and consistency of strategy within the various parts of the supply chain.

- CFOs help to set the right growth priorities and pace of growth; they support and challenge the rationale for new investment, apply data analytics to support and challenge business decisions and ensure that tax is considered as part of operational decisions.

- Monitoring and enhancing performance through the establishment of appropriate KPIs that are aligned to the broader organisation (this will be discussed in more detail in section 6).

- Managing risk and business continuity; the CFO has the opportunity to work with procurement and treasury to determine the extent to which risk is owned and managed by the company, and to what extent it is pushed further down the supply chain.

Illustration 25 – Technology and business partnering

Data and analytics present CFOs with a significant opportunity to drive a more collaborative, business partnering relationship with the supply chain. Robust information and insight are central to any business partnering relationship. The CFO's access to financial information from across the business allows them to create a credible single version of the truth to drive decisions and performance measurement.

6 Key performance indicators

6.1 Introduction

 Critical success factors (CSFs) are the vital areas 'where things must go right' for the business in order for them to achieve their strategic objectives.

 Key performance indicators (KPIs) are the measures which indicate whether or not the CSFs are being achieved.

The achievement of the KPIs should be measured and any necessary corrective action taken.

Illustration 26 – CSFs and KPIs for supply chain management

The operations function will identify CSFs for its supply chain and may establish that it is critical for them to achieve a high level of quality, minimal level of waste and a reduction in supply chain costs.

The function will use techniques such as TQM, Kaizen, lean, JIT and reverse logistics management to optimise their performance in these areas.

KPIs will be used to indicate whether or not the CSFs are being achieved.

The **finance function will work with the operations function** to establish appropriate KPIs. So, for example:

- Defect/error rate, % product returns, amount spent on warranties will be used in a TQM environment

- Target costs will be used in a Kaizen environment

- Waste measurement and lean techniques will go hand in hand

- Inventory measurement will be important in a JIT environment

- % returns, reuse/recycling of returns will be used to monitor and measure the effectiveness of a reverse logistics strategy.

Characteristics of good KPIs include:

- KPIs should cascade from strategy to tactics, and to operational level.

- KPIs should cover all perspectives in supply chain management such as cost information and financial performance, quality of the supply chain, flexibility, resource utilisation, innovation, sustainability and competitiveness. This coverage will give a complete and well balanced view of

  - internal/external performance

  - short-term and long-term performance and

  - financial performance and non-financial performance.

- KPIs should be challenging but achievable and should enable employees to understand the performance measures they have control over and should motivate them to achieve KPIs through the establishment of appropriate rewards.

- KPIs should be SMART, i.e. **s**pecific, **m**easurable, **a**chievable, **r**elevant and **t**ime-bound.

- KPIs should be extended to include supply chain partners, because the objective of SCM is to create a supply chain that is much more competitive than the alternative supply chain providers of that product or service.

6.2 Examples of KPIs for operations

Appropriate KPIs may include:

- Supply chain costs per unit sold
- Time taken to deliver a customer order
- Percentage on-time delivery to a customer
- Percentage of customer orders fulfilled
- Percentage defect rate (supplies and customer orders)
- Percentage wastage rate
- Quality costs (individual KPIs for prevention, detection, internal failure and external failure costs)
- Labour utilisation rate
- Asset utilisation rate
- Warehousing costs
- Transport costs
- Queues and waiting times
- Working capital ratios such as inventory days, payable days and receivable days and the length of the cash operating cycle:
  - Inventory days = Inventory ÷ Cost of sales × 365
  - Receivables days = Receivables ÷ Sales × 365
  - Payables days = Payables ÷ Purchases × 365
  - Cash operating cycle = Inventory days + Receivables days – Payables days

Test your understanding 15

Ali is constructing some KPIs to measure whether or not the firm's CSFs are being met. He has been told that these KPIs should be SMART. **Which of the SMART criteria is not being met in the following KPI?**

KPI: Reduce the time taken to deliver a customer's order by three days. (the current lead time for deliveries is two weeks).

A Specific

B Measurable

C Achievable

D Relevant

E Time-bound

Test your understanding 16

Calculate the cash operating cycle using the extracts from the financial statements below:

Statement of Profit or Loss

		$000
Sales		400
Cost of Sales		
opening inventory	12	
purchases	245	
closing inventory	15	
		242
Gross Profit		158

Statement of Financial Position (extract)

	$000
Inventory	15
Trade receivables	45
Cash	78
Payables	35

6.3 How the finance function manages operations using KPIs

Introduction

The finance function plays an important role in the performance management of the operations function, implementing a performance management approach that gives a complete and well balanced view of all supply chain activities.

Information to impact framework revisited

We can understand how the finance function helps manage operations through the use of KPIs by looking at the **information to impact framework** (as discussed in Chapter 2):

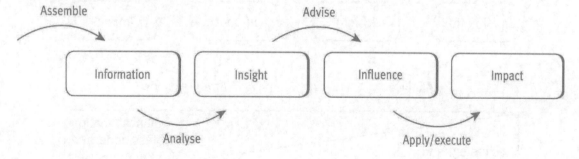

Finance function activity	Explanation of how the finance function helps manage operations through the use of KPIs
Assembling information	The finance function works with operations to establish a set of appropriate KPIs (as per the characteristics in section 6.1). It then **assembles** data from a range of internal and external sources and processes this data to turn it into useful KPI information. This information is then **reported** to those people who need it within the organisation and across the supply chain.
Analysing for insights	The finance function analyses the KPI information to draw out patterns and relevant **insights** for those who use the information. This **questioning** may require individual KPIs to be broken down into several different performance measures so that the root cause of any deviations between the actual KPI and the target KPI can be established.
Advising to influence	The finance function then: • communicates these insights and • contributes an objective and responsible perspective helping to **develop solutions** to any operational problems or areas for improvement identified to **influence** decision making in the operations function.
Applying for impact (also called 'execute')	The finance function applies the information to harness value for the operations function through its **impact**. **Solutions are deployed** such as changes to the operational strategy and future KPIs.

Impact of technology

In Chapter 2 we discussed the impact of technology and automation on the information to impact framework.

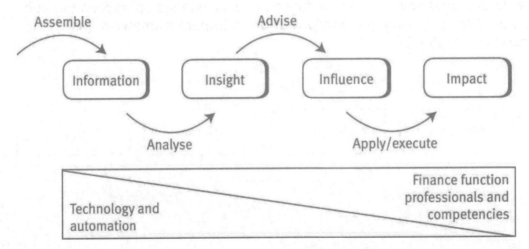

If we now consider this in relation to how the finance function manages operations through the use of KPIs we can see that:

- **Technology and automation** will play an important role in all of the activities of the finance function but will have the largest impact on the 'assembly' and 'analysis' activities.

  – Successful companies operate an enterprise data warehouse that acts as a single source to **assemble** 'clean' data (in-house data is seamlessly integrated with data from supply chain partners) and reports this in the form of a supply chain dashboard that is accessible and adaptable for relevant users across the supply chain and the organisation.

  – This integrated technology can draw out patterns and relevant insights for those who use the information, reducing the **analysis** role of the finance function.

- This will 'free up' the resource of the finance function professionals who can now place greater focus on the '**advising**' and '**applying/executing**' activities. However, even in these activities, technology will take on a role. For example, predictive algorithms may be used for advanced business intelligence and to determine timely corrective actions along the end-to-end supply chain.

Illustration 27 – Technological developments

Advances in technology offered by the 4th Industrial Revolution are giving organisations an opportunity to enhance performance management in the operations function. For example:

- Easier **linking of internal supply chain data with external sources** such as financial information about suppliers to improve supply chain risk management.

- Ongoing **digitisation of supply chains** and resulting exponential growth in data from connected devices (such as delivery vehicles).

- Use of **web mining** to report only the most relevant data and to quickly react to new events.

- A shift to real-time data enabled by sensors covering different locations.

- The most common use of **data visualisation** is in creating a dashboard to display the key performance indicators of a business in a live format, thus allowing immediate understanding of current performance and potentially prompting action to correct or amend performance accordingly.

- Increasing use of **predictive measures** to (for example) forecast sales, detect product quality issues, evaluate maintenance requirements and produce sound 'what-if' scenarios.

- **Improved analytics capabilities** (for example, using cloud technology) allowing for fast processing and analysis of large amounts of data.

Test your understanding 17

The finance function helps manage operations through the use of KPIs.

Match the following KPI activities to the relevant stage in the 'information to impact framework'.

Assembling information	Deploying solutions such as developing future KPIs
Analysing for insights	Helping to develop solutions to any operational problems
Advising to influence	Establishing the cause of any deviations between actual and target KPIs
Applying for impact	Establishing a set of appropriate KPIs

Test your understanding 18

Which of the following statements is/are correct?

I   Technology will have the largest impact on the assemble and analysis activities of the finance function

II Technology facilitates easier integration of internal supply chain data with external sources

III By analysing KPIs, the finance function can guarantee that CSFs are met

IV A primary feature of the interaction between finance and operations is performance management

A   All of them

B   I and IV

C   I only

D   I, II and IV

7 Chapter summary

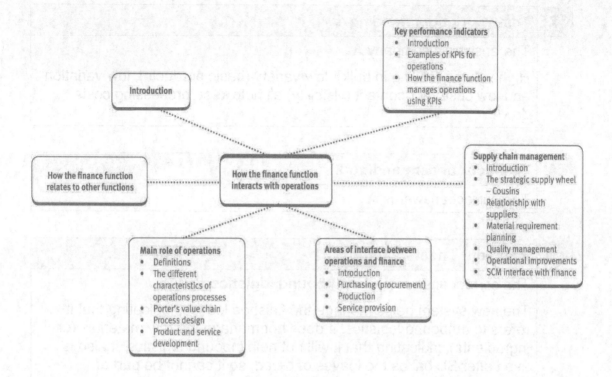

Introduction

Key performance indicators
- Introduction
- Examples of KPIs for operations
- How the finance function manages operations using KPIs

How the finance function relates to other functions

How the finance function interacts with operations

Supply chain management
- Introduction
- The strategic supply wheel – Cousins
- Relationship with suppliers
- Material requirement planning
- Quality management
- Operational improvements
- SCM interface with finance

Main role of operations
- Definitions
- The different characteristics of operations processes
- Porter's value chain
- Process design
- Product and service development

Areas of interface between operations and finance
- Introduction
- Purchasing (procurement)
- Production
- Service provision

Test your understanding answers

Test your understanding 1

The answer is company **A**

High volume (selling in bulk), low variety (basic products), low variation and low customer contact (visibility) all help keep processing costs down.

Test your understanding 2

The correct answer is **A**

Test your understanding 3

The correct answer is **C – outbound logistics**

The new system helps manage the finished loaves, indicating that it refers to outbound logistics. It does not manage the raw materials (or ingredients), indicating that it will not help inbound logistics. It also is used after BB bakes the loaves of bread, so it cannot be part of operations. The system does not affect marketing or procurement of the bread.

Test your understanding 4

The correct answer is **A**

B relates to marketing, C relates to production and D relates to human resource management.

Test your understanding 5

The correct answer is **A**

Note that provision of services would be unlikely to affect the sale of physical units, so inventory turnover would be unaffected.

Test your understanding 6

The correct answer is **B**

By definition.

Test your understanding 7

Statement	True/False?
The co-ordination of activities from the supplier(s) of raw materials at one end of the supply chain to the customer at the other end is known as supply chain management	True
Cost savings are the only advantage of supply chain management	False. Supply chain management can also add value to an organisation, for example in improved customer services.
The objective of SCM is to achieve synergies that benefit the customers at the end of the supply chain	False. The objective of SCM is to achieve synergies that benefit every player along the chain.
Cousins' supply wheel is a model used to look at the traditional supply function	False. Cousins' model examines supply in a strategic way. Successful organisations in today's competitive environment have recognised that supply should be viewed as a strategic issue.
Cousins' supply wheel has five spokes	True. The spokes are: Organisation structure, Performance Measures, Relationships with suppliers, Cost Benefit, and Competences.

Test your understanding 8

The correct answers is **A, B and C**

Answer D – improved quality is not guaranteed and therefore this is not an advantage.

Answers E and F – these are disadvantages.

Test your understanding 9

Higher quality can help to increase revenue and reduce costs:

- Higher quality improves the perceived image of a product or service. As a result, more customers will be willing to buy the product/service and may also be willing to pay more for the product/ service.

- A higher volume of sales may result in lower unit costs due to economies of scale.

- Higher quality in manufacturing should result in lower waste and defective rates, which will reduce production costs.

- The need for inspection and testing should be reduced, also reducing costs.

- The volume of customer complaints should fall and warranty claims should be lower. This will reduce costs.

- Better quality in production should lead to shorter processing times. This will reduce costs.

Test your understanding 10

The correct answer is **B and E**

Prevention costs are those incurred in order to prevent poor quality.

Answer A – inspection of raw materials is an appraisal cost.

Answer C – returns from customers are an external failure cost.

Answer D – machine breakdown repairs are internal failure costs.

Test your understanding 11

Tail off – after an initial burst of enthusiasm, top management fails to maintain interest and support.

Deflection – other initiatives or problems deflect attention from TQM.

Lack of buy-in – managers pay only 'lip service' to the principles of worker involvement and communication.

Rejection – TQM does not fit in with the organisational culture and is therefore rejected.

Test your understanding 12

Advantages of JIT

- Lower stock holding costs means a reduction in storage space which saves rent and insurance costs.

- As stock is only obtained when it is needed, less working capital is tied up in stock.

- There is less likelihood of stock perishing, becoming obsolete or out of date.

- Avoids the build-up of unsold finished products that can occur with sudden changes in demand.

- Less time is spent checking and re-working the products as the emphasis is on getting the work right first time.

The result is that costs should fall and quality should increase. This should improve the company's competitive advantage.

Disadvantages of JIT

- There is little room for mistakes as little stock is kept for re-working a faulty product.

- Production is very reliant on suppliers and if stock is not delivered on time or is not of a high enough quality, the whole production schedule can be delayed.

- There is no spare finished product available to meet unexpected orders, because all products are made to meet actual orders.

- It may be difficult for managers to empower employees to embrace the concept and culture.

- It won't be suitable for all companies. For example, supermarkets must have a supply of inventory.

- It can be difficult to apply to the service industry. However, in the service industry a JIT approach may focus on eliminating queues, which are wasteful of customers' time.

Test your understanding 13

Technique	Explanation
Statistical Process Control	A method for measuring and controlling quality during a process.
Just in Time	A system whose objective it is to produce or procure products or components as they are required by the customer or for use, rather than for inventory.
Total Quality Management	The continuous improvement in quality, productivity and effectiveness obtained by establishing management responsibility for processes as well as outputs.
Six sigma	An approach to achieve a reduction in the number of faults that go beyond an accepted tolerance limit.
Lean thinking	A philosophy that aims to systematically eliminate waste.
Reverse logistics	The return of unwanted or surplus goods, materials or equipment back to the organisation.
Kaizen	The philosophy of continuous improvement via small incremental steps.

Test your understanding 14

The correct answers are **A, B, E, F & H**

The other two wastes to be eliminated under lean thinking are waiting and defective units.

Test your understanding 15

The correct answer is **E** time-bound. There is no mention of by when the KPI needs to be achieved. Just because it mentions a number of days, does not make it time-bound.

The KPI is straight forward and, hence, specific, the time to deliver can be easily measured. Three days reduction seems achievable. The KPI is relevant to the CSF as delivery waiting times will be important to the customer.

Test your understanding 16

Receivables Days	$\dfrac{45}{400} \times 365 =$	41 days
Inventory Days	$\dfrac{15}{242} \times 365 =$	23 days
Payables Days	$\dfrac{35}{245} \times 365 =$	52 days
Cash operating cycle	41 + 23 – 52 =	12 days

Test your understanding 17

Assembling information	Establishing a set of appropriate KPIs
Analysing for insights	Establishing the cause of any deviations between actual and target KPIs
Advising to influence	Helping to develop solutions to any operational problems
Applying for impact	Deploying solutions such as developing future KPIs

Test your understanding 18

The correct answer is **D**

Option III is not correct as there is no guarantee that the CSFs will be met.

How the finance function interacts with sales and marketing

Chapter learning objectives

Lead	Component
E2: Describe how the finance function interacts with sales and marketing.	Describe: (a) Main role of sales and marketing (b) Areas of interface with finance (c) Key performance indicators

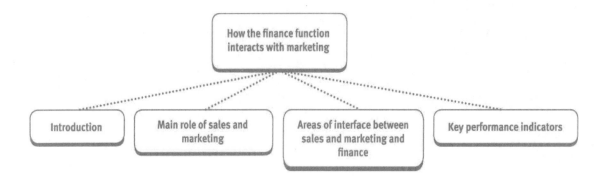

1 Introduction

In Chapter 9 we described the finance function's relationship with operations. In this chapter we will continue to describe how the finance function plays its role by interacting with the rest of the organisation and, more specifically here, the organisation's sales and marketing function.

We will begin by discussing the main role of the sales and marketing function; understanding the marketing environment, the marketing mix and the main techniques of sales and marketing.

We will then discuss the areas of interface with finance; understanding how the finance function interacts with sales and marketing and the role of big data analytics.

The final part of this chapter will discuss how the finance function helps to manage the sales and marketing function through the use of key performance indicators (KPIs).

2 Main role of sales and marketing

2.1 Introduction

 Marketing is defined by the Chartered Institute of Marketing (CIM) as 'the management process that identifies, anticipates and supplies customer needs efficiently and profitably.'

The key emphasis of the sales and marketing function is thus on **customer needs**.

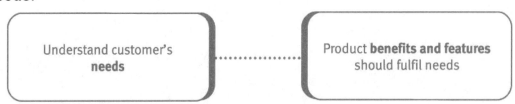

Four possible approaches to selling a product

There are four possible approaches to selling a product:

Marketing orientation: starts by understanding customers' needs and then produces products with benefits and features to fulfil these needs.

Production orientation: focus is on high volume production to achieve low unit cost.

Product orientation: focus is on continual improvement of products assuming customers simply want the best quality for their money.

Sales orientation: uses aggressive promotional policies to entice the customer.

Sales forms but a part of the entire marketing process and philosophy. The sales aspect of marketing will be most prominent in an organisation that rejects the marketing orientation in favour of an alternative approach. Under these circumstances, the sales team will be obliged to 'find' customers and persuade them to buy the products that have been made. This may be an unenlightened approach, but it still exists in some industries.

Benefits of a marketing orientation

As CIM point out:

"It is all about getting the right product or service to the customer at the right price, in the right place, at the right time. Business history and current practice both remind us that without proper marketing, companies cannot get close to customers and satisfy their needs. And if they don't, a competitor surely will."

Test your understanding 1

Marketing is mainly concerned with which of the following?

A   Increasing sales revenue

B   Streamlining production

C   Anticipating and meeting customer needs

D   Maximising profit

The market planning process

A marketing action plan will be needed to ensure the effectiveness of the sales and marketing processes.

The following is an example of the different components that could be included in this plan:

Step 1: Situation analysis

A number of techniques can be used. These include:

SWOT analysis – the organisation needs to understand its own strengths (S) and weaknesses (W) together with an appreciation of the wider environment in which it operates, i.e. the opportunities (O) and threats (T).

PESTEL analysis – The organisation should review the external environment for opportunities that may allow it to further meet their customers' needs. This analysis divides the business environment into six related sub-systems – Political, Economic, Social, Technological, Environmental/Ecological factors and Legal. Each of these factors can be applied to the marketing function.

Note: PESTEL will be discussed in section 2.2 below.

Step 2: Review mission and objectives

The organisation will already have a mission statement and a set of objectives in place. These will underpin the marketing objectives.

Step 3: Set marketing objectives

Marketing objectives should be consistent with the organisation's overall mission and objectives.

Marketing objectives should be SMART – specific, measurable, achievable, relevant and time bound. For example, acquire 50,000 new online customers this financial year at an average cost per acquisition of $30 with an average profitability of $5.

Step 4: Devise an appropriate marketing strategy

There may be a gap between the current performance and the performance required to achieve the marketing objectives set. The organisation needs to consider how to close the gap. The following techniques can be used:

- **Market research** will be required to understand the organisation's activities and to provide a basis for effective marketing decisions to be made.

- **Segmentation** – the market should be segmented, for example by age, social class or income. The needs of each segment should be established using market research.

- **Targeting** – the most attractive segments in terms of profitability and growth should be targeted using an appropriate marketing mix.

- **Positioning** – an appropriate positioning strategy, for example differentiation or cost leadership should be chosen for each market segment.

- **Marketing mix** – the organisation should use the marketing mix to determine the correct marketing strategy.

Note: Each of these ideas will be explored in more detail in sections 2.3 and 2.4 below.

Step 5: Implementation

The marketing action plan should then be implemented and appropriate KPIs established (section 4).

Step 6: Review

The plan should be monitored to gauge its success (or otherwise) and to identify any necessary changes required to achieve the marketing objectives set.

Note: The market planning process sometimes shows the marketing mix as a separate step (step 5) and then implementation as step 6. However, the process will be the same.

2.2 Understanding the marketing environment

The marketing environment is the content in which the organisation exists. The environment can have a considerable impact on the organisation.

The **macro environment** includes all the factors that influence an organisation but are outside of their control. Organisations will need flexible marketing practices to respond to this dynamic environment.

One popular technique for analysing the macro environment is **PESTEL** analysis:

PESTEL factor	Explanation
Political	Political factors can have a direct effect on the way an organisation operates. Decisions made by government affect our everyday lives. For example, the instability of many governments in less developed countries has led a number of companies to question the wisdom of marketing in those countries.
Economic	All businesses are affected by economic factors nationally and globally. For example, within the UK, the climate of the economy can dictate consumer expenditure on luxury goods.

Social	Forces within society such as family, friends and the media affect our attitude, interests and opinions and, in turn, will influence our purchases. For example, within the UK people's attitudes are changing towards their diet and health. Over the last 5 years, the UK has seen a massive increase in demand for vegan food.
Technological	This is an area in which change takes place very rapidly and the organisation needs to be constantly aware of what is going on. For example, new technology has resulted in the production of new products, such as hybrid cars. These cars have improved fuel economy and reduced emissions.
Environmental/ Ecological	These have become increasingly important in recent years and influence a marketing orientated organisation in a number of ways. For example, using the example above, demand for vegan food has increased not only for health reasons but also due to the negative environmental impact of meat and dairy farming and fishing.
Legal	Laws and regulations governing businesses are widespread. These include laws on health and safety, information disclosure, the dismissal of employees, vehicle emissions, the use of pesticides and many more. For example, the UK smoking ban in public places has resulted in UK tobacco companies exploring new products, such as the legal, electronic cigarette (although these may also be banned in public in the near future), and new markets outside of the UK.

Test your understanding 2

Describe the changes that may be made to the marketing approach of a supermarket if the country goes into recession.

Social factors

According to Johnson and Scholes the following social influences should be monitored:

- **Population demographics** – a term used to describe the composition of the population in any given area, whether a region, a country or an area within a country.

- **Income distribution** – will provide the marketer with some indication of the size of the target markets. Most developed countries, like the UK, have a relatively even distribution spread. However, this is not the case in other nations.

- **Social mobility** – the marketer should be aware of social classes and the distribution among them. The marketer can use this knowledge to promote products to distinct social classes within the market.

- **Lifestyle changes** – refer to our attitudes and opinions to things like social values, credit, health and women. Our attitudes have changed in recent years and this information is vital for the marketer.

- **Consumerism** – one of the social trends in recent years has been the rise of consumerism. This trend has increased to such an extent that governments have been pressured to design laws that protect the rights of the consumer.

- **Levels of education** – the level of education has increased dramatically over the last few years. There is now a larger proportion of the population in higher education than ever before.

2.3 Understanding the marketing mix

 The marketing mix is the set of controllable variables that a firm blends to produce desired results from its chosen target market.

The 7 Ps

The traditional marketing mix (4 Ps):	Elements
Product	This includes product features, durability, design, brand name, packaging, range, after-sales service, warranties and guarantees.
Place	Distribution channels and intermediaries, transportation and storage.
Promotion	Advertising, personal selling, public relations, sales promotion, sponsorship, direct marketing, e.g. direct mail and telephone marketing.
Price	Price level, discounts, credit policy, payment methods.

Additional 3 Ps for the service industry:	Elements
People	The role of employees in the service industry is particularly important because of the inseparability of the service from the service provider. Staff must be selected, trained and motivated to meet the needs of the target customer.
Processes	These are the systems through which the service is delivered. For example, the teaching methods used in a university or the speed and friendliness of service in a restaurant.
Physical evidence	Required to make the intangible service more tangible. For example, brochures, testimonials and the appearance of staff and of the environment.

The extension of the traditional marketing mix to include the three additional Ps acknowledges that there are fundamental differences between products and services and therefore services marketing assumes a different emphasis to product marketing. However, although the extended mix is particularly relevant to service organisations, product based organisations would also do well to consider these aspects, particularly the competence of people and process efficiency.

Features of service organisations

Service organisations have certain distinguishing features that should be considered:

- Services are **intangible** and it is more difficult to measure their quality than it is for a physical product. Customers may be more reluctant to make a purchase due to uncertainty regarding what they will receive. Tools such as testimonials and brochures may help to address this problem.

- Services are consumed immediately and **cannot be stored**. Meeting customer needs depends on staff being available. Therefore, anticipating and responding to levels of demand is a priority.

- **Heterogeneity** – maintaining consistent, standard output can be difficult, for example due to the high level of staff and human intervention. The marketing policy could address this, e.g. through effective staff selection and standards for customer service and care.

- **Inseparability** of the service from the provider will again reinforce the need for high quality employee selection and training.

- Services **do not result in the transfer of propert**y and so it will be necessary to convince the customer of the benefits of what they are paying for. A tangible symbol of ownership, such as a certificate, may be used.

Each element of the traditional marketing mix will be reviewed in turn:

Product

There are two main product issues to consider:

- Product definition – The main issue regarding product is to define exactly what the product should be. This can be done on three levels:

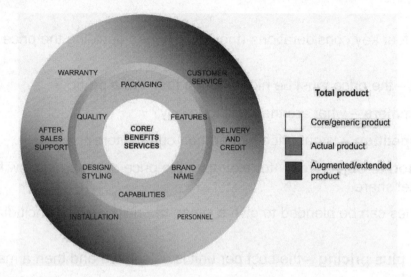

- Product positioning – With all of these factors the question of product positioning is critical – how does our product compare with the offerings of competitors? Is our product better? If so, in what way?

 Illustration 1 – Product definition

A new car could be specified as follows:

- Core/generic product – personal transportation.

- Actual product – range of engine sizes, different body shapes offered, etc.

- Augmented product – manufacturer's warranty or dealer's discounted service contract.

 Product – further considerations

The **core product** – what is the buyer really buying? The core product refers to the use, benefit or problem-solving service that the consumer is really buying when purchasing the product, i.e. the need that is being fulfilled.

The **actual product** is the tangible product or intangible service that serves as the medium for receiving core product benefits.

The **augmented product** consists of the measures taken to help the consumer put the actual product to sustained use, including installation, delivery and credit, warranties, and after-sales service.

A product, therefore, is more than a simple set of tangible features. Consumers tend to see products as complex bundles of benefits that satisfy their needs. Most important is how the customer perceives the product. They are looking at factors such as aesthetics and styling, durability, brand image, packaging, service and warranty, any of which might be enough to set the product apart from its competitors.

Pricing

There are four key considerations (the '4 Cs') when deciding the price of a product:

- **Cost** – the price must be high enough to make a profit.

- **Customers** – what are they willing to pay?

- **Competition** – is our price higher than competitors?

- **Corporate objectives** – for example, the price could be set low to gain market share.

These issues can be blended to give a range of pricing tactics, including the following:

- **Cost plus pricing** – the cost per unit is calculated and then a mark-up added.

- **Penetration pricing** – a low price is set to gain market share.

- **Perceived quality pricing** – a high price is set to reflect/create an image of high quality.

- **Price discrimination** – different prices are set for the same product in different markets, for example, peak/off-peak rail fares.

- **Going rate pricing** – prices are set to match competitors.

- **Dynamic pricing** – prices are altered in line with demand, for example this is used widely in the hotel and airline industries.

- **Price skimming** – high prices are set when a new product is launched. Later the price is dropped to increase demand once the customers who are willing to pay more have been 'skimmed' off.

- **Loss leaders** – one product may be sold at a loss with the expectation that customers will then go on and buy other more profitable products.

- **Captive product pricing** – this is used where customers must buy two products. The first is cheap to attract customers but the second is expensive, once they are captive.

Test your understanding 3

Companies with high costs will find it difficult to compete on the basis of price and would be well advised to:

A compete on the Internet

B develop brand loyalty amongst customers

C employ high pressure sales techniques

D develop new products

Promotion

Promotion is essentially about market communication. The primary aim is to encourage customers to buy the products by moving them along the **AIDA** sequence:

Awareness ⌦ Interest ⌦ Desire ⌦ Action

Towards this organisations will use a combination of different promotional techniques as part of their 'promotional mix', including:

- Advertising – for example, placing adverts on the Internet, TV, in newspapers, on billboards, etc.
- Sales promotion techniques – for example, 'buy one get one free'.
- Personal selling – for example, telesales.
- Public relations (PR) – building good relationships and a good corporate image, for example, by sponsoring sports events.

Test your understanding 4

Identify the advantages and disadvantages of following methods of promotion:

(a) Advertising

(b) Sales promotion

(c) Personal selling

(d) Public relations

Advertising

There are two polar opposite views on advertising:

- Advertising is ineffective and a waste of money, only adding to company (and hence customer) costs. Brands such as Rolls Royce and Zara do not see a need to use advertising in their promotional campaigns relying instead on other sources of information in order to form positive attitudes towards their products. In any case some might think that advertising demeans a particular product or company. In some cases, advertising may seem unethical. Lancaster and Withey (2005) conclude that some brands may be strong enough to sell on their own merits only if they are long established and have strong brand-loyal users.

- Advertising is so powerful and effective as to be essential. Consumers, it could be argued, will rarely purchase unadvertised brands so by not advertising, a company will be at a serious disadvantage compared to its competitors. The results of advertising campaigns have been undeniably successful including those for brands such as Walkers Crisps and John Lewis.

Some **new forms** of marketing communication include:

Type of marketing communication	Explanation
Viral	Encourages individuals to pass on a marketing message to others, so creating exponential growth in the message's exposure in the same way computer viruses grow.
Guerrilla	Relies on well thought out, highly focused and often unconventional attacks on key targets. This form of marketing is often low cost and has allowed organisations with small promotional budgets to be very effective.
Experiential	An interactive marketing experience aimed at stimulating all the senses, for example road shows, street theatre, product trials. The next time the consumer sees the product, it should trigger a range of positive memories making it the first choice.
Digital	The promotion of products or brands via one or more forms of electronic media, for example using email, social media, the organisation's website or Google search.

Type of marketing communication	Explanation
Search engine marketing	A form of digital marketing that involves the promotion of an organisation's website by increasing its visibility in search engine results pages, such as Google.
Social media marketing	A form of digital marketing, social media marketing refers to the process of gaining traffic or attention through social media sites.
Postmodern marketing	A philosophical approach to marketing which focuses on giving the customer an experience that is customised to them and in ensuring they receive marketing messages in a form they prefer.

 New forms of marketing communication

Viral marketing

A good example of viral marketing is Dove's 'choose beautiful' campaign which involved a video where women had to choose which door to use when entering a building – one was labelled 'beautiful' and the other 'average'. The campaign concludes with all women wishing they had chosen beautiful like some of their peers, reinforcing Dove's idea of real beauty and what that means.

Guerrilla marketing

A good example of guerrilla marketing is when a leading men's magazine projected the image of the model Gail Porter on the Houses of Parliament in London. It was a stunt that was talked about by a huge number of people. It was an attempt to get people to vote for the magazine's 'world's sexiest women' poll and the results were outstanding.

Experiential marketing

Carlsberg unveiled a billboard in Brick Lane, London, named 'Probably the best poster in the world' that had an actual working tap attached to the centre where people could pour themselves a pint of beer.

Place

A key decision under 'place' is between:

- **Selling direct** – here the manufacturer sells directly to the ultimate consumer without using any intermediaries. For example, rather than booking a holiday through a travel agent, the internet has enabled customers to go directly to hotel websites or airline websites and book their accommodation and flights themselves.

- **Selling indirect** – here there is a longer supply chain. The channel strategy could comprise a mixture of retailer, distributors, wholesalers and shipping agents. For example, food distribution will often involve distributors and retailers to get the product from farmer to consumer. Using the example above, customers could use online travel websites (such as Expedia) to book their holidays from a range of options that the website has sourced from flight and hotel reservation systems.

Variations in marketing mix settings

Different companies put different emphasis on each of the four components of the marketing mix.

For example, some companies place all the focus on making a good quality product; other companies place the emphasis on making it at a cheap price or emphasise the promotion and advertising to sell it. A manufacturer of desks might wish to sell to both the consumer market and the industrial market for office furniture. The marketing mix selected for the consumer market might be low prices with attractive dealer discounts, sales largely through discount warehouses, modern design but fairly low quality and sales promotion relying on advertising by the retail outlets, together with personal selling by the manufacturing firm to the reseller. For the industrial market, the firm might develop a durable, robust product that sells at a higher price; selling may be by means of direct mail-shots, backed by personal visits from salespeople.

An interesting comparison can be made between different firms in the same industry; for example, Avon and Elizabeth Arden both sell cosmetics but, whereas Avon relies on personal selling in the consumer's own home, Elizabeth Arden relies on an extensive dealer network and heavy advertising expenditure.

2.4 The main techniques of marketing

The marketing strategy discussed in section 2.1 touched upon the following marketing techniques:

- market research (this includes data gathering techniques and methods of analysis)

- market segmentation

- market targeting and

- market positioning.

These will be explored in turn below.

Market research

 Market research is the systematic **gathering**, recording and **analysing** of information about problems relating to the marketing of goods and services. These problems will all relate to what customers and potential customers want, need and care about.

Data **gathering** techniques can be divided into two main types:

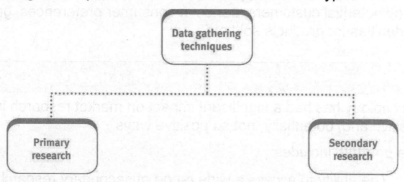

Data gathering technique	Examples
Secondary (desk) research – this is data that is already available and is therefore usually quicker and cheaper than carrying out primary research. However, the data may not be accurate and may not meet the exact needs of the organisation.	• Internal sources – accounts information, production records, order information, organisational website information, loyalty card information etc. Often sourced using an organisation's database. • External sources – such as the internet, trade and technical journals, published statutory reports, market research agency data etc.
Primary (field) research – this involves the collection of new (primary) information direct from respondents. As such, it is usually more expensive than desk research and is only performed if desk research fails to answer the questions asked. The sample chosen should be representative of the population in question.	• Questionnaires – can be done online, face to face, over the telephone or by self-completion. • Interviews – focus on a small group of individuals. • Focus groups – a trained moderator leads group discussion, such as feedback on a new product. Can be online or face to face. • Trial testing – for example, out of three chocolate bars which would you choose? • Observation – for example, use cameras to determine on average how long it takes to serve customers in a restaurant.

The data gathering techniques discussed above will be used to collect two main types of data:

- **Quantitative** (i.e. numerical) data – such as the total market size, market share percentage, segment information such as age and gender, location of existing/potential customers etc.

- **Qualitative** (i.e. non-numerical) data – such as the values and beliefs of existing/potential customers, trends in consumer preferences, growth opportunities for products sold etc.

Illustration 2 – Technology used in market research

Technology has had a significant impact on market research in both positive and, potentially, not so positive ways.

The **positive** includes:

- The ability to access a wide range of secondary research (research conducted by others) online.

- The ability to conduct qualitative research activities such as sentiment analysis and consumer perception analysis through social media monitoring.

- Organisations can now also conduct focus groups online through technology allowing us to interact with people across wide geographic boundaries.

- Business insight can be gained faster and more comprehensively than before.

However, the use of technology for market research is not without its **disadvantages**. For example, online research can give the false impression that it is as statistically reliable as traditional research. It certainly can be, but much of what passes as statistically reliable, quantitative research, these days really isn't. Organisations need to understand how to tell what is, and isn't, reliable or valid. That's not to say that qualitative research can't be helpful. It can. Organisations just need to know what they are dealing with.

The data gathered will be recorded and then **analysed** to provide insights that will help to achieve the goals of the research. Large quantities of data must be summarised and presented in such a way that clearly communicates the most important features and conclusions. (**Note:** The role of big data analytics and its use in the marketing process will be discussed in section 3.3).

The organisation may use an automated platform tailored to the specific needs of the organisation to do this. This technology will enable the organisation to filter, sort, highlight and present visually (for example, using pie charts or bar charts) the data.

Illustration 3 – Market research and analysis techniques for websites and apps

Market research and data analysis technology can be used to improve the performance of an organisation's website or app helping to track the behaviour of individual users, gather insights, test new ideas and tie the activities back to revenue.

Some examples of tools used include:

- Click analysis – tracks the actions of individual users within the website or app. For example, an e-commerce site may monitor items added to a shopping cart by visitors or a new app that relies on advertising revenue may monitor view time and clicks.

- Visual behaviour tools – reveal where users spend time looking at a screen (for example, through the use of number of taps and swipes on a mobile). Data may be presented as a heat map that highlights the most heavily trafficked or clicked areas.

- Search engine optimisation (SEO) tools – help the organisation understand how likely their site and content are to show up in online search results.

- Dashboard tools – consolidate market research into one interface so that the data can be quickly manipulated to gain insight.

Market segmentation

Market segmentation is the sub-dividing of the market into homogenous groups to whom a separate marketing mix can be focused.

A market segment is a group of consumers with distinct, shared needs.

Why segment the market?

- The key objective is to say that people falling into a particular segment are more likely to purchase the product than most.

- The company will choose a particular segment or segments to target. The total marketing budget can be split based on the likely return from each segment.

- The organisation may be able to identify new market opportunities or can try to dominate a particular segment because it will have a better understanding of customers' needs in each segment.

Kotler suggested that segments must meet **three criteria**. They should be:

- **Measurable** – it must be possible to identify the number of buyers in each market segment so that their potential profitability can be assessed. For example, the size of the segment of people aged 30–40, or who are married with children, can be accurately calculated but information about the number of people who are environmentally conscious is not readily available.

- **Accessible** – it must be possible to reach potential customers via the organisation's promotion and distribution channels. For example, some potential customers may be inaccessible if they are tied to other suppliers by long-term supply contracts.

- **Substantial** – small market segments may prove unprofitable to target.

There are a number of **different bases for segmentation**. Possible bases include:

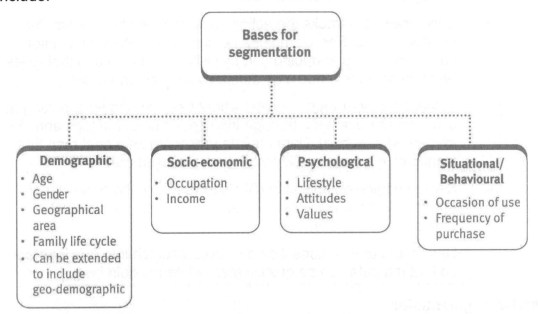

Bases for segmentation

Demographic

Market segments are frequently based on age, gender, geographical location or family life cycle.

This can be highly relevant with some products, for example, certain brands of breakfast cereal have regular sales to families with young children (for example, Coco Pops), whereas other brands (for example, Bran Flakes) sell almost entirely to adults.

In other areas, demographic influences seem to have little effect. For instance, own-label products are believed to sell equally to high and low income families and single people and across all age groups.

Family life cycle segmentation divides customers by their position in the family life cycle:

Life cycle stage	Characteristics	Examples of products purchased
Bachelor	Financially well off. Fashion opinion leaders. Recreation orientated.	Cars, holidays, basic furniture, kitchen equipment.
A couple with no children	Still financially well off. Very high purchase rate, especially of durables.	Cars, furniture, houses, holidays, refrigerators.
A couple or individual with a very young child/children	Liquid assets low. Home purchasing at a peak. Little money saving.	Kitchen appliances, baby foods, toys, medicines.
A couple or individual with an older child/children	Better off. Some partners work. Some children work part time. Less influenced by advertising.	Larger size grocery packs, foods, cleaning materials, bicycles.
A couple or individual with a child/children almost old enough to leave home	Better off still. Purchasing durables.	New furniture, luxury appliances, recreational goods.
A couple or individual with a child/children who have left home	Satisfied with financial position.	Travel, luxuries, home improvements.
An ageing individual or couple who are not working	Drastic cut in income. Stay at home.	Medicines, health aids.

Geo-demographic segmentation combines demographic and geographic variables. This is a recent, but powerful, development in which geographical segmentation is undertaken at a much more localised level and linked to other demographic factors.

Socio-economic

One of widely used forms of segmentation in is socio-economic. While such class-based systems may seem out of date, the model is still widely used, especially in advertising. Socio-economic class is closely correlated with press readership and viewing habits, and media planners use this fact to advertise in the most effective way to communicate with their target audience.

Psychological

Lifestyle segmentation may be used because people of similar age and socio-economic status may lead quite different lifestyles. Marketers have segmented the market using terms such as 'Dinkies' (double income, no kids).

Attitudes and values can be harder to measure but can prove to be a useful basis for segmentation. For example, individuals may have a value based on caution and therefore purchase a safe, reliable car.

Situational (or behavioural)

Occasion of use – a product may be bought at different times for different uses. For example, workers may expect a lunchtime meal in a restaurant to be fast and good value for money, whereas those same individuals may be willing to pay more in the evening for a more relaxed dining experience.

Frequency of purchase – frequent buyers may be more demanding with regards to product features and may be more sensitive to price changes.

Test your understanding 5

Explain five variables that you think would be useful as a basis for segmenting the market for cars.

Targeting

Targeting is the process of selecting the most lucrative market segment(s) for marketing the product.

Having segmented the market, the organisation can now decide how to respond to the differences in customer needs identified and will reach a conclusion as to which segments are worth targeting.

The organisation may choose a number of different approaches. For example, the market for package holidays can be split into a variety of different segments – the family market, the elderly market, the young singles market, the activity holiday market, the budget holiday market, etc.

It would be virtually impossible to provide one single holiday package that would satisfy all people in the above markets. Because the people in the different segments will have different needs and wants, a holiday company has a choice in terms of its marketing approach. It can go for:

- **Concentrated marketing** (sometimes referred to as niche or target marketing) specialises in one of the identified markets only, where a company knows it can compete successfully. For example, Saga holidays offer a variety of holidays for the older market niche only.

- **Differentiated marketing** (sometimes called segmented marketing) – the company makes several products each aimed at a separate target segment. For example, Virgin Holidays offers a variety of family holidays, honeymoon packages and city breaks, each of which is targeted at a different group. Many retailers have developed different brand formats to target different groups.

- **Undifferentiated marketing** (sometimes called mass marketing) – this is the delivery of a single product to the entire market. There is little concern for segmentation. The hope is that as many customers as possible will buy the product. When Henry Ford began manufacturing cars he offered any colour 'as long as it's black'.

Positioning

 Positioning involves the formulation of a definitive marketing strategy around which the product would be marketed to the target audience.

After the target market has been chosen, marketers will want to position their products in relation to the competitors for that segment. A variety of techniques are available.

For example, Porter identified four positioning strategies:

	Low cost	High cost
Broad target	**Cost leadership** – the organisation aims to be the lowest cost producer in the industry.	**Differentiation** – the organisation produces products which are different and appeal to customers on the grounds of, say, quality or design.
Narrow target	**Cost focus** – the pursuit of a cost leadership strategy but focused on one particular segment only	**Differentiation focus** – the pursuit of a differentiation strategy but focused on one particular segment only

Test your understanding 6
Undifferentiated marketing involves an organisation in offering:
A   products based on market research
B   a single product to the market as a whole
C   multiple products to the market as a whole
D   single products to segmented markets

Test your understanding 7
Segmentation involves identifying target markets that must be:
A   measurable, accessible and substantial
B   acceptable, feasible and suitable
C   undeveloped, undiscovered and undifferentiated
D   aligned to core competences

Test your understanding 8
Which of the following phrases explains concentrated marketing?
A   The company produces one product for a number of different market segments
B   The company introduces several versions of the product aimed at several market segments
C   The company produces one product for a mass market
D   The company produces one product for a one segment of the marketplace

3   Areas of interface between sales and marketing and finance

3.1 Introduction

The way in which finance interacts with sales and marketing will be explored in greater depth below. However, it is useful to begin by thinking about some basic ways in which the two areas interact:

Budgeting	Finance will discuss the likely sales volume of each product with the sales and marketing team, in order to produce the sales budget.
Advertising	Finance will help sales and marketing in setting a budget, and in monitoring whether it is cost effective. For example, they could help in measuring new business generated as a result of different advertising campaigns.

Pricing	Finance will have input into the price that is charged. Often products are priced at cost plus a percentage. Even if sales and marketing determine the price based on market forces they need to consult with finance to ensure that costs are covered.
Market share	Finance can provide marketing with information on sales volumes for each product, to help the marketing department in determining market share.
KPIs	Finance will establish and monitor the KPIs for the sales and marketing function.

3.2 How the finance function interacts with sales and marketing

Introduction

- Finance and sales and marketing should interact to achieve organisational goals and their own individual functional goals.

- Traditionally, there may have been antagonism between the two functions over issues such as pricing and cost control.

- The modern approach is for the two functions to collaborate and to work in partnership.

- Effective interaction will be based on close working teams which possess a shared vision for the organisation and an appreciation of each other's specialisms.

- Technology is assisting this collaboration through the use of tools such as cloud computing, data analytics and blockchain.

The finance function has a unique end to end view of the organisation and is considered a trusted advisor. As a result, there are a number of areas where the CFO (and their team) has an opportunity to enhance performance through business partnering with the sales and marketing. Two of these areas will be explored below:

- product/service development
- product/service life-cycles and costing

Product/service development

Organisations need to continually look for new or improved products or services, to achieve or maintain competitive advantage in their market.

The stages of product/service development are as follows:

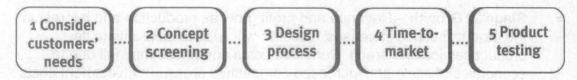

1 Consider customers' needs … 2 Concept screening … 3 Design process … 4 Time-to-market … 5 Product testing

> **Test your understanding 9**
>
> M Ltd are in the process of designing a new product to fit with the rapidly changing environment.
>
> **Which THREE of the following are activities that M may undertake during the first three stages of product development?**
>
> A   Interviewing customers to determine what they want
>
> B   Analysing social media to gain an insight into customer tastes
>
> C   Testing the product to ensure it is durable
>
> D   Using computer aided design (CAD) to build a prototype
>
> E   Ensuring the product is released ahead of the competition

Given the rapidly changing nature of the modern consumer's preferences and expectations, this initial process of development can make or break an organisation. The finance function will work collaboratively with the sales and marketing function to evaluate new product/service lines or innovations. They have a sharp eye for the economic upside (or otherwise!) of a product/service.

Product/service life-cycles and costing

After product/service development most products/services go through a number of stages in their existence:

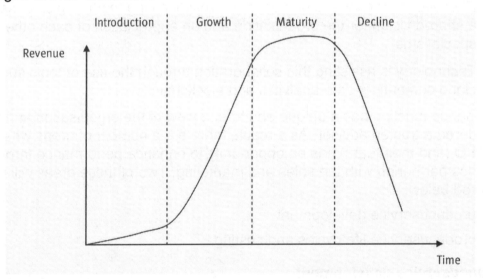

- **Stage 1: Introduction** – A small number of individuals will be prepared to pay a high price for a new, innovative product/service, for example, the latest mobile phone model. Revenues will be low and expenditure (including marketing costs) high.

- **Stage 2: Growth** – Revenue and profit grow as production and interest in the product/service increases. The firm will seek to differentiate its product/service and brand. Purchase costs and prices may fall due to economies of scale and increased competitive pressure. Investment costs will still be high.

- **Stage 3: Maturity** – This is the longest and most successful stage of the life cycle. Costs settle down into a pattern of repeat or replacement costs. Growth slows or halts due to high levels of competition. The price may be cut in order to attract a new group of customers.

- **Stage 4: Decline** – Few people will purchase the product/service at the end of the life cycle as superior alternatives replace it and promotional activity will drop. The firm will look to exit the market and find profitable alternatives.

The finance function will interact with the sales and marketing function in two main ways:

- **Life-cycle costing** – this considers the costs and revenues of a product/service over its whole life (including product/service development) rather than one accounting period. Therefore, the full cost incurred prior to, during and after production will be considered to ensure that the costs can be covered and/or any possible steps are taken to reduce the costs.

- **Balanced portfolio** – products/services at different stages in the lifecycle have different implications for resource requirements, risk and strategy. This would emphasise the importance of the finance function's involvement in portfolio management, helping to inform decisions about the organisation's overall product/service offering.

  For example, having too many products/services in the development stages will put a strain on finances as they will all require significant investment in marketing. On the other hand, if all products/services are at the maturity stage, then there may be a question mark over the organisation's long-term future – how long will it be before they move into the decline phase?

  An appropriate balance of existing products/services in a mature market, together with investment in new products in the introduction and growth stages is best.

Test your understanding 10	
Are the following statements about the product life-cycle true or false?	
Statement	**True/False?**
Economies of scale will be greatest during the introduction stage	
The growth stage is the longest stage	
Prices tend to increase during the maturity stage as this is when demand is highest and therefore, revenue can be maximised	
Product costs tend to be lowest during the later stages of the lifecycle	
All businesses will have a product at each stage of the lifecycle	

Illustration 4 – The use of technology in the life-cycle

Blockchain offers the prospect of designing a data structure from the perspective of the product; meaning that in a single chain all vital data about that product over its whole life-cycle can be captured. An accurate record of say, inventory levels, costs and revenue is available by examining the current state of the block.

The internet of things (IoT) connects devices over the internet. Its applications can be used in the life-cycle in several ways:

- Maintenance and service – sensors can provide data on products for servicing purposes. This should help optimise future service schedules and reduce maintenance costs.

- Requirements management – providing visibility into how customers are using products. Knowing that some product functions are not in use and injecting this information in product modifications and future requirement analysis is of huge advantage.

- Product performance monitoring – providing real performance data from, say, the engine and other parts of a car, airplane, computer or even a toothbrush. This data helps inform future decisions.

3.3 Big data analytics in marketing

Introduction

Big data and data analytics have been discussed in detail in Chapters 5-8.

Illustration 5 – Big data analytics

An organisation and its sales and marketing function face a number of challenges in using its big data. For example, a lack of insight for targeted campaigns or an inability to support data growth.

Value is extracted from big data by the process of data analytics.

For example, **Google Analytics** tracks many features of website traffic.

Hadoop software allows the processing of large data sets by utilising multiple servers simultaneously. It enables instant analysis of social sentiment and customer feedback across digital, face-to-face and phone interactions.

The result should be a reduced time to obtain customer insight, an ability to make changes to campaigns or adjust product roll outs based on real-time customer reactions and an ability to offer incentives and new services to retail and grow its customer base.

Unlocking the potential value of big data using real-time data analytics and its significance to an organisation's sales and marketing function presents a huge opportunity to gain unique insight which can be used to improve competitive position and potentially gain competitive advantage over rivals. The finance function will work collaboratively with the sales and marketing function to provide this insight.

Examples of big data analytics in marketing

- **Market segmentation and customisation** – The volume and variety within big data enables organisations to create highly specific segments within its markets and to tailor its products and services precisely to meet those needs in real-time.

Illustration 6

Biscuit manufacturer, Oreo

Many marketers consider Oreo's famous 'You can still dunk in the dark' marketing campaign during Super Bowl in New Orleans to be a landmark event in real-time marketing. During the third quarter of the game, the Superdome experienced a partial power outage, darkening the stadium and suspending play for 34 minutes. During this time, Oreo cleverly took advantage of the situation and tweeted its message out to thousands of loyal followers, receiving over 10,000 re-tweets and 20,000 likes on Facebook.

- **Product/service development** – Organisations can use data on customer behaviour and social trends to create new products/services to meet customers' needs or to enhance existing products/services so that they meet these needs more exactly.

Illustration 7

Motor insurance

The availability of real-time location data, from satellite sensors and satellite navigation systems, can enable motor insurance companies to refine the pricing of their insurance policies according to where, and how, people drive their cars.

Health and life insurance

Health and life insurance company, Vitality, is offering its customers the opportunity to link their activity tracking device or app to their online Vitality profile. Points are earned for completing eligible activities such as a target number of steps, a gym visit or a park run. Customers can then redeem their points for treats such as Starbucks coffee or cinema visits.

- **Decision making** – The sophisticated analytics tools can also be used to improve decision making. For example, a retailer may use algorithms to optimise decisions about inventory levels and pricing (i.e. dynamic pricing) in response to current and predicted sales. Real-time data visualisation technologies (for example, dashboards) allow managers to adjust tactics based on, for example, live sales or inventory data.

Illustration 8

Dynamic pricing in action

The chances are that you've already seen dynamic pricing in action, even if you haven't realised you're being specifically targeted in this way. Perhaps you've viewed a flight or a holiday several times on a website but when you finally return to book it the price has jumped. Or maybe you've added an item to your basket on Amazon but a week later when you go to actually click 'buy' the price has changed.

This kind of dynamic pricing is the result of ever increasing quantities of data giving retailers and service providers more insights into their own supply and customer desires than ever before. They can increase the price when demand rises or supply falls, or they can fill those last seats and sell out a service by dropping the price as the deadline comes closer. Some retailers can even work out how likely you are to make a purchase and either drop the price to give you an extra incentive to buy or hike it because they know you're ready to pay.

- **Obtaining customer feedback** – Organisations now have access to huge amounts of customer feedback in real or almost real time. For example, identifying what customers are saying in social media about an organisation's products or its customer service could help the organisation identify potential changes that may be needed.

Test your understanding 11

Using the options below, complete the following statements concerning big data analytics in marketing:

Tailoring products and services precisely to meet customers' needs in real-time is known as_____

Using algorithms to optimise decisions such as those about pricing is known as _____ pricing

What a consumer is saying about the product on social media can be a useful way of obtaining_____

Options to choose from:

- Hadoop
- Criticism
- Feedback
- Dynamic
- Static
- Customisation
- Analytics

4 Key performance indicators (KPIs)

4.1 Introduction

In section 6 of Chapter 9 we:

- defined KPIs
- discussed their use in managing the operations function
- identified relevant KPIs for operations
- discussed how the finance function manages operations using KPIs and
- discussed the impact of technology in this area.

Much of this discussion can also be applied to the sales and marketing function and can therefore be referred back to.

In this section we will briefly discuss how the finance function helps to manage the sales and marketing function through the use of KPIs before identifying some relevant KPIs for sales and marketing.

4.2 How finance helps to manage sales and marketing using KPIs

- The sales and marketing function will identify its relevant CSFs (i.e. the vital areas where things must go right for the function in order for them to achieve their strategic objectives).

- The KPIs are the measures that indicate whether or not the sales and marketing function is achieving these CSFs. KPIs are essential to the achievement of these objectives since 'what gets measured gets done', i.e. the things that are measured get done more often than the things that are not measured.

- The finance function works with the sales and marketing function to:

    - **identify** appropriate KPIs
    - **assemble** KPI data and information
    - **analyse** this for insight

- give **advice** to the sales and marketing function based on this insight and

- **apply** what has been learned to impact the achievement of the objectives of the sales and marketing function and the organisation as a whole.

- **Technology** will act as a key enabler in this, particularly in the 'assembly' and 'analysis' tasks.

Illustration 9 – KPI dashboards
One of the most common technologies used in this area is performance dashboards. The dashboard displays the KPIs of the sales and marketing function in a live format, thus allowing immediate understanding of current performance and potentially prompting action to correct or amend performance accordingly.
The dashboards assist with data visualisation. The simple and visually appealing layout can be understood by non-technical users. With just a few clicks interactive and versatile views can be built, providing, at a glance, relevant information and insights for different users.
This will 'free up' the resource of the finance function who can now spend more time on the 'advising' and 'applying' activities – a shift that makes better use of their skills and expertise.
Note: It would be useful to spend a few minutes looking at examples of sales and marketing dashboard images on the internet.

4.3 Examples of KPIs for sales and marketing

Example activity	Possible KPI
Overall sales and marketing activity	Growth in sales volume/revenue
	Market share
	Gross margins
	Customer retention rate
	Cost of customer acquisition
	Marketing spend per customer
	Customer lifetime value
Promotion	Promotion cost
	Awareness levels
	Website traffic to conversion %
	Social media reach (for example, Twitter followers)
	Email marketing performance (for example, unsubscribe rate)
	Sales team response times

Example activity	Possible KPI
Product/service	Product development time/cost
	Product life-cycle costs
	Repurchase rate
	Brand value
	Warranty claims
Pricing	Price relative to industry average
	Price elasticity of demand
Place	Transport costs
	Storage costs

Test your understanding 12

Match the following KPIs to the element of the marketing mix that it could measure.

A   Brand value

B   Packaging cost

C   Lead times

D   Price elasticity of demand

E   Social media activity

F   Number of 'clicks to buy'

Choose from the following options:

1   Product

2   Price

3   Place

4   Promotion

5 Chapter summary

```
                        ┌─────────────────────────┐
                        │ How the finance function │
                        │ interacts with marketing │
                        └─────────────────────────┘
```

Introduction

Main role of sales and marketing
- Introduction
- Understanding the marketing environment
- Understanding the marketing mix
- The main techniques of marketing

Areas of interface between sales and marketing and finance
- Introduction
- How the finance function interacts with sales and marketing
- Big data analytics in marketing

Key performance indicators
- Introduction
- How finance helps manage sales and marketing using KPIs
- Examples of KPIs for sales and marketing

Test your understanding answers

Test your understanding 1

The correct answer is **C**

The key focus of marketing is customer needs.

Test your understanding 2

The changing needs of the population must be reflected in the product offerings. For example:

- The supermarket may reduce its range of luxury items in favour of lower priced, basic products.

- Special offers may be made on products, for example, discounts, buy one get one free offers, additional loyalty points on products.

- The supermarket may introduce more 'restaurant style' meals to reflect the trend that fewer people are eating out.

Test your understanding 3

The correct answer is **B**

The key focus of successful marketing is customer needs and therefore developing brand loyalty amongst customers would assist in this.

Test your understanding 4

Method	Advantages	Disadvantages
(a) Advertising	• Reach a large number of potential customers. • Low cost for each potential customer.	• Total cost can be very high. • Difficult to evaluate effectiveness.
(b) Sales promotion	• Can help gain new users. • Counteract competition. • Clear out surplus stock.	• Can be costly. • May not win customer loyalty.

Method	Advantages	Disadvantages
(c) Personal selling	• Can focus on needs of individual customer. • A talented salesperson can be very persuasive.	• Can be seen as pushy. • High cost per potential customer.
(d) Public relations	• Low or no cost. • Can be targeted. • Unbiased opinion.	• Negative review may damage reputation.

Test your understanding 5

Gender

It would be useful to segment the market based on gender. Females may prefer a car that is smaller, is available in bright colours and comes with fashionable accessories. Males, on the other hand, may prefer a more masculine looking and powerful car.

Age

The age of the consumer will be of upmost importance. Teenage drivers may prefer a cheaper model, whereas drivers in their 20s, with more disposable income, may prefer a more expensive and stylish model.

Lifestyle

There may be a number of different lifestyles that could be targeted. Each group will have quite different needs. For example, a leisure user may be more interested in the style and design of the car where as a commuter may want a safe, reliable car.

Income

The level of income will impact the make and the model that the user can afford and any optional extras that may be purchased.

Family life cycle

The life cycle stage will be important. For example, bachelors may prefer a higher priced, sporty, stylish model where as those with a young and growing family may prefer a safe, reliable and family orientated people carrier.

Test your understanding 6

The correct answer is **B**

Test your understanding 7

The correct answer is **A**

Test your understanding 8

The correct answer is **D**

Test your understanding 9

The correct answers are A, B and D

The first three stages are:

1   Consider customer's needs,

2   Concept screening, and

3   Design process

Interviewing customers and analysing social media will help to understand the customer's needs. Building a prototype is part of the design process.

The final two stages are:

1   Time to market and

2   Product testing

Test your understanding 10

Statement	True/False?
Economies of scale will be greatest during the introduction stage	False, economies of scale are greatest when higher volumes of the product are sold.
The growth stage is the longest stage	False, each stage can vary in length. However, it is the maturity stage that tends to be the longest.
Prices tend to increase during the maturity stage as this is when demand is highest and therefore, revenue can be maximised	False, prices tend to decrease during the maturity stage, partially in order to attract new customers to prolong the maturity phase.

Statement	True/False?
Product costs tend to be lowest during the later stages of the lifecycle	True
All businesses will have a product at each stage of the life-cycle	False, whilst a business may aim to have balanced portfolio, there is no guarantee that they will have products at each stage.

Test your understanding 11

Tailoring products and services precisely to meet customers' needs in real-time is known as **customisation**.

Using algorithms to optimise decisions such as those about pricing is known as **dynamic** pricing.

What a consumer is saying about the product on social media can be a useful way of obtaining **feedback**.

Test your understanding 12

A   Brand value – **product**

B   Packaging cost – **product**

C   Lead times – **place**

D   Price elasticity of demand – **price**

E   Social media activity – **promotion**

F   Number of 'clicks to buy' – **promotion**

How the finance function interacts with human resources

Chapter learning objectives

Lead	Component
E3: Describe how the finance function interacts with human resources.	Describe: (a) Main role of human resources (b) Areas of interface with finance (c) Key performance indicators

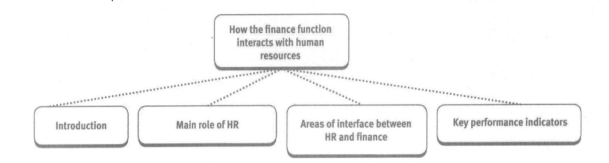

1 Introduction

In this chapter we will continue to describe how the finance function plays its role by interacting with the rest of the organisation (syllabus area E) and, more specifically here, the organisation's human resources (HR) function.

We will begin by discussing the main role of the HR function; understanding the different HR activities that exist. An effective HR function will view employees as a hugely valuable resource within the organisation and as a potential source of .competitive advantage.

We will then discuss the areas of interface with finance before moving on to the final part of the chapter which will discuss how the finance function helps to manage the HR function through the use of key performance indicators (KPIs).

2 Main role of HR

2.1 Introduction

 The HR function is responsible for human resource management within the organisation. Human resource management (HRM) is the creation, development and maintenance of an effective workforce, matching the requirements of the organisation to the environment and responding to that environment.

Note: That although many aspects of HRM are likely to be the responsibility of the HR function, there will also be some responsibility of line managers in charge of employees' day-to-day work.

The HR plan

 The HR plan is a strategy developed in the context of the organisation's overall strategic plan.

A typical plan will look forward 3-5 years and aims to identify and close the gap between the demand for labour and the supply of labour within the organisation.

Stages of HR planning

Stage 1: Strategic analysis
- The organisation's strategic objectives will have implications regarding the number of employees and the skills required over the planning period (e.g. development of a new product or expansion into a new market)
- The broader strategic environment should also be considered (e.g. trends in population growth, pensions, education and employment rights of women)

Stage 2: Internal analysis
- An 'audit' of existing staff should be carried out to establish the current numbers and skills
- Also consider:
  - Turnover of staff and absenteeism
  - Overtime worked and periods of inactivity
  - Staff potential

Stage 3: Identify the gap between supply and demand
- Shortages or excesses in labour numbers and skills deficiencies should be identified

Stage 4: Put plans into place to close the gap

Adjustments for shortfall
- Internal: Transfers, promotions, training, job enlargement, overtime, reduce labour turnover
- External: Fill remaining needs externally. Consider suitability and availability of external resource

Adjustments for a surplus
Consider use of natural wastage, recruitment freeze, retirement, part time working and redundancy

Stage 5: Review
Measure the effective use of the human resource and their contribution towards the achievement of the organisation's objectives

Test your understanding 1

The economic situation in a country (or specific area of a country) may have a marked effect on the ability of an organisation to attract suitable candidates.

Is this statement:

A   True?

B   False?

Test your understanding 2

How can an organisation plan rationally in an unstable environment?

The HR cycle

A common approach to viewing the different HR activities is as a cycle:

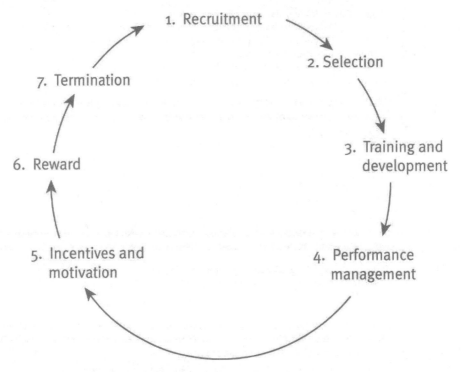

The first six of these activities will be discussed below.

2.2 Recruitment

 Recruitment involves attracting a field of suitable candidates for the job.

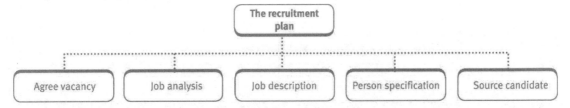

The best recruitment campaign will attract a small number of highly suitable applicants, be cost effective, be speedy and show courtesy to all candidates.

 Illustration 1 – Recruitment in a downturn

In periods of economic recession, recruitment would appear to be less important, as large numbers of people will be looking for employment, meaning a field of candidates should be easy to attract.

However, even in times of high unemployment, organisations must ensure they only hire the correct people with the skills and abilities that they need. This can become more difficult when there are larger numbers of applicants.

Assessing the need to recruit

When considering recruitment, there are two questions that managers must address. The first is whether there is really a job, and the second is whether there is someone suitable who is already employed by the organisation. There are many alternatives to recruitment, for example:

- Promotion of existing staff (upwards or laterally)

- Secondment (temporary transfers to another department, office, plant or country) of existing staff, which may or may not become permanent

- Closing the job down, by sharing out duties and responsibilities among existing staff

- Rotating jobs among staff, so that the vacant job is covered by different staff, on a systematic basis over several months

- Putting the job out to tender, using external contractors.

Agree vacancy – A vacancy may arise due to growth in the organisation, a change of direction or because an employee leaves the organisation.

Job analysis – This is the detailed study and description of the tasks that make up the job.

Job description – After a full job analysis has been carried out, a job description can be drawn up.

A job description is a broad statement of the purpose, scope duties and responsibilities of the job.

A typical job description will tend to include:

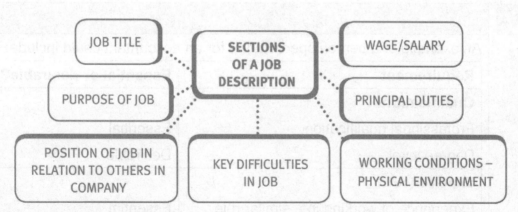

Test your understanding 3

Prepare a job description for a London based role as a Finance Director in an internet media company which is about to become a public company.

Person specification – Once management have a job description, they can attempt to define the key attributes and qualities that the jobholder should ideally have. Prospective candidates can then be compared to this specification as part of the selection process.

Alec Rodgers devised a seven-point plan which suggests the content of a person specification. You can remember this using the acronym **BADPIGS**.

Category	Example
B – Background/ circumstances	Details of previous work experience and circumstances – for example, criminal record or flexible working requirements.
A – Attainments	Details of qualifications and any relevant experience.
D – Disposition	The individual's nature (for example, can work calmly under pressure) and goals (for example, future ambitions).
P – Physical make-up	Personal appearance and level of health.
I – Interests	General interests and hobbies will be important. For example, being a member of a football team demonstrates teamwork skills.
G – General intelligence	Not necessarily academic qualifications but may refer to practical intelligence such as problem solving ability or whether the candidate is of average intelligence (or otherwise).
S – Special attributes	Skills such as the ability to speak another language or IT skills.

Illustration 2 – Person specification for an accountant

An example of a person specification for an accountant could include:

Requirement	Essential or desirable?
Qualifications	
Professional qualification	Essential
Degree level	Desirable
Experience	
Experience of working in a similar role	Essential
Experience of dealing with clients	Desirable

Requirement	Essential or desirable?
Skills and competencies	
Excellent communication skills	Essential
Ability to present complex information	Essential
Excellent numerical skills	Essential
Team player	Desirable
Ability to work flexibly	Desirable
Personal attributes	
Self-motivated	Essential
Able to use own initiative	Essential
Attention to detail	Essential
Prepared to learn new skills	Desirable
Other	
Ability to use Microsoft Word and Sage	Essential
Willing to participate in client meetings	Essential

Test your understanding 4

The purpose of a person specification is to provide details of:

A   Organisational size and diversity of activity

B   The types of responsibilities and duties to be undertaken by the post holder.

C   Personal characteristics, experience and qualifications expected of a candidate

D   Individual terms of engagement and period of contract

Test your understanding 5

Are there any circumstances when discrimination on the basis of physical make-up is acceptable?

Source candidates – this stage involves persuading relevant candidates to apply for the role the organisation wishes to fill.

The following methods may be used to make contact with and to secure the application of appropriate candidates:

- internal sourcing
- internet and social media
- recruitment consultants

- newspaper and specialist journal advertising
- radio and television advertising
- job centres
- job fairs.

> **Illustration 3**
>
> Care must be taken not to transgress one of the laws relating to discrimination, as in the case of a job advertisement seeking 'a female Scottish cook and housekeeper', which was barred both on the grounds of race and sex discrimination.

2.3 Selection

 Selection is aimed at choosing the best person for the job from the field of candidates sourced via recruitment.

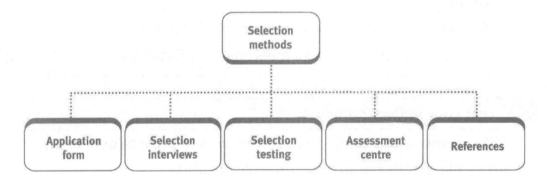

Application form

Application forms are used to obtain relevant information about the applicant and allow for comparison with the person specification of the job.

They should also give the applicants some ability to express themselves beyond the limited factual remit of the form.

A Curriculum Vitae (CV) may be requested alongside the application form. This details the individual's unique skills, character, experience and achievements.

Selection interviews

Once the least appropriate candidates have been rejected using their application forms, the remaining applicants can be interviewed.

The purpose of an interview is to:

- find the best person for the job

- ensure that the candidate understands what the job involves and what the career prospects are

- make the candidate feel that they have been treated fairly in the selection process.

There are various types of interview that an organisation may use, including:

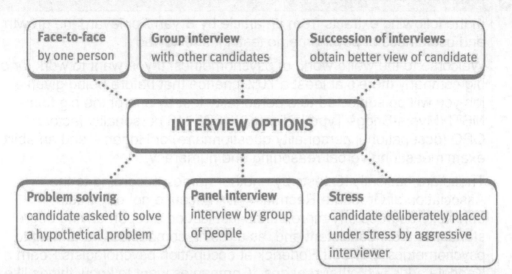

Test your understanding 6

(a) What are the key advantages and disadvantages of interviews as a way of selecting candidates?

(b) For each of the interview options, identify one advantage and one disadvantage.

Test your understanding 7

A has been asked to attend a job interview. He has been told that he will be interviewed by the Finance Director first, followed by the HR Director.

What type of interview is A going to experience?

A   Group

B   Panel

C   Stress

D   Succession

Selection testing

Testing can be undertaken either before or after the interview has taken place.

The two basic types of test are:

- **Proficiency and attainment** – these are used to examine the applicant's competences, skills and abilities in areas that will be required in the job they have applied for.

- **Psychometric** – these are more general and test psychological factors, such as aptitude, intelligence and personality.

Psychometric testing

In the following extracts from an article by Bryan Appleyard the growth and usefulness of psychometric testing is reviewed:

Welcome to the weird world of psychometrics. If you want to work for a big company there's at least a 70% chance that before being given a job you will be subjected to a personality test by one of the big four – MBTI (Myers-Briggs Type Indicator), 16PF (16 personality factors), OPQ (occupational personality questionnaire) or Hogan – and an ability exam measuring verbal reasoning and numeracy.

These are basically IQ tests by another name...according to the Association of Graduate Recruiters, it's because nobody trusts university degrees any more. It has just issued a report saying degree standards are inconsistent and, as a result, companies are turning to psychometrics. But Ceri Roderick at occupation psychologists Pearn Kandola adds two other reasons. 'Companies want to know things like the motivational characteristics of recruits and the technology is now available to do these things.' There's also a fourth reason: the need to compete for quality recruits. 'There's a war for talent,' says Professor David Bartram of the British Psychological Society (BPS), 'companies are fighting to get the best people.' All of which means there is now a rapid proliferation of psychometrics consultancies, most of them offering candidates the chance to do all the tests online....

Sceptics think the whole enterprise is misguided. In America a book – The Cult of Personality by Annie Murphy Paul – has cast doubt on the intellectual credibility of psychometrics...

In support of Paul's book the author Malcolm Gladwell questions the very idea of measuring personality: 'We have a personality in the sense that we have a consistent pattern of behaviour. But that pattern is complex and that personality is contingent: it represents an interaction between our internal disposition and tendencies and the situations that we find ourselves in.'...

But are Gladwell and Paul right to question the whole theory on which they are based? The history of psychometrics marches hand in hand with the history of IQ testing. Alfred Binet, the French psychologist, produced the first modern IQ test in 1905 and Walter Dill Scott subjected 15 engineering graduates to the first psychometric test in 1915. Both ideas were inspired by the conviction that there could be no reason why the human mind should be impervious to scientific investigation. .

Psychometrics works, but only if the tests are properly applied, rigorously interpreted and accompanied by traditional interviews. This means that they do not necessarily speed up the recruitment process. They might, however, help weed out unsuitables in advance, a huge benefit at a time when all companies are swamped with applicants for attractive jobs.

Source: Appleyard, B. (2007) Want a job? Let's play mind games.

Assessment centres

Assessment centres involve candidates being observed and evaluated by trained assessors as they are given a selection of pre-programmed exercises or trials. These exercises may include:

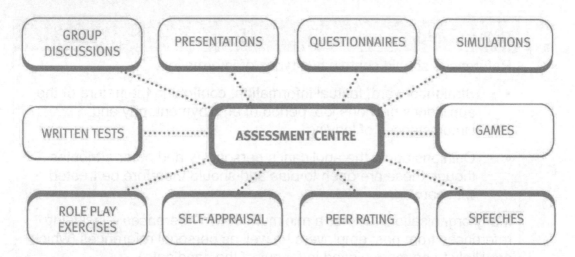

Assessors will be looking for evidence that candidates have certain abilities that are important in the job they have applied for. These criteria will change from job to job, but may include leadership or communication skills, for example.

Assessment centres

The assessment centre is really a combination of many forms of selection. Groups of around six to ten candidates are brought together for one to three days of intensive assessment. As well as being multi-method, other characteristics of assessment centres are that they use several assessors and they assess several dimensions of performance required in the higher-level positions.

The advantages of assessment centres include:

- A high degree of acceptability and user confidence.

- Avoidance of a single-assessor bias.

- Reliability in predicting potential success (if the system is well conducted).

- The development of skills in the assessors, which may be useful in their own managerial responsibilities.

- Benefits to the assessed individuals, including experience of managerial/supervisory situations, opportunity for self-assessment and job-relevant feedback and opportunities to discuss career prospects openly with senior management.

References

The purpose of references is to confirm facts about the employee and increase the degree of confidence felt about information given during the other selection techniques.

References

References should contain two types of information:

- Straightforward, factual information, confirming the nature of the applicant's previous job, period of employment, pay and circumstances of leaving.

- Opinions about the applicant's personality and other attributes, though these are open to bias and should therefore be treated with caution.

Many organisations ask for a minimum of two references – including references from past employers as well as personal references (which are likely to be more biased in favour of the candidate).

References, while useful, have to be viewed with caution. Allowances must be made for:

- prejudice (favourable or unfavourable)

- charity (withholding detrimental remarks)

- fear of being actionable for libel (although references are privileged, as long as they are factually correct and devoid of malice).

What happens next?

Once a suitable candidate has been found, a **job offer** can be made. It may be necessary to **negotiate** over some aspects of the employment contract, such as pay or hours of work.

On starting work with the organisation, the employee should be effectively assimilated into the organisation through a process of **induction**.

Illustration 4

The average UK employee turnover rate is 15% and the average cost of employee turnover is £6,300 for each employee. A major reason why employees leave within the first six months to a year is a poorly planned induction process. Therefore, there are significant savings to be made from implementing an effective induction process.

2.4 Staff development and training

Introduction

Often the terms 'training' and 'development' are used inter-changeably. However, there are differences between the two:

 Training is the planned and systematic modification of behaviour through learning events, programmes and instruction which enable individuals to achieve the level of knowledge, skills and competence to carry out their work effectively.

 Development is the growth or realisation of a person's ability and potential through conscious or unconscious learning and educational experiences.

It is often argued that development is therefore more general, more future-oriented and more individually-oriented than training.

Organisations should view training and development of staff as an investment.

Test your understanding 8
What are the benefits, for both the learner and the organisation, of training and development?

The training and development process

Due to the obvious importance of training and development, a systematic approach should be taken in order to maximise its effectiveness. To help with this, organisations may find it helpful to view training and development as a step-by-step process.

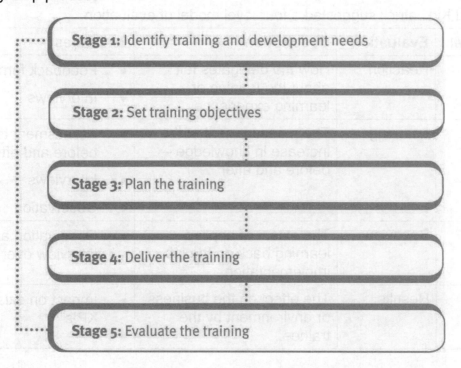

Stage 1: Identify training and development needs

Stage 2: Set training objectives

Stage 3: Plan the training

Stage 4: Deliver the training

Stage 5: Evaluate the training

Stages in training and development

- **Identifying training (or development) needs** – this could include an investigation into the organisation's current performance as well as mapping the corporate skills base. It should drill down to the level of the individual to target specific needs.

- **Setting training (or development) objectives** – as with all objectives these should have clear, specific, measurable targets in relation to the standard of behaviour required in order to achieve a given level of performance.

- **Planning the training (or development)** – this covers who provides the training, where the training takes place and divisions of responsibilities between trainers, line managers or team leaders and the individual personally.

- **Delivering/implementing the training (or development)** – a combination of formal and on-the-job training programmes will be used.

- **Evaluating training (or development)** – assessment of cost versus benefit using feedback forms, end of course tests, assessment of improved performance in the work place and impact on corporate goals.

Evaluating the training (or development)

To ensure training and development are effective, learning processes need to be evaluated (stage 5).

Donald Kirkpatrick suggested a four level model of evaluation.

Level	Evaluation	Description	Examples
1	Reaction	How the delegates felt about the training or learning experience	• Feedback forms • Interviews
2	Learning	The measurement of the increase in knowledge – before and after	• Assessment tests before and after • Interviews • Observation
3	Behaviour	The extent of applied learning back on the job - implementation.	• Observation and interview over time
4	Results	The effect on the business or environment by the trainee.	• Impact on existing KPIs

The evaluation should be completed by line managers in conjunction with the delegates themselves. Once completed, collated 'results' need to be interpreted by HR professionals and/or line managers to inform future decisions.

2.5 Performance management

Introduction

 Performance management is used to assess and ensure that the employee is carrying out their duties which they are employed to do in an effective and satisfactory manner, which is contributing to the overall objectives of the organisation.

Organisations follow four main steps when managing the performance of employees:

- **Set targets** – at the start of the period, the manager and employee should agree on which SMART goals and targets the employee is going to work towards.

Setting targets

The targets usually include:

- Areas that the employee needs to improve (perhaps where the employee is currently making mistakes)

- Targets that link in to the overall business goals (such as increasing activity by five percent)

- Development and training targets that will benefit the employee (and the business) and therefore increase motivation.

It is important that employees understand and agree to these targets. If they do not 'buy into' them, they will not put any effort in to accomplishing the goals set – especially if they do not feel that the targets are achievable. This can lead to demotivation.

- **Monitor** – during the period, the manager should monitor employee performance and provide regular feedback. Managers can offer rewards for good performance and support and help where it looks as though the employee is failing to meet their targets.

- **Review** – at the end of the period, the manager and employee will usually have a formal appraisal where they discuss the employee's performance and investigate how successful the employee has been at meeting the pre-agreed targets (appraisal is discussed in more detail below).

- **Action plan** – the manager and employee then agree on new targets that will be set for the coming period.

Appraisal

 Appraisal is the systematic review and assessment of an employee's performance, potential and training needs.

Illustration 5 – Appraisal

Karl works for a call centre and is set targets for the number of calls he takes in the year, the number of customers who say they were satisfied with his performance and the number of complaints he receives in the year.

At the end of the year, the appraisal will allow both Karl and his manager to compare his actual performance against these targets. Any areas where he deviates from the targets (in either a positive or negative way) can be discussed and are likely to form the basis of Karl's annual bonus and pay rise for next year.

Any areas that Karl is struggling with, or would like to gain additional skills and knowledge in, can be used to identify training and development opportunities for the coming year.

Finally, the appraisal can then be used to agree what Karl's targets will be for next year.

Test your understanding 9

Which of the following is an objective of the appraisal process to an employer?

A   It enables them to identify underperforming employees for punishment

B   It helps the business to recruit the best possible employees

C   It helps to identify employees' skills gaps

D   It reinforces management authority over employees

If not handled carefully, appraisals can cause demotivation for employees. Various studies have indicated that criticism of employees can have a negative effect on their goal achievement and self-confidence.

Lockett suggested that there are six main barriers to effective appraisals.

Barrier	Example
Confrontation	• Feedback is badly delivered. • Differing views regarding performance.
Judgement	• Appraisal is seen as a one-sided process – the manager is judge, jury and counsel for the prosecution.
Chat	• Lack of will from either party. • No outcomes set.
Bureaucracy	• Purely a 'form filling exercise'. • No purpose or worth.
Annual event	• A traditional ceremony carried out once or twice a year.
Unfinished business	• No follow up. • Points agreed not actioned.

2.6 The role of incentives and practices relating to motivation

Introduction

 In an organisation, **motivation** refers to the willingness of individuals to perform certain tasks or actions. It is the incentive or reason for them behaving in a particular way.

In practice, motivation is taken as meaning how hard an employee is willing to work in their job. It goes beyond employees merely following rules and orders and looks at how **dedicated** they are.

> **Test your understanding 10**
>
> **What are the benefits for:**
>
> • the organisation
>
> • the individual employee and
>
> • the teams they work in
>
> **of having motivated staff members?**

As there are so many advantages to having motivated workers, motivation is a key issue for most organisations.

Unfortunately, motivation is difficult to measure directly, meaning that managers have to look at other factors that may indicate the level of motivation within the organisation, often including staff turnover or productivity levels.

However, remember that these factors could also be caused by issues other than employee motivation. For instance, low productivity could be caused by poor working practices within the organisation, rather than unhappy staff.

Illustration 6 – Maslow's hierarchy of needs

A well know theory of motivation is Maslow's hierarchy of needs.

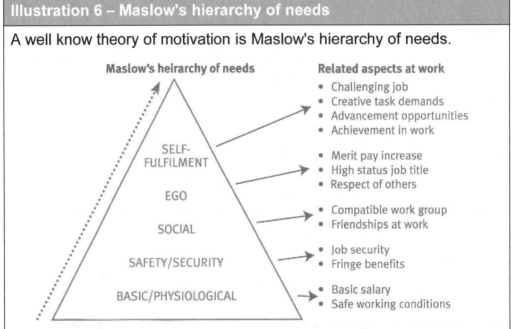

Maslow stated that people's wants and needs follow a hierarchy. As employees become progressively more highly paid, monetary rewards become less important as other needs such as recognition and an ability to achieve one's potential become more important.

There are a number of different incentives and practices that can be used to assist in the motivation of employees. The role of the **psychological contract**, **employee involvement** and the use of **workforce flexibility** will be discussed below. The use of an appropriate **reward system** will be discussed separately in section 2.7.

The psychological contract

 The psychological contract outlines the perceptions of the employee and the employer regarding what their mutual obligations are towards each other.

Unlike the employment contract, the psychological contract is highly subjective, not written down and not legally binding.

Key elements include the following:

	Employee	Employer
What do they want?	Want their needs to be satisfied	Want employee to work hard. Will have a set of expectations for each employee
What are they willing to give?	Will offer their energies and talents	Payment, benefits and other outcomes, e.g. a promotion

In order for managers to **motivate** and retain employees, they must understand the importance of the psychological contract and fulfil their side of the bargain.

Illustration 7

Kate has worked as a trainee accountant with the same company for the past two years. She is ambitious and enjoys her work. Her manager asks her to produce a report that is outside of her normal role.

The report turns out to be difficult and time consuming and she has to put in long hours to complete the report on time as well as carrying out her normal work.

She meets the deadline and sends the report to her manager. However, she receives no acknowledgement. The next day she finds out that her manager has successfully presented the findings of the report to his boss and has taken the credit for the report.

Kate is angry and has decided that she will never do any extra work for her boss again and has even started looking for another job due to the breach of her psychological contract.

Employee involvement

Employees should be empowered to contribute to the organisation. Relying on all employees for their ideas, intelligence and commitment to make the organisation successful should increase employee motivation and have positive financial benefits for the business.

Illustration 8 – Talent management at Apple

Apple's amazing product success is, in part, due to their (sometimes unusual) approach to talent management.

- Apple has an ability to move into and dominate completely unrelated industries. This is only possible because of extraordinary talent, the way it manages it and the creation of a culture that after succeeding in one task, employees will immediately move onto something different.

- A lean talent management approach enables Apple to achieve exceptional levels of employee productivity. Tight deadlines and lean schedules force everyone to work together and solve problems early on.

- The rewards and recognition programme is extremely attractive creating a performance culture and an element of internal competition.

- Rather than a work/life balance, Apple makes it clear that it is looking for extremely hard-working and committed individuals; the idea being that the satisfaction and reward achieved by the employee for their hard work is huge.

Illustration 9 – Employee empowerment and quality

Quality in operations management was discussed in Chapter 9. Many of the quality practices rely on the empowerment of employees. For example:

- In **TQM,** employees are expected to seek out, identify and correct quality problems and are responsible for achieving targets.

- With **Kaizen,** employees are encouraged to come up with small improvement suggestions on a regular basis.

- A **lean** culture will require a multi-skilled and flexible workforce.

- Highly skilled and well trained staff will be required for effective operation of a **JIT** system.

Workforce flexibility

- **Flexible working arrangements** – these can be used to increase employee motivation. Flexibility in work patterns can be achieved in many ways:

Type of flexible working arrangement	Explanation
Remote working/teleworking	Technology has enabled employees to work away from the office, usually at home
Flexitime	The need to work a standard set of hours but less restriction on when these hours are worked
Shift system	Working outside of normal working day patterns
Compressed week	Standard hours within fewer days in a shift rotation
Job sharing	Two employees share a standard hour week
Part-time	Fewer hours than the standard weekly number

Flexible working arrangements encompass one type of flexibility within organisations. Other types of flexibility are:

- **Task or functional flexibility** – employees have the ability to move between tasks as and when is required. This will allow an organisation to react to changes in production requirements and levels of demand and should result in better skilled and motivated employees.

- **Financial flexibility** – this is achieved through variable systems of rewards, for example bonus schemes or profit sharing. By linking rewards to performance, a number of improvements in performance should be realised.

2.7 Reward systems

A reward system refers to all the monetary, non-monetary and psychological payments that an organisation provides for its employees in exchange for the work they perform.

The aims of a reward system

Reward is not simply a benefit for the employee and a cost for the employer. Rather it is a fundamental aspect of HRM:

- It should support the overall strategy.
- It is a vital part of the psychological contract being adhered to.
- It influences the success of recruitment and retention policies.
- It must conform to relevant laws and regulations.
- It must be affordable.
- It affects motivation and performance management and should be managed accordingly.
- It must be administered efficiently and correctly.

Methods of reward

Rewards can be divided into three categories:

- **Basic pay** – this is the minimum amount that the employee receives for working in the organisation. It can be determined in a number of ways, such as an hourly rate or an annual salary.

- **Performance-related pay** – pay is based on the level of performance. Rewards may be based on individual, group or organisational performance, all of which aim to motivate employees to work harder. SMART objectives should be set for employees so that it is clear the level of performance they are trying to achieve.

Illustration 10 – Types of performance-related pay

There are a number of different types of performance-related pay:

- **Individual performance-related pay** – a pay rise or bonus is given to an employee on achievement of pre-agreed objectives or based on the assessment by a manager (as part of their appraisal). Advantages include the ability to align individual objectives with organisational goals and the controllability of rewards by the employee. However, such schemes may result in a lack of teamwork and in tunnel vision (sole concentration on areas which are measured and rewarded).

- **Group performance-related pay** – rewards are based on the achievement of group targets. Encourages teamwork but may not be seen as fair by employees.

- **Knowledge contingent pay** – for example, an accountant may receive a bonus or pay rise on passing their CIMA exams.

- **Profit-related pay** – part of the employee's remuneration is linked to organisational profit. Can motivate employees to increase company profit and increase loyalty but may lead to short termism and lack of motivation if employees feel they have no control over organisational profit.

- **Share options** – they are often given to senior managers and should motivate them to increase share price. However, there is an argument that many of the factors that influence share price will be outside of the manager's control or that (previously risk averse) managers could be tempted to take risks in the hope of increasing the share price.

- **Commission** – normally used for sales staff and is based on a percentage of their sales. Can motivate staff but may lead to short termism and manipulation of results.

- **Piecework schemes** – a price is paid for each unit of output.

> • **Benefits** – a wide range of rewards other than wages or pensions, such as company cars or health insurance. These can provide additional incentives at a lower cost and can be designed in a flexible way to suit the individual employee.

3 Areas of interface between HR and finance

3.1 Introduction

In Chapters 9 and 10 we discussed the interaction between the operations function/sales and marketing function and finance. Much of the discussion below overlaps with what has already been said in that finance, as a trusted advisor, should collaborate with the other function to achieve organisational goals and their own individual functional goals.

3.2 Interaction between HR and finance

- **Traditionally**, the HR function and the finance function worked independently:

  - Finance very much viewed people as a cost whereas HR viewed people as an asset.

  - Collaboration between the functions was limited to, for example, establishing a budget for a reward programme.

- The **modern** approach is to view people as one of the greatest assets an organisation has. Finance and HR need to work more closely with the 'people as assets' as their focus.

> ### Illustration 11 – Interaction between HR and finance
>
> Fulfilling these responsibilities will require data analysis and financial projections from the finance function. For example, an increase in salary, bonus payments or benefits will result in an increased cost for the organisation but this cost needs to be considered in the context of the increased benefit to the organisation due to, say, increased motivation and productivity and reduced staff turnover. The finance function can provide this '**information**' and can then use it for '**insight**', '**influence**' and '**impact**'.

Illustration 12 – AI to replace doctors?

In the past, doctors were viewed as one of the greatest assets in the medical world, with highly prized training, skills and experience. However, there is a view that even in organisations that have previously viewed their employees as their key asset, technology will be able to replace many of the roles they previously carried out.

One example of this technology is the use of artificial intelligence (AI) systems in medicine. AI systems stimulate human intelligence by learning, reasoning and self-correction. Already this technology shows potential to be more accurate than doctors at making diagnoses in specialist areas such as radiology and intensive care and at performing surgery.

Having said that, it is still widely thought that machines will never be able to replicate the inter-relational quality of the therapeutic nature of the doctor-patient relationship and that doctors will still be viewed as the greatest asset in the treatment of patients.

- Technology is freeing both functions from day-to-day duties in their respective fields. This combined with the increasingly competitive and fast changing global environment is leading to the functions having an increased role in the strategic direction of the organisation and an opportunity to work in a more joined-up way.

- Both functions will have overlapping responsibilities. For example, they must consider:

  - The cost and benefit of recruiting and selecting new employees

  - The impact of HR policies, such as reward policies, on the profitability of the business.

Test your understanding 11

Which of the following is an example of co-ordination between HR and the finance function?

A   Establishing credit terms

B   Determining sales prices

C   Allocating costs

D   Calculating reward packages

3.3 How technology is helping this interaction

- New technology has resulted in better joined up systems creating better information.

- Some examples of this technology usage are illustrated below.

Illustration 13 – How the cloud is fuelling this collaboration

Sharing a finance and HR cloud system, integrating enterprise resource planning and human capital management systems will:

* Make it quicker and easier to track and to forecast key HR information

* Will aid collaboration to make effective decisions that will help achieve functional and organisational objectives.

Illustration 14 – Analytics technology fuelling better collaboration

Advances in analytics technology have helped in quantifying different HR activities or to measure the impact of a HR programme.

By demonstrating the value of investing in different HR activities, through measures such as employee satisfaction scores, HR and finance can work together to ensure they have the right information for responsible decision-making.

4 Key performance indicators (KPIs)

4.1 Introduction

In section 6 of Chapter 9 we:

* defined KPIs

* discussed their use in managing the operations function

* identified relevant KPIs for operations

* discussed how the finance function manages operations using KPIs and

* discussed the impact of technology in this area.

Much of this discussion can also be applied to the HR function and can therefore be referred back to.

In this section we will briefly discuss how the finance function helps to manage the HR function through the use of KPIs before identifying some relevant KPIs for HR.

4.2 How finance helps to manage HR using KPIs

Let's begin by recapping our discussion from Chapter 10 but this time in the context of the HR function.

* The HR function will identify its relevant CSFs.

* The KPIs are the measures that indicate whether or not the HR function is achieving these CSFs.

- The finance function works with the HR function to:

  - **identify** appropriate KPIs

  - **assemble** KPI data and information

  - **analyse** this for insight

  - give **advice** to the HR function based on this insight and

  - **apply** what has been learned to impact the achievement of the objectives of the HR function and the organisation as a whole.

- **Technology** will act as a key enabler in this, particularly in the 'assembly' and 'analysis' tasks.

Illustration 15 – KPI dashboards

As discussed in Chapter 10, one of the most common technologies used in this area is performance dashboards. The dashboard displays the KPIs of the HR function in a live format, thus allowing immediate, visual understanding of current performance and potentially prompting action to correct or amend performance accordingly.

Separate dashboards may be used for areas such as:

- The recruitment and selection process – identifying bottlenecks and opportunities in the hiring process; in order to improve efficiency, reduce lost revenue and minimise costs

- Rewards – ensuring the system is fair (for example, females are not at a disadvantage compared to males) and competitive (for example, by benchmarking against competitor salaries)

- Employee turnover rate – to help prevent valued employees leaving the business and to minimise hiring and training costs.

Note: It would be useful to spend a few minutes looking at examples of HR dashboard images on the internet.

4.3 Examples of KPIs for HR

Example activity	Possible KPIs
Recruitment and selection	Cost per employee hired
	Selection method conversion rate
	Time to fill a position
	Female to male ratio
Training and development	Training and development costs
	Impact of training on existing KPIs
	Training feedback

Performance management	Appraisals completed on time
	Appraisal action plan agree and followed up
Motivation	Turnover rate
	Employee absenteeism
	Employee productivity
	Employee satisfaction scores
	Flexible working arrangements offered
Reward systems	Cost of rewards
	Competitiveness of reward system
	Adherence to laws and regulations

Test your understanding 12

Match the following CSFs of the HR function to the most appropriate KPI.

CSF	KPI
Diversity of workforce	Employee turnover
Motivated workforce	Training and development costs
Fair remuneration	Female to male ratio
Efficient recruitment process	Competitiveness of reward system
Suitably skilled workforce	Time to fill a position

Test your understanding 13

Fernando is constructing some KPIs to measure whether or not the firm's HR CSFs are being met. He has been told that these KPIs should be SMART.

Which of the SMART criteria is not being met in the following KPI?

KPI: 90% of all staff appraisals to be completed by the end of January each year (last year 50% of appraisals were completed by the end of January).

A   Specific

B   Measurable

C   Achievable

D   Relevant

E   Time bound

Test your understanding 14 – KPI Case Study Question

Pop Up Limited

Pop Up Limited (PUL) is a business that provides a platform for pop up shops to run themselves a little more efficiently. Many pop-up shops have virtually no management experience and so 'fly by the seat of their pants a little', making mistakes along the way.

PUL provides an accounting system linked to a point-of-sale (POS) system along with the necessary equipment to record transactions. It also provides a performance management system to ensure that the staff have a clearer idea what is expected of them from the start.

PUL ask owners to complete an on line form and questionnaire and from that, the basic understanding of the business is gleaned. Key performance targets are then generated and allocated to all staff members taking into account their individual roles. It is common that each staff member be allocated one KPI and the system will measure against this KPI every day, reporting to the owner accordingly.

Required:

Identify and explain three errors of the KPI setting process outlined above.

(15 marks)

5 Chapter summary

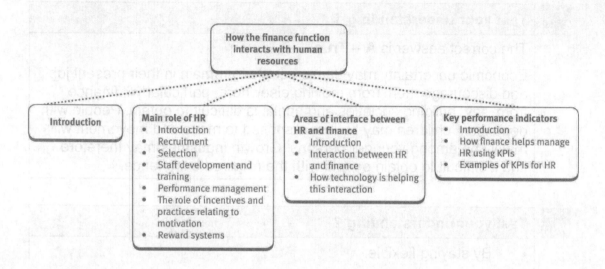

How the finance function interacts with human resources

Introduction

Main role of HR
- Introduction
- Recruitment
- Selection
- Staff development and training
- Performance management
- The role of incentives and practices relating to motivation
- Reward systems

Areas of interface between HR and finance
- Introduction
- Interaction between HR and finance
- How technology is helping this interaction

Key performance indicators
- Introduction
- How finance helps manage HR using KPIs
- Examples of KPIs for HR

Test your understanding answers

Test your understanding 1

The correct answer is **A – True**

Economic uncertainty may cause people to remain in their present job and discourage them from moving elsewhere, particularly if finance from, say, building societies and banks is difficult to obtain. People with dependent children may be less disposed to move and movement will mainly be among younger persons. Growth industries may therefore find it difficult to obtain people with the required experience.

Test your understanding 2

- By staying flexible.
- By taking greater account of external factors.
- By more sophisticated monitoring and control mechanisms.
- By planning in shorter time frames.

Problems in achieving plans might to a degree be predictable and in the past have also centred on:

- Retention, especially when employees are well trained or have specialist skills
- Slow promotion leading to staff turnover
- Unexpected vacancies arising in senior positions or vital skills areas.

Test your understanding 3

- Finance Director required **(job title)**.
- At least five years post qualified experience **(special requirements)**.
- Experience of a dynamic industry **(special requirements)**.
- Understanding of investor relations and pre-flotation requirements **(special requirements)**.
- Ability to manage change and form own department **(special requirements)**.

- Role includes **(brief description of role)**:
  - Planning, monitoring and control of business and financial strategy.
  - Reporting and accounting as per the legal requirements.
  - Management of strategy for and liaison with stock market business press and the business analyst community.

- Excellent package including competitive salary and share options **(remuneration)**.

- Responsible for a growing team of 18 people **(number of staff directly supervised)**.

- Report directly to the Managing Director **(responsible to)**.

- Located in London with approximately 20% travel to other European locations **(location and special attributes, for example, shift systems, willingness to travel)**.

Test your understanding 4

The correct answer is **C**

Test your understanding 5

Discrimination may be acceptable in certain circumstances, for example:

- Army soldiers must be fit, healthy and be able to carry heavy kit.

- Firemen must be a certain height so that they can reach the equipment.

- An Italian restaurant can choose to recruit only Italian waiters and waitresses.

Test your understanding 6

(a)

Advantages of the interview technique	Disadvantages of the interview technique
• Places candidate at ease. • Highly interactive, allowing flexible question and answers. • Opportunities to use non-verbal communication.	• Too brief to 'get to know' candidates. • Interview is an artificial situation. • Halo effect from initial impression.

• Opportunities to assess appearance, interpersonal and communication skills. • Opportunities to evaluate rapport between the candidate and the potential colleagues/bosses.	• Qualitative factors such as motivation, honesty or integrity are difficult to assess. • Prejudice – stereotyping groups of people. • Lack of interviewer preparation, skill, training and practice. • Subjectivity and bias.

(b)

Interview option	Advantage	Disadvantage
Face-to-face by one person	Good for establishing rapport between interviewer and candidate	Can be subject to bias
Group	A good opportunity to compare candidates	One candidate may dominate
Succession	Allows for a range of opinions about the candidate	Opinions about the candidate may vary and conflict
Panel	Allows comparison of the candidate in real time	May be more suited to confident candidates
Problem solving	Good for identifying relevant problem-solving skills	May be more suited to confident candidates
Stress	Good for judging how the candidate reacts under stress	Putting excessive stress on an individual may be considered unethical

Test your understanding 7

The correct answer is **D**

Test your understanding 8

The benefits for the learner and the organisation include:

For the individual:

- Improved skills and (dependent on the type of training) qualifications

- Increased confidence and job satisfaction.

For the organisation:

- Increased motivation of employees, leading to higher productivity

- Increased competence and confidence, meaning higher quality and fewer mistakes

- Low staff turnover, saving the organisation time and money

- Skilled workforce, leading to more innovation and a better customer experience.

Test your understanding 9

The correct answer is **C**

The appraisal process is certainly not designed to find employees that need to be punished and only applies to existing employees, meaning that it will not help the organisation with its recruitment. It is also designed to improve communication between managers and employees, not reinforce the differences between them.

Test your understanding 10

Having motivated staff members has a range of benefits – from the perspectives of both the organisation and the individuals or teams themselves. These include:

Organisation perspective	Individual perspective	Team perspective
Harder working employees	Greater job satisfaction	Increased co-operation
Fewer mistakes and errors	Improved health, due to less stress	More commitment to team needs
Less waste of time and resources	Improved career prospects	Better ideas generation and evaluation

More suggestions and ideas generated	Finding the job more interesting and enjoyable	
Increased job satisfaction and therefore lower staff turnover		
More customer satisfaction due to better service from staff		

Test your understanding 11

The answer is **D, calculating the rewards package**

Test your understanding 12

The CSFs should be matched to the KPIs as follows:

CSF	KPI
Diversity of workforce	Female to male ratio
Motivated workforce	Employee turnover
Fair remuneration	Competitiveness of reward system
Efficient recruitment process	Time to fill a position
Suitably skilled workforce	Training and development costs

Test your understanding 13

The answer is **Achievable**. It will be very difficult to increase this completion rate by 40%.

Test your understanding 14 – KPI Case Study Question

The PUL system has a number of flaws and only three are required:

Lack of discussion

It is sensible that KPIs are discussed with staff members in advance, but this is not the case here. This discussion would flush out practical problems that might exist and would ensure the employee fully understood what was expected of them. It is generally accepted that discussion and agreement prevent dictated standards. Employees will often buy in to targets more readily if they feel that they have had an input to them. This is clearly not the case here.

Incorrect level of difficulty

Equally, without due discussion, the level of difficulty set for the KPI could be wildly wrong. Setting a target that is too difficult can demotivate an employee meaning that they resent the target (and the employer who set it) and underperform. There is plenty of evidence to suggest that the level of output achieved is sub-optimal in this situation.

Equally the level of target could be too easy. Whilst this is then easily achieved an employee will often have a lack of respect for the setter as they will think of them a fool to set such an easy target. They may even feel patronised. As above, the output actually achieved will be suboptimal in most cases as the employee stops pushing once the target is reached.

Single KPI

Setting only one KPI keeps things simple and this may well have been the intention. However, single KPIs are notoriously easy to manipulate. Suppose a target is simply to make more sales volume. A staff member could quickly realise that this is achievable by deep discounting prices. This will destroy margin. Without a second KPI, perhaps on price level or margin achieved the consequences of a volume only target could be dire.

Unfairness between different members of staff

There is no evidence that the targets set are compared in terms of level of difficulty from one staff member to another. Resentment can quickly fester if a staff member feels unfairly treated.

12

How the finance function interacts with IT

Chapter learning objectives

Lead	Component
E4: Describe how the finance function interacts with IT.	Describe:
	(a) Main role of IT
	(b) Areas of interface with finance
	(c) Key performance indicators

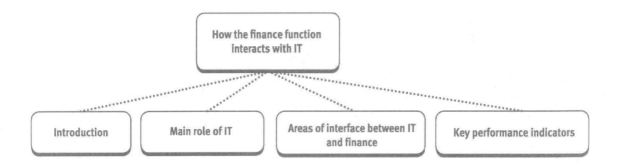

1 Introduction

In this chapter we will complete our discussion of how the finance function plays its role by interacting with the rest of the organisation (syllabus area E) and, more specifically here, the organisation's information technology (IT) function.

We will begin by discussing the main role of the IT function; understanding how IT systems can be used to support the rest of the organisation, how these systems can be best organised and managed and the costs and benefits of information systems.

We will then discuss the areas of interface with finance before moving on to the final part of the chapter which will discuss how the finance function helps to manage the IT function through the use of key performance indicators (KPIs).

2 Main role of IT

2.1 IT systems support

The role of information systems in organisations

Organisations need information systems to enable them to capture and generate the information that managers need for **planning, control** and **decision-making**.

The hunger for information has never been greater than for today's organisations, likewise the value of information systems that deliver this information has never been so keenly felt. It follows that information technology (IT) and information systems (IS) assume increasing managerial importance within the modern organisation.

As has been discussed in earlier chapters, IT is becoming a strategic weapon which many organisations are using to improve their competitive position. This can come in many forms. For example, using IT can improve efficiency and reduce costs in order to compete better, it can help the organisation react more quickly to the changing environment or it can create new opportunities etc.

Before discussing the role of IT in more detail, it is useful to understand a few key **definitions**.

Information systems (IS) refer to the provision and management of information to support the running of the organisation.

 Information technology (IT) is the supporting equipment (hardware) that provides the infrastructure to run the information systems.

 The **IT function** is responsible for planning, evaluating, installing, operating and maintaining the hardware, software, networks and data centres required by the organisation.

 A **management information system** (**MIS**) converts internal and external data into useful information which is then communicated to managers at all levels and across all functions to enable them to make timely and effective decisions for planning, directing and controlling activities.

There are a number of key types of MIS:

Type of MIS	Explanation
Executive information system (EIS)	An EIS gives senior management access to internal and external information. Information is presented in a flexible, user-friendly, summarised form with the option to 'drill down' to a greater level of detail.
Decision support system (DSS)	A DSS aids managers in making decisions. The system predicts the consequences of a number of possible scenarios and the manager then uses their judgement to make the final decision.
Transaction processing system (TPS)	A TPS is mainly used by operational managers to make decisions. It records all the daily transactions (for example, payroll or purchases) of an organisation and summarises them so they can be reported on a routine basis.
Expert system	Expert systems hold specialist knowledge, for example on law and taxation, and allow non-experts to interrogate them for information, advice and recommended decisions. Can be used at all levels of management.

Illustration 1 – EIS

A typical report from an EIS would combine many types of data on the same screen and make it easier for senior management to understand the performance of the business.

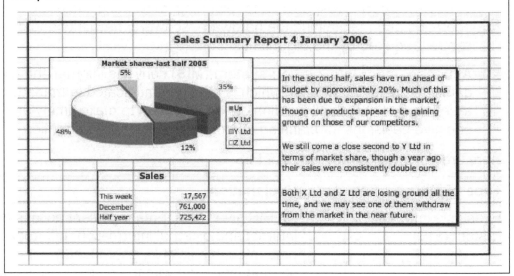

Illustration 2 – DSS

A supermarket chain is planning to start selling its goods online, but is uncertain of whether it is appropriate for the organisation.

A DSS would gather information about the company itself – does it have the resources to start selling online?

It will also provide information about the online groceries market, such as the size of the market and who the competitors are.

The DSS will then present this information in a way that is easy to understand, helping the management to make the decision.

Illustration 3 – Expert systems

An accountant could use an expert system (ES) to calculate a client's personal tax liability.

The accountant will input the relevant information about the client's circumstances. The ES will then access its database of rules and regulations about personal tax, decide which rules apply to the client and then use them to calculate a tax liability.

How IT enables knowledge management between the functions

In Chapter 7 we discussed how:

- The finance function can use data and information to assist sales and marketing to better understand customers and to develop customer value proposition

- The finance function can use data and information to assist operations in enhancing operational efficiency

- The finance function can partner with other areas of the organisation to create value from digital assets.

As part of this discussion, we covered some really good and relevant examples of how IT enables knowledge management between functions.

Here we will look more specifically at knowledge management systems and how these enable knowledge management between the functions.

Knowledge is an important organisational resource. There is a difference between:

- **Data** – raw facts

- **Information** – processed, organised data

- **Knowledge** – an application of a cognitive process to the information so that it becomes useful.

There are two broad types of knowledge:

- **Explicit knowledge** – is knowledge that the company knows it has, for example customer information.

- **Tacit knowledge** – is personal knowledge and expertise held by people within the organisation that has not been formally documented, for example knowledge gained through the experiences of employees within the organisation.

Knowledge management is the process for the acquisition, sharing, retention and utilisation of knowledge.

In, what is increasingly referred to as a knowledge-based economy, it is evident that sufficient management attention should be given to this valuable organisational asset.

Organisations hold a huge volume and variety of information in different systems and people and therefore a knowledge management strategy is needed to unlock the value of this asset and improve organisational performance.

An important part of this strategy will involve a technology-based solution (a knowledge management system).

Knowledge management systems refer to any type of IT that helps to capture, store, retrieve and use knowledge to enhance the knowledge management process.

Examples include:

- Groupware – refers to technology designed to help people collaborate. Examples include email, file sharing technology and video/audio conferencing.

- Intranets – a private network within the organisation allowing the sharing of information and resources with employees.

- Extranets – an extension of an intranet to include suppliers, customers and other business partners.

- Data warehouses and data mining.

- Decision support systems (DSS).

- Content management systems – these make it easier to create content (for example, using templates), to edit content, to track changes allowing for version control and allow for collaborative and parallel work on content.

- Document management systems – often part of a content management system. They assist with, for example, the indexing and retrieval of documents.

It is important to note that although technology is an important part of knowledge management, it may simply increase the volume and management of unfocused data and analysed information if **appropriate people skills and organisational processes focused on the conversion of this data/information into knowledge are not established**.

Test your understanding 1
The best working definition of information from the options below would be:
A   Facts you can work with
B   Facts
C   Facts useful to the operations manager
D   Facts useful to the decision maker

2.2 IT infrastructure

Introduction

 IT infrastructure consists of the core networks, databases, software, hardware and procedures managed by the IT function.

The modernisation of IT infrastructure is necessary to take advantage of innovations such as data visualisation, AI and blockchain, which will all require the analysis of huge amounts of data.

In this section, we will discuss the ways of organising and managing IS in the context of the wider organisation including:

- The emergence of new technology
- Enabling transformation
- Geographically dispersed teams
- Enhancing internal and external relationships
- Ethical and social issues with IS and data.

Each of these will be explored in turn.

The emergence of new technology

Advancements in technology (as discussed in Chapter 5) are allowing organisations to do much more than they have in the past. However, many organisations are struggling with the pace of change, constantly having to react rather than lead with technological innovation.

There are a number of factors that influence the extent and the pace of technology adoption by organisations. These include:

- Technical feasibility
- The cost of developing, implementing and maintaining the new technology
- The economic benefits of the new technology
- The availability of labour skills to implement and use the new technology
- Regulatory and social acceptance.

By implementing an up to date and flexible IT infrastructure, the organisation can manage many of these factors – enabling technical feasibility, minimising costs and maximising the economic benefit and having the appropriate labour skills present – thus allowing them to embrace new technology and the opportunities it presents.

Enabling transformation

Technology is no longer viewed mainly as a vehicle for improved productivity but is seen as a key component of business transformation.

Illustration 4 – Cloud technology

The cloud is one transformational technology of IT infrastructure. Previously, organisations that wanted to increase their capability would have had to invest in new equipment which was time consuming and expensive.

Organisations are at different stages of their digital transformation but having a good IT infrastructure in place can enable organisational transformation in a huge variety of ways, such as:

- The adoption of new ways of working across the **business** and the **industry**.

Illustration 5 – BPR

BPR enabling new ways of working across the business

A company manufactures high quality women's clothing in its factory. The company is organised into traditional functional departments most of which have their own unreliable spreadsheet-based systems for planning and reporting. As a result, the company often fails to produce accurate, timely and consistent data to monitor its own performance, which contributes to failures in achieving the performance targets set by its retail customers.

The market is highly competitive. Retailers, who are the company's customers, have two key demands: they want lower prices to pass on to consumers and they also require suppliers to meet performance targets relating to lead times and quality.

To help them comply with the retailers' demands, the company have decided to use BPR to re-engineer the production process. It will close down all of their own manufacturing facilities and outsource all production to overseas suppliers, who have much larger factories and lower costs.

IT will act as a key enabler in this re-engineering. To mitigate the cost of shipping goods over long distances, the company have invested in sophisticated software to consolidate orders so that each shipping container is completely full before despatch from their suppliers. Purchase invoice processing will also be automated by the integration of information systems into the suppliers' bespoke systems.

The changes will mean that staff from the company's functional departments will reorganise into multi-disciplinary teams, each serving major customer accounts. Each team will perform all aspects of account management from taking sales orders and procurement through to arranging shipping and after sales service.

Illustration 6 – Disruptive technology

Disruptive technology and new ways of working across the hospitality industry

Airbnb, which was founded in 2008, is an online website. It allows hosts to post their homes on the site for short-term rent. Airbnb do not own the homes, it just acts as a broker and takes commission on every property that is rented. Innovative technology has been used, such as the use of cloud-based platforms to collect payments and the incorporation of the latest technology to allow hosts to set the optimum price for their accommodation.

Earlier, it was only focusing on low-value customers, but eventually, it started focusing on high value customers as well. Renters can select homes or apartments on the basis of location and the money they want to pay. Airbnb is tough competition to the hotels and other accommodation providers in the hospitality industry who are not able to match Airbnb on price, household comforts and the local experience offered.

- Productivity improvements

Illustration 7 – Technology improving farming productivity

In the United Kingdom, farm subsidies keep farmers' incomes from sagging but there is a real need for direct application of digital and other technologies to increase farm productivity and address increasingly visible climate change impacts. Some examples of how technology can be used to improve farm productivity include:

- Geographic information systems for agricultural mapping enabling better management of soil and irrigation.

- Digital technology can guide crop and input selection, provide weather, disease and pest-related advice, and real-time data on domestic and export markets.

- Multi-source data capture and analysis

Illustration 8 – Big data analytics use by supermarkets

In Chapter 5, we discussed big data and data analytics:

- Big data describes data sets so large and varied they are beyond the capability of traditional data-processing.

- Data analytics is the process of collecting, organising and analysing large sets of data to discover patterns and other information which an organisation can use for future decisions.

A supermarket can analyse this multi-source big data to improve its targeting of customers:

For example, a supermarket is able to take data from your past buying patterns, its internal inventory information, your mobile phone location data, social media as well as weather information to send you a voucher for barbeque food; but only if you own a barbeque, the weather is nice, you are within 3 miles of one of their stores and the barbeque food is in stock.

- The creation of shared service capability – shared service centres were discussed in Chapter 3. Globalisation and **technological advances** have meant that much of the routine processing of the organisation's functions (for example, the finance function) could be carried out by a shared service centre (i.e. the centralisation of this routine processing into one place).

- Digitisation of information

Illustration 9 – Digitisation within the NHS

The National Health Service (NHS) provides healthcare for all citizens in the United Kingdom. It is the fifth largest employer in the world. The government has committed billions of pounds to creating a 'paperless' NHS, recognising that making the best use of IT will deliver huge benefits and improved outcomes for patients.

Digitisation is planned across the whole NHS, for example:

- The creation of electronic records for all patients (so patients will no longer have to repeat their medical history)

- The creation of online booking and prescription ordering services

- Access to healthcare apps for patients (for example, allowing patients to send real-time data to their healthcare providers on long-term conditions such as high blood pressure or diabetes)

- Options for patients to choose to speak to a doctor online or via video link.

However, digitisation is a huge challenge due to antiquated systems, the vast scale of the task and insufficient funding. However, although the modernisation is fraught with difficulty, it continues to make progress in an attempt to move the NHS forward.

- Flexible working practices (see discussion below)
- Virtual organisations (see discussion below).

Geographically dispersed teams

Technology developments have enabled the creation of new ways of working. Two significant changes include an increase in **remote working** (sometimes called homeworking or teleworking) and the formation of **virtual teams**:

- **Remote working** – IT developments (such as email and the internet), have enabled employees to work away from the office (for example, at home). The advantages and disadvantages for the organisation may include:

Advantages	Disadvantages
• Lower infrastructure costs	• Difficulties in co-ordinating staff
• Increased employee motivation and productivity	• Loss of control of staff
• Increased commitment to the organisation	• Dilution of organisational culture
• Attracting individuals because of the availability of such conditions	• Less commitment to the organisation
• Reduced absenteeism and staff turnover	• Extra labour costs, for example providing employees with equipment

Test your understanding 2

Consider your own employment. Would you like or dislike working from home? Discuss the reason for your opinion on this issue.

- **Virtual teams**

  Before discussing virtual teams, it is useful to understand what is meant by a virtual organisation. This is because virtual teams are a key component of a virtual organisation.

  A **virtual organisation** outsources most or all of its functions to other organisations and simply exists as a network of contracts, with very few, if any, functions being kept in-house.

Illustration 10 – Amazon, a virtual company

Many internet companies are examples of networks – Amazon being perhaps one of the best known on-line retailers.

- Amazon operates its website but relies on external suppliers, book publishers, warehouses, couriers and credit card companies to deliver the rest of the customer experience.

- These partners are also expected to provide Amazon with information on, for example, stock availability, delivery times and promotional material.

- The customer feels that they are dealing with one organisation, not many.

Test your understanding 3

Which of the following statements regarding virtual organisations is incorrect?

A   Virtual organisations occur when some or all elements of the organisation's functions are outsourced to third party organisations

B   Information technology is usually a vital requirement for virtual organisations

C   Virtual organisations usually face higher overhead costs

D   Virtual organisations have more flexibility than traditionally structured organisations

As mentioned, virtual teams are a key component of virtual organisations.

A **virtual team** is a group of people who interact through independent tasks guided by a common purpose and work across space, time and organisational boundaries with links strengthened by IT.

They are essentially teams of people who are not present in the same office or organisation.

The following challenges face virtual teams:

Challenge	Explanation
Forming a team	It may be difficult to establish a cohesive and trusting team.
Knowledge sharing	It may prove more difficult due to the absence of face to face contact.
Processes and goals	It may be more difficult to establish clear decision making processes and goals.
Leadership	This may be more difficult since individuals will be working at different times, in different locations and in different ways.
Cultural differences	Team members will be from different backgrounds and cultural differences may make working together more difficult.
Morale	Some team members may find this way of working isolating.

Test your understanding 4

Identify the ways in which the challenges faced by virtual teams can be overcome.

Enhancing internal and external relationships

Information systems provide an opportunity to build stronger relationships with stakeholders and to improve internal efficiency by providing convenient, easy to use, communication channels. For example, intranets and extranets, shared databases (these may utilise the cloud), email and live chat features.

Illustration 11 – Enhancing relationships with customers

One example of a system that can be used to enhance relationships with stakeholders (in this case, customers) is a **customer relationship management (CRM)) system**.

CRM is the process the organisation uses to:

- Identify, attract and win new customers

- Retain existing customers

- Entice past customers back.

CRM systems refer to the technology that is used to gather the information needed to achieve the above (i.e. CRM). CRM systems range from simple spreadsheets and databases containing information about the customer to more complex online applications which are fully integrated with the organisation's other systems. A CRM system may include the following features:

Feature	Benefit
A central database that is accessible by all employees to view and update customer data.	Improved customer service, loyalty and retention.
Analysis of customer data including customer segmentation (existing and potential customers).	Improved marketing campaigns through customised targeting.
Customer web-based ordering.	Reduced order cost and customer service cost.
Identifying and tracking potential customers.	A wider customer base and more focused prospect tracking.
Reports generated with up-to-date information including revenue forecasting and trend analysis.	Better and more timely decision making.

Ethical and social issues with IS and data

In Chapter 6 we discussed how the increased use of technology impacts ethical and social considerations. In the context of IT infrastructure, the organisation must manage its information systems and data with these ethical and social issues in mind, including:

- **Data protection and data privacy** – the amount of personal data available to and used by organisations means that the privacy, sensitivity and security of this data is a very significant consideration in modern business. A business must ensure it is compliant with all legislation but there are also considerations from an ethical and social responsibility point of view in terms of what is right and wrong in the eyes of the public.

Illustration 12 – IT infrastructure and legal, ethical and social issues

An organisation must manage its information systems in the context of the legal, ethical and social issues that exist with IS and data:

Example of an issue	Possible intervention
Legal issue – data may be used or handled in an unlawful way, for example resulting in unauthorised access of data.	In the UK, the organisation's IS must be set up to comply with GDPR principles. This will ensure that the organisation's data is used lawfully. Data controllers within the organisation may be used to ensure that these adequate GDPR safeguards are in place.
Ethical issue – goes beyond legal requirements and considers what is right or wrong for the organisation to do. For example, just because an organisation's IS will allow the collection and analysis of an employee's social media presence, it may not be considered ethical to do so.	Organisations may create a written code of ethics and instruct employees to follow them. In the context of the example given here, it may contain a broad or more specific statement regarding the use of the organisation's IS to monitor an employee's social media presence.
Social issue – an organisation should make choices that are for the best of the society in which it operates (see illustration below).	The IT infrastructure within the organisation should be set up to collect, analyse and share data in an appropriate way. So, for example, a pharmaceutical company may align its systems so that it can easily share data and analysis with university research teams.

Illustration 13 – Social issues

In Chapter 6, we said that pharmaceutical companies may hold huge amounts of data and analysis from clinical trials. It may not make financial sense but from a societal point of view the company should consider donating this data and analysis to, say, universities for research purposes that could benefit society.

For example, in 2014, Johnson and Johnson agreed to give all of its clinical trial data to Yale University to help advance science and medicine.

- **Corporate digital responsibility (CDR)** – as discussed in Chapter 6, CDR is a voluntary commitment by organisations to go beyond mere compliance with legislation, when it comes to how they handle technology and data. The social and ethical issues discussed above will be relevant here. The organisation's IT infrastructure should be aligned to it CDR strategy.

2.3 The costs and benefits of IS

Introduction

When an organisation sees a possibility for introducing a new IS, an evaluation of the new system should be made to decide whether the potential benefits are sufficient to justify the costs.

 Cost-benefit analysis (CBA) can be used to assess the expected costs and benefits of the IS.

The **costs** of a new IS are:

Initial costs	Running costs
• Costs to design and develop system if software is bespoke.	• Cost of labour time to run the system.
• Purchase price of software if it is not bespoke.	• Cost of materials, for example replacement parts.
• Purchase cost of new hardware.	• Cost of service support, for example IT helpdesk.
• Cost of testing and implementation of the new system.	• Other ongoing costs such as the cost of quality or security adherence/failure.
• Training costs.	

The **benefits** of a new IS include:

- Speed – for example, in dealing with repetitive tasks such as data collection and payroll processing.

- Accuracy – the IS should reduce the incidence of human error and better information should be produced.

- Volume – the IS should be able to handle much larger volumes of data, 24 hours per day.

- Complexity – once systems are computerised and integrated, they can generally handle a greater level of complexity than humans.

- Collaboration – the IS can enable collaboration across the organisation due to better access and sharing of real-time information.

- Presentation – the IS may display information in as 'user-friendly' way as possible.

- Lower costs – all of the above benefits mean that IS have become highly cost-effective providers of 'good' information.

The **finance function can assist the IT function** in this cost-benefit analysis.

We will now look more specifically at **the different costs and benefits of information systems** including:

- Privacy and security

- Systems architecture

- Data flows

- Big data information management.

Privacy and security

As discussed already, IS are exposed to privacy and security issues. The organisation must safeguard the privacy and security of data (considering legal, ethical and social factors and a wider sense of CDR) as well as ensuring complete and accurate processing of data.

There are different privacy and security risks that exist, together with solutions as to how the organisation can tackle each risk. Each of the solutions will have an associated **cost** (i.e. to implement the solution) and **benefit** (i.e. mitigation of the risk).

Potential threat	Solution
Natural disasters – for example, fire or flood	• Fire procedures – fire alarms, extinguishers, fire doors, staff training and insurance cover. • Location, for example, not in a basement area liable to flooding.

Chapter 12

Potential threat	Solution
	• Physical environment – for example, air conditioning and dust controls. • Back up procedures – data should be backed up on a regular basis (ideally in real-time) to allow recovery. • Business continuity planning – to decide which systems are critical to the organisation continuing its activities.
Malfunction – of computer hardware or software	• Network design – to cope with periods of high volumes. • Back up procedures and business continuity planning (as above).
Unauthorised access, usage, damage or theft	• Personnel controls – includes segregation of duties, policy on usage and compliance with regulations such as GDPR, hierarchy of access. • Access controls – such as passwords and time lock-outs. • Computer equipment controls – to protect equipment from theft or destruction.
Viruses – a small program that once introduced into the system spreads extensively. Can affect the whole computer system	• Anti-virus software – should be run and updated regularly to prevent corruption of the system by viruses. • Formal security policy and procedures, for example, employees should only download files or open attachments from reputed sources. • Regular audits to check for unauthorised software.

359

Potential threat	Solution
Hackers – deliberate access to systems by unauthorised persons	• Firewall software – should provide protection from unauthorised access to the system from the Internet. • Passwords and user names – limit unauthorised access to the system. • User awareness training and a formal security policy so that employees are aware of the risks that exist and how best to mitigate them. • Data encryption – data is scrambled prior to transmission and is recovered in a readable format once transmission is complete.
Human errors – unintentional errors from using IS	• Training – adequate staff training and operating procedures. • Controls ensuring only valid data is input/processed and that all data is processed.
Human resource risk – for example, repetitive strain injury (RSI), headaches and eye strain from computer screens, tripping over loose wires	• Ergonomic design of workstations should reduce problems such as RSI. • Anti-glare screens reduce eye strain. • Cables should be in ducts.

Illustration 14 – WikiLeaks

WikiLeaks is a not-for-profit organisation created to protect whistle blowers and journalists who have sensitive information to communicate to the public. WikiLeaks has dominated the news because of its steady drip feed of secret documents. For example:

• In 2010, the site released almost 400,000 secret US military logs detailing its operations in Iraq, 90,000 classified military records giving an insight into military strategy in Afghanistan and posted a video on its website showing a US Apache helicopter killing at least 12 people during an attack in Baghdad in 2007.

- In 2016, during the US presidential election, thousands of emails from Hilary Clinton's personal server were published by WikiLeaks. Some proved embarrassing and detracted from her campaign. Many were utilised by her opponent Donald Trump as part of his ultimately successful campaign.

Illustration 15 – Virus infection in the NHS

The NHS (National Health Service) faced a week of chaos after hackers demanding a ransom infiltrated the health service's computer system.

Operations and appointments were cancelled and ambulances diverted as up to 40 hospital trusts became infected by a ransomware (malicious software) attack demanding payments to regain access to vital medical records.

The attack was part of the biggest ransomware attack in history with 57,000 infections in 99 countries being observed.

Systems architecture

 The **systems architecture** is the way the systems infrastructure is organised together to support the organisation's functions and its overall goals.

The development of **network** technology has facilitated the transfer of information between different parts of the business. Organisations connect their computers together in **local area networks** (LANs), enabling them to share data (for example, via email) and devices (such as printers). **Wide area networks** (WANs) are used to connect LANs together, so that computer users in one location can communicate with computers users in another location.

There are **two broad approaches to systems architecture** – a centralised architecture or a decentralised architecture:

 A **centralised** systems architecture is when the whole IT function or the entire IS is based out of a single, central location.

 A **decentralised** systems architecture is when the IT function or the IS is spread out throughout the organisation's location.

The **costs and benefits of a decentralised approach** are as follows:

Costs	Benefits

• Higher costs due to duplication of equipment and effort:
 	
  – analysis, design and implementation of IS
 	
  – data gathering and administration
 	
  – operation, support and maintenance of IS.
 	
• Barriers to sharing data between different parts of the organisation, for example, due to unaligned IS.
 	
• Inconsistent data, for example, one version of the data may be more reliable or up to date.
 	
• Loss of control at a central level may result in common goals not being worked towards.
	• Better ability to meet local needs.
	
	• Fewer staff relying on a single system.
	
	• Less reliance on a few key staff who plan, develop and run the systems.
	
	• Technology tends to be less complex making problems easier to diagnose.
	
	• Security breaches will have less of an impact.
	
	• Efficiencies since time is saved not having to collect information locally, process it and collate it centrally and then feedback down to a local level.

The **costs and benefits of centralised systems architecture are the opposite of those above**.

It is worth noting that an organisation may decide to **outsource IS** – the scope ranging from outsourcing of the development of a single system to total outsourcing when the vast majority of the organisation's IS and IT services and capabilities are outsourced.

Data flows

 Data flow is the movement of data through a process or system. It includes:

- Data inputs (raw data)
- Data processing (turning the raw data into meaningful information)
- Data outputs ('good' information, i.e. accurate, timely, relevant, concise and cost effective, is produced for the user)
- Data storage.

There will be **costs** associated with data flows, i.e. the cost of collecting the data, processing the data, data output costs and the cost of the storage of data (much of this will rely on effective network technology). There will also be an upfront cost for the production of a data flow diagram – this is a model used to map out the entire process of data movement.

However, there are **benefits** of having good data flows in place. As discussed in Chapter 5, understanding the potential value of data and its significance to an organisation presents a real opportunity to gain unique insight which can be used to improve competitive position and potentially gain competitive advantage over rivals.

Big data information management

Big data and data analytics was discussed in previous chapters. Effective big data information management will unlock the potential value of big data but this will also come at a cost to the organisation:

The **benefits**, as discussed in Chapter 7, are:

- Enhanced transparency

- Performance improvement

- Market segmentation and customisation

- Improved decision making

- Possible product innovation

- Effective risk management and control.

Illustration 16 – Big data information management at Netflix

Netflix has over 100 million users worldwide. The company uses information gathered from analysis of viewing habits to inform decisions on which shows to invest in. Analysing past viewing figures and understanding viewer populations and the shows they are likely to watch allows the analysts to predict likely viewing figures before a show has even aired. This can help to determine if the show is a viable investment.

However, there are **costs** associated with big data information management:

- The **cost** of establishing the hardware and software needed. In addition, there will be a need to constantly **update** or **maintain** it in order to achieve competitive advantage.

- There may be **technical difficulties,** and therefore associated costs, with integrating existing data warehousing and, for example, Hadoop systems.

- **Incorrect data** (poor veracity) may result in incorrect conclusions being made. For example, data collected from social media may not be accurate. This wastes times and can result in poor and costly decisions.

- It is important to recognise that just because something can be measured, this does not necessarily mean it should be. There is a risk that **valuable time is spent measuring relationships that have no organisational value**.

- The **security of data** is a major concern in the majority of organisations and if the organisation lacks the resources to manage data then there is likely to be a greater risk of leaks and losses. There can be a risk to the data protection of organisations as they collect a greater range of data from increasingly personal sources (for example, Facebook). Current laws and regulations on the storage of personal information must be complied with to avoid legal action and/or reputational damage. This will all come at a cost.

- The nature of much of the data means that there is a risk that it will become **outdated and irrelevant very quickly** resulting in the need to constantly monitor databases.

- The **availability of skills** to use big data systems, which is compounded by the fact that many of the systems are rapidly developing and support is not always easily and readily available. There is also an increasing need to combine data analysis skills with a deep understanding of the industry being analysed and this need is not always recognised. Recruitment and training of the right staff and provision of competitive remuneration to these staff can prove costly.

3 Areas of interface between IT and finance

3.1 Introduction

In Chapters 9 to 11, we discussed the interaction between the operations function/sales and marketing/HR function and finance. Much of the discussion below overlaps with what has already been discussed, in that finance, as a trusted advisor, should collaborate with the other function to achieve organisational goals and their own individual functional goals.

3.2 Interaction between IT and finance

- **Traditionally**, the IT function and the finance function worked independently:
  - Finance very much viewed IT as a cost whereas the IT function viewed it as an asset
  - Collaboration between the functions was limited to, for example, establishing a budget for a new IT system.

- The **modern** approach is to view IT as one of the greatest assets an organisation has. Given the central role that technology plays in supporting modern business and their finance functions, the finance function and the IT function need to form a productive partnership. Examples of why the two functions need to interact include:
  - **Smarter investment in IT** – whether the business needs to implement a company-wide system or a solution that's for the finance function alone, the expert guidance of the IT function on which technology will help the company achieve its strategic goals and increase competitiveness will be of huge benefit to the finance function.

- **Information security and compliance** – when it comes to data privacy and security, the finance function can work with the IT function on many fronts, including creating access policies and minimising the threat of data theft and loss.

- **Data analytics** – organisations of all sizes are working to find ways to turn their data into actionable business intelligence. The finance function wants to make sure that only the most relevant and accurate data is used for decision making. This requires the business to apply the right combination of technologies, processes and strategies. The IT function is well equipped to lead and shape these activities.

- **Cost-benefit analysis** (as discussed in Section 2.3).

4 Key performance indicators (KPIs)

4.1 Introduction

In section 6 of Chapter 9 we:

- Defined KPIs

- Discussed their use in managing the operations function

- Identified relevant KPIs for operations

- Discussed how the finance function manages operations using KPIs and

- Discussed the impact of technology in this area.

Much of this discussion can also be applied to the IT function and can therefore be referred back to.

In this section we will briefly discuss how the finance function helps to manage the IT function through the use of KPIs before identifying some relevant KPIs for IT.

4.2 How finance helps to manage IT using KPIs

Let's begin by recapping our discussion from Chapter 10 but this time in the context of the IT function.

- The IT function will identify its relevant CSFs.

- The KPIs are the measures that indicate whether or not the IT function is achieving these CSFs.

- The finance function works with the IT function to:
    - **Identify** appropriate KPIs
    - **Assemble** KPI data and information
    - **Analyse** this for insight
    - Give **advice** to the IT function based on this insight and
    - **Apply** what has been learned to impact the achievement of the objectives of the IT function and the organisation as a whole.
- **Technology** will act as a key enabler in this, particularly in the 'assembly' and 'analysis' tasks.

4.3   Examples of KPIs for IT

Type of activity	Possible KPIs
Operational activities – KPIs are used to monitor the day to day activity and effectiveness of the IT function.	<ul><li>Ticket response rates for IT issues sent to IT support</li><li>Resolution rates</li><li>System/technology downtime</li><li>Customer feedback/experience</li></ul>
Transformational activities – KPIs are used to measure the impact of IT initiatives in terms of better and more informed decision making.	<ul><li>Cost of new technology</li><li>Time saved using new technology</li><li>IT spend per employee</li><li>IT utilisation</li><li>Security adherence/breaches</li></ul>
Strategic activities – KPIs are used to monitor the progress of the IT function towards long-term strategic goals.	<ul><li>New/improved business opportunities using technology</li><li>Revenue generated by using new technology</li><li>Technology leading to competitive advantage</li><li>IT function as a leader in the market place</li></ul>

Test your understanding 5

Lamp Limited is introducing a new information system and given it is a large project the project manager has decided to set some key performance indicators for the team after discussion with them.

The project manager is concerned that the benefits from the project exceed the costs of it and that the project is completed on time with all the deliverables (outputs) of suitable quality.

Three KPIs have been selected for scrutiny and you have been asked to comment.

KPI	Background
Volume of transactions Capable of processing up to 6,000 transactions per hour	This is an increase of 80% over the previous system
Labour Total labour spend on the project must not exceed $100,000	This is based on the original specification and scope of the project
Deliverables All originally specified deliverables (outputs) must be 100% delivered	This is based on the original specification and scope of the project

Required:

For each KPI listed above comment on the positives and the negatives you can identify in the measure suggested and comment on whether and how this measure could be manipulated.

(15 marks)

5   Chapter summary

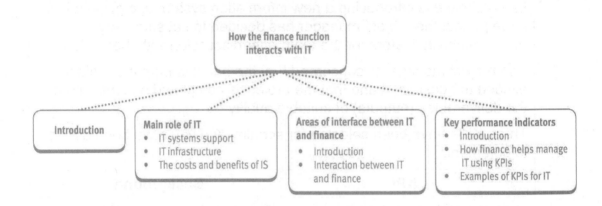

Test your understanding answers

Test your understanding 1

The best answer here is **D**

Test your understanding 2

Advantages

- Reduced travel time and hence cost savings.

- Reduction in stress due to the removal of the daily commute and the removal of the distractions of a busy office.

- Better work/life balance due to the removal of the daily commute and potential opportunities to work more flexible hours than the traditional '9 to 5'.

- Control – employees may feel an improved sense of control if they have more flexibility to decide their working patterns and hours.

- Employment opportunities for disadvantaged individuals, for example disabled people may now find it possible to work due to the removal of travel and the office environment.

Disadvantages

- May not suit those with poor personal motivation or who are not self-starters.

- May be distracted at home, for example by family members.

- Loss of learning/sharing of ideas from face to face contact.

- Loss of social interaction and stimulation.

- Difficultly in separating home and work life – an inability to 'switch off' from work may lead to 'burn out' or damaged personal relationships.

Test your understanding 3

The correct answer is **C** – virtual organisations usually have lower overhead costs.

Test your understanding 4

The challenges faced by virtual teams can be overcome by:

- training in technology and teamwork

- spending time getting to know each other, for example, team identity, jokes, occasional face to face meetings, team trips out

- clear roles and responsibilities

- detailed and timely feedback between the leader and team members

- regular and predictable communication matters. The benefits should be maximised, for example, the use of email, video conferencing, social networking sites and blogs could all assist in overcoming some of the challenges. Time zone differences may mean that managers and employees may have to accept that response times may not be immediate

- paying attention to cultural differences. This may require training in cross-cultural appreciation

- choosing dependable and self-reliant employees but managers should still be on hand to offer support

- valued staff should be made to feel wanted and a sense of loyalty to the firm instilled

- managers may need to view their role differently, the emphasis being on co-ordination rather than leadership

- clear communication from managers of information coming from higher up in the organisation to ensure that employees are fully informed and share the organisation's vision.

Test your understanding 5

Volume of transactions

Positive aspects

This measure is clearly very specific and should be measurable. It could be that the capacity of the system may never be fully utilised and so the 6,000 could never be reached and which case the actual data may show a number less than this target, without there being any underperformance.

Negative aspects

It is unclear whether an 80% increase is achievable, although system upgrades do tend to result in big increases in potential speeds in the modern IT world.

There is no quality aspect and speed alone may not be what is needed or preferred.

Manipulation

The number of transactions processed in a given time space is a very factual matter and without any element of judgement it is more difficult to manipulate.

A determined employee could duplicate transactions in order to get this figure higher but that would result in the need for reversal and the likelihood of being caught.

Total labour spend

Positive aspects

Providing a financial constraint is clearly relevant and this measure is clear and measurable. However, this is set based on the agreed specification and scope of the project and if these change at all during the project then this limit might have to be revisited.

Negative aspects

Setting cash limits can constrain decisions during the project. "We can't do (sensible thing) because we will spend more than was allowed". This can have very damaging effects on the project outcomes.

If the scope changes and the target is not adjusted it will become either too lenient, or more likely too harsh.

Manipulation

Costs incurred could be wrongly categorised to either another cost heading or another project thus under recording the cost in this project

Deliverables

Positive aspects

This is a clear target that is incapable of being misunderstood. It is relevant as the quality of work was a concern of the project manager.

Negative aspects

One questions the achievability of 100% perfection, if a target is too difficult it can be ignored or become a demotivating factor. You could also question its desirability. If delivering perfection gets expensive the costs might exceed the benefits here.

Manipulation

Other than just lying it is harder to see how this measure could be manipulated. Either the system delivers, or it doesn't. However, if some of the deliverables have elements of subjectivity (the "good" appearance of a document) then it is possible to "stretch" the definition a little and say it delivers when some might believe it does not.

Index

Index